Handbook of Stroke

Handbook of Stroke

David O. Wiebers, M.D.
Chair, Division of Cerebrovascular Diseases, and Consultant,
Departments of Neurology and Health Sciences Research, Mayo Clinic
and Mayo Foundation; Professor of Neurology, Mayo Medical School;
Rochester, Minnesota

Valery L. Feigin, M.D., D.Sc.
Visiting Scientist, Departments of Neurology and Health Sciences
Research, Mayo Clinic and Mayo Foundation, Rochester, Minnesota

Robert D. Brown, Jr., M.D.
Consultant, Department of Neurology, Mayo Clinic and Mayo
Foundation; Assistant Professor of Neurology, Mayo Medical School;
Rochester, Minnesota

Foreword by

Jack P. Whisnant, M.D.
Consultant Emeritus, Department of Health Sciences Research, Mayo
Clinic and Mayo Foundation; Emeritus Professor of Neurology, Mayo
Medical School; Rochester, Minnesota

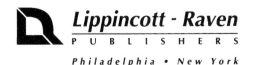

Lippincott - Raven
P U B L I S H E R S
Philadelphia • New York

Acquisitions Editor: Nancy Megley
Manufacturing Manager: Dennis Teston
Production Manager: Jodi Borgenicht
Production Editor: Anthony Pomes
Cover Designer: Vanessa Corzano
Indexer: Nancy Newman
Compositor: Focus/Graphics
Printer: R. R. Donnelley & Sons Company

Printed in the United States of America

9 8 7 6 5 4 3 2

Library of Congress Cataloging-in-Publication Data
Wiebers, David O.
    Handbook of stroke / David O. Wiebers, Valery L. Feigin,
Robert D. Brown, Jr. ; foreword by Jack P. Whisnant.
      p.   cm.
    Includes bibliographical references and index.
    ISBN 0-316-94760-1
    1. Cerebrovascular disease—Handbooks, manuals, etc. I. Feigin,
Valery L. II. Brown, Robert D., Jr. (Robert Duane), 1961–
III. Title.
    [DNLM: 1. Cerebrovascular Disorders. WL 355 W642h 1997]
RC388.5.W463 1997
616.8'1—dc20
DNLM/DLC
for Library of Congress

To our wives,
Andrea, Tatiana, and Julie,
for their unfailing love and understanding
and their compassion for all life

Contents

Foreword

During the first half of the twentieth century, little scientific attention was given to understanding the clinical characteristics of patients with different types of stroke, and no attention was directed at differentiating mechanisms. The nosologic term for stroke in mortality statistics in the early part of the century was *apoplexy,* from the Greek, "to strike down." The derivation of the generic clinical term *cerebrovascular accident* is unclear to me. This term helped to promote the idea that patients with stroke were victims and that somehow the disorder was providential, therefore not something that was subject to intervention by physicians or scientists. In teaching hospitals, patients with stroke were not considered appropriate for teaching of residents and students about disease. Patients with stroke either were not admitted to an acute care hospital or were admitted to a nonteaching service for maintenance care.

The last half of this century began with a few clinicians calling attention to the importance of stroke as a clinical problem and providing leadership in efforts to understand the mechanisms of the disorders that produce stroke. These early efforts led to increasing interest by clinicians, which soon attracted clinical and laboratory research attention to this clinical disorder.

Clinicians now recognize the importance of differentiating types of stroke and the pathophysiologic substrate when possible. Imaging studies have greatly enhanced the precision of the neurologist and others in determining the type of stroke. The further responsibility of the clinician is to assess the patient for management options, either medical or surgical.

Successful treatment up to the present time has centered around appropriate management of risk factors and comorbid conditions to prevent stroke. Recent attention has focused on protecting and preserving the integrity of brain tissue after ischemia has developed and on lysing thrombi in arteries that may have been the cause of the ischemia. The usefulness of either of these approaches has yet to be proved. The need now is for clinicians to be aware of the urgent need for attention if these treatments of stroke are to be effective or even to be adequately tested.

Handbook of Stroke has been produced by experienced clinicians who have presented the topics in a unique fashion, following the thought processes that experienced neurovascular clinicians use. The emphasis on the importance of what can be learned from the history is almost unique in recent literature on stroke. The authors use six clinical management algorithms that are helpful to clinicians of all types. Telephone triage is important for appropriate patient care, and the authors have addressed it clearly.

Development of effective treatments for stroke aimed at preventing death and reducing impairment of function will require knowledgeable clinicians who put a high priority on attending to the care of patients with stroke as soon as the stroke is evident.

I know the three authors well through personal interaction, and I am pleased that they have produced a volume that emphasizes the importance of clinical assessment of patients with stroke.

Jack P. Whisnant, M.D.

Preface

To help facilitate the goals of preventing cerebrovascular disorders and improving the care of patients with these conditions, all health care providers must build for themselves and continually update a solid foundation of information based on sound concepts, systems, and classifications. To these building blocks, all of us may then add our own components of personality and style when interacting with individual patients to create what we know as the art of medicine.

There is something particularly fulfilling about assisting colleagues by providing important information or building blocks that can contribute to the care of patients. It is a win-win situation in which both patients and physicians benefit and feel fulfillment. It was this potential for benefit and fulfillment that formed the impetus for our writing *Handbook of Stroke,* and it is our sincere hope that those who use this book will find it helpful as both a learning resource and a quick reference manual advancing the comprehensive care of patients.

We are greatly indebted to numerous persons who played major roles in developing and completing this book. From a professional standpoint, we recognize our numerous colleagues and trainees who provided us with a source for exchange of ideas, learning, and camaraderie. We express particular gratitude and indebtedness to Jack P. Whisnant, M.D., our beloved mentor and colleague, whose unselfish guidance and generosity over the years have been particular blessings. We only wish it were possible for all physicians to work with someone like Jack during the course of their careers.

We also gratefully acknowledge the outstanding contributions of LeAnn Stee, Roberta Schwartz, Dorothy Tienter, and Dianne Kemp for their editorial support at the Mayo Clinic; Nancy Megley, Tammerly Booth, Anne Holm, Anne Miller, Nancy Newman, Cate Rickard, and Vanessa Corzano for their editorial support; Marcia Tolmie, Denise Farr, Denise Gravenhof, and Melissa Albrecht for their secretarial support; Bob Benassi for his artistic expertise in illustrating the book; Glenn Forbes, M.D., and John Huston, M.D., for their radiologic expertise and assistance in providing radiographs; and Rita Jones, R.D., for her valuable assistance on dietary and nutritional issues.

We also express our deepest thanks to our parents for teaching us the importance of caring for others, for developing our desire for knowledge, and for instilling within us the courage to dream and the will to succeed. We also deeply thank our other cherished family members for all they have done for us. Finally, we thank our patients for their role in inspiring us to write this book and for allowing us the opportunity to experience the profound satisfaction of assisting them.

D. O. W.
V. L. F.
R. D. B.

Handbook of Stroke

Clinical and Laboratory Assessment of Patients with Cerebrovascular Disease

Notice

The indications and dosages of all drugs in this book have been recommended in the medical literature and conform to the practices of the general medical community. The medications described do not necessarily have specific approval by the Food and Drug Administration for use in the diseases and dosages for which they are recommended. The package insert for each drug should be consulted for use and dosage as approved by the FDA. Because standards for usage change, it is advisable to keep abreast of revised recommendations, particularly those concerning new drugs.

Systematic Clinical Assessment

The clinician must call on comprehensive clinical assessment skills to provide the patient with an accurate and efficient diagnosis. Because many processes other than cerebrovascular disease may cause neurologic symptoms, differential diagnosis is important. A detailed clinical history and systematic neurologic, neurovascular, and general examinations are important aspects of the clinical assessment of patients with suspected cerebrovascular disease.

Although the clinical evaluation of patients with different forms of cerebrovascular disease varies somewhat (for example, with altered levels of consciousness or intellectual disturbances), most parts of the clinical assessment are uniform.

Questions to Ask

It is important for the clinician to use a systematic approach to evaluate the patient with a potential cerebrovascular problem. In patients with transient neurologic dysfunction, it is useful to discuss in great detail from beginning to end at least one spell with the patient to clarify the diagnosis. For virtually all patients in whom cerebrovascular disorders are suspected, it is useful to direct the interview step-by-step to facilitate answering four fundamental questions:

1. Is the problem vascular?
2. Is the vascular problem one of hemorrhage or ischemia?
3. If the problem is hemorrhagic, what are the location and cause?
4. If the problem is infarction, what is the arterial or venous distribution, and what is the underlying mechanism for the ischemia?

IS THE PROBLEM VASCULAR?

The answer to the first question is based primarily on the temporal profile of the patient's presenting symptoms. The classic vascular profile involves sudden onset with rapid progression to maximal deficit (instantaneously or in seconds). All the affected areas of the body are involved from the onset. The **rapid onset and evolution** usually apply to all types of cerebrovascular episodes, regardless of the total duration of symptoms. The prototype for brief ischemic spells is the **transient ischemic attack** (TIA), defined as a temporary episode of **focal** ischemic neurologic dysfunction that completely resolves within 24 hours. It is important to distinguish TIA from an episode of generalized cerebral ischemia (syncope) and from spells such as seizures or migraine, both of which may appear as episodes of transient focal neurologic dysfunction. The temporal profile of focal seizures generally involves progression and evolution within a few minutes (approximately 2–3 minutes), whereas the focal deficit that sometimes occurs with migraine usually builds or moves during 15 to 20 minutes (for example, increasing scintillating scotomata or marching numbness starting in one hand) before subsiding and is often associated with localized headache, normally occurring after the focal neurologic deficit.

Another distinguishing characteristic of vascular spells is that most tend to produce negative phenomena (for example, weakness, deadness, visual loss), but focal seizures tend to produce positive phenomena (for example, tonic-clonic movements, tingling, visual hallucinations, scintillating scotomata), and migraine may produce either phenomena (more commonly, positive).

There are rare exceptions to these guidelines. Some TIAs may present with rhythmic jerking of the arm or leg, often occurring when the patient arises from a sitting or lying position. A contralateral high-grade carotid stenosis is often detected (the so-called shaky TIA). Likewise, seizures may present with speech arrest, or weakness may occur after a seizure (Todd's paralysis).

When a focal ischemic deficit persists for longer than 24 hours but resolves within 3 weeks, the episode is considered a minor ischemic stroke, but it is termed a **reversible ischemic neurologic deficit** (RIND). Deficits persisting longer than 3 weeks are called **cerebral infarctions (ischemic strokes).**

An exception to the usual rapid evolution of ischemic cerebrovascular events occurs in patients who have increasing neurologic deficit for as long as 72 hours after the onset of symptoms. These patients are classified as having **progressing cerebral infarction,** a phenomenon that is more common in strokes involving the vertebrobasilar system. In this situation, the clinician should carefully consider the possibility of an underlying mass lesion (for example, subdural hematoma, neoplasm, or abscess), demyelinating disease, or a superimposed encephalopathy.

IS THE VASCULAR PROBLEM ONE OF HEMORRHAGE OR ISCHEMIA?

Having determined that the problem is vascular, the clinician must next attempt to distinguish whether the main process is one of hemorrhage or ischemia. Overall, ischemic strokes comprise approximately 80% to 85% of all strokes; intracerebral hemorrhage and subarachnoid hemorrhage comprise approximately 10% and 5% of all strokes, respectively.

The onset of symptoms with headache or stiff neck favors a hemorrhagic process, as does early decreased level of consciousness in a patient with a presumed supratentorial lesion. Ischemia is more likely if the symptoms are consistent with neurologic dysfunction from a single arterial territory or if improvement occurs rapidly or early in the clinical course. Although the distinction between hemorrhage and ischemia is seldom difficult clinically, there are exceptions, and sometimes the two occur simultaneously (such as hemorrhagic infarction). Computed tomography has revolutionized the clinician's ability to distinguish between hemorrhage and infarction in emergency situations and thus has resolved virtually all cases in which uncertainty exists. Ischemic lesions appear as normal areas or as areas of decreased attenuation within the first several hours after the onset of symptoms, whereas hemorrhagic lesions usually appear immediately as areas of increased attenuation. Rarely, magnetic resonance imaging may provide additional help with the distinction between hemorrhage and ischemia.

IF THE PROBLEM IS HEMORRHAGIC, WHAT ARE THE LOCATION AND CAUSE?

If the problem is hemorrhagic, the clinician must attempt to define the type, location, and cause of the hemorrhage to facilitate proper management (Table 1-1). It is important to determine location because this usually helps define the cause of the hemorrhage. The five commonly defined locations, proceeding from external to internal, are (1) epidural and (2) subdural hematomas, both usually caused by head trauma; (3) subarachnoid hemorrhage, usually caused by aneurysm or arteriovenous malformation; (4) intracerebral and (5) intraventricular hemorrhages, both often a result of hypertension, arteriovenous malformation, or aneurysm (Fig. 1-1).

IF THE PROBLEM IS INFARCTION, WHAT IS THE ARTERIAL OR VENOUS DISTRIBUTION, AND WHAT IS THE UNDERLYING MECHANISM FOR THE ISCHEMIA?

If the problem is ischemic, the clinician should first attempt to define the location of the process within the patient's central nervous system. This involves localizing the neurologic dysfunction to one or more vascular territories and requires some knowledge of neuroanatomy, including the cerebral circulation. The **first step in localization** is to distinguish generalized ischemia (syncope, anoxic encephalopathy) from focal cerebral ischemia (TIA, reversible ischemic neurologic deficit, cerebral infarction, progressing cerebral infarction). Differentiation is particularly important because of the vastly different implications of the two ischemias in terms of cause, management, and prognosis. If the problem is focal (or multifocal), the **second step in localization** involves distinguishing anterior circulation (carotid system) from posterior circulation (vertebrobasilar system) processes. From there, the clinician can further subdivide the ischemic lesion into individual or multiple vascular territories by relating the clinical findings to the functional anatomy of the cerebral vessels (see Appendixes A-1 and A-2). If a patient has multiple vascular spells, it is important to know whether all spells are similar (stereotyped) and to review at least one spell in great detail.

After localization of the process is clarified, one should next consider the underlying mechanism. Major categories of cerebral ischemic events relating to underlying pathophysiology, proceeding

Table 1-1. Locations and associated causes of intracranial hemorrhage

Location	Cause
Epidural	Head trauma, tear in meningeal artery
Subdural	Head trauma, tear in bridging vein
Subarachnoid	Aneurysm or arteriovenous malformation
Intracerebral	Hypertension, arteriovenous malformation, aneurysm, amyloid angiopathy, primary and metastatic neoplasms, infections, hematologic disorders, use of anticoagulant or thrombolytic agents
Intraventricular	Hypertension, aneurysm, arteriovenous malformation, hematologic disorders, use of anticoagulant or thrombolytic agents (often an extension of deep intracerebral hemorrhage)

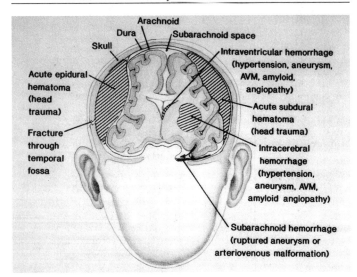

Fig. 1-1. Locations of intracranial hemorrhage. AVM = arteriovenous malformation.

from proximal to distal in the arterial system, are (1) **cardiac disease**, (2) **large vessel disease** (craniocervical occlusive disease), (3) **small vessel disease** (intracranial occlusive disease), and (4) **hematologic disease** (see Table 8-1). Another common but somewhat less clinically useful way to categorize ischemic stroke subtypes is to use the categories of **thrombotic infarction,** in which a locally decreased blood supply is caused by a blockage formed in situ in an artery; **embolic infarction,** referring to a blockage caused by a piece of material that has broken free from a more proximal site; and **lacunar infarction,** which is frequently, but not always, caused by thrombosis of one of the small penetrating branch arteries.

Historical Evaluation of Key Signs and Symptoms

A detailed history is the most important part of the evaluation of a patient with cerebrovascular disease. **Approximately 80% of cerebrovascular diagnosis is based on historical information.** Initial attention should be directed toward identifying and characterizing (1) the patient's **chief complaints** or **main symptoms;** (2) the **time of onset** and possible **precipitating events;** (3) the features of the **circumstance of onset,** including the patient's activities, the **temporal profile** of the **onset of symptoms,** and the rapidity with which maximal deficit developed (a typical vascular profile involves sudden onset with rapid progression to maximal deficit with all the affected areas of the body involved from the onset); (4) the presence of focal or generalized **neurologic deficit** at the onset; alterations of **level of consciousness** at onset; (5) the presence of **headache, vomiting, or seizure activity** (focal or generalized); and (6) the **chronologic course of neurologic symptoms** after onset.

Frequently, the patient may not remember the precise details of the early temporal course and other important historical details. In this case, family members are often the best source of the information. The patient should be asked what is specifically meant by certain words used to describe symptoms (for example, "dizziness," "headache," and "poor vision") because these terms have a wide range of different meanings with different implications for diagnosis and management.

This chapter describes several symptoms that are particularly pertinent to patients with cerebrovascular disorders and addresses their application to the diagnosis of these conditions.

Headache

Sudden severe headache described by the patient as "like being hit over the head by a hammer" (or some similar description) is suggestive of **subarachnoid hemorrhage**. This headache is usually associated with neck stiffness (meningismus) and may be localized to the posterior neck. However, as many as 30% of all subarachnoid hemorrhages present atypically, and a minor subarachnoid hemorrhage, especially in elderly persons, may not present with severe headache, stiff neck, or catastrophic onset. In these cases, any element of abruptness in a new character of headache should always raise the possibility of subarachnoid or other intracranial hemorrhage.

Localized or pulsating headache associated with slowly progressive focal neurologic deficit may occur with growing intracranial **arteriovenous malformations** (which may produce pulsatile tinnitus with or without cranial bruit) **or aneurysms**. Aneurysms of the internal carotid artery (intracavernous part or near the petrous apex) may produce facial or retro-orbital pain. Aneurysms of the middle cerebral artery (lateral fissure) are sometimes associated with retro-orbital pain; aneurysms of the posterior cerebral artery are associated with retro-orbital or occipital pain; and aneurysms of the basilar artery cause hemifacial pain.

The headache of **intracerebral hemorrhage** is usually sudden in onset and often associated with a progressive focal neurologic deficit, vomiting, and altered consciousness.

Patients with **cerebral infarction** uncommonly (20%) have headache at the onset of the episode (more commonly with embolic ischemic lesions). Occasionally, a patient with a large cerebral infarction may experience headache (caused by cerebral edema) beginning as long as a few days after the onset of stroke. However, this type of headache is usually temporary; more severe or persistent headache warrants further investigation for other underlying causes such as tumor, abscess, vasculitis, or hemorrhagic infarct. **Transient ischemic attack** seldom produces substantial headache.

Severe hypertension with diastolic blood pressures of more than 110 mm Hg may be associated with headache, but mild hypertension rarely causes headaches. Severe headache caused by abrupt increases in blood pressure may occur in patients with **acute hypertensive encephalopathy** (often associated with neurologic deficits resulting from cerebral edema, hemorrhage, or vasospasm).

Headache caused by **chronic increased intracranial pressure**, as occurs with cerebral tumor, is often present when the patient awakens in the morning and may be **brought on** with increased Valsalva maneuvers or lowering the head below the level of the heart. In contrast, almost any type of headache may be **worsened** by Valsalva maneuvers, lowering the head below the level of the heart, or excessive stress or tension.

Headache resulting from **venous circulatory dysfunction** (for example, intracranial venous sinus thrombosis) usually results from increased intracranial pressure and has a tendency to be present when the patient awakens and to be brought on or enhanced by Valsalva maneuvers, supine position, or lowering the head below the level of the heart. Occasionally these disorders are associated with central nervous system infection and produce fever and headache as a result of meningeal irritation.

The headache of **temporal (cranial) arteritis** is characterized by severe, persistent pain associated with enlarged, beaded, tender, erythematous, or pulseless temporal arteries and jaw claudication. Scalp tenderness is characteristic, and it is often very difficult for patients to comb their hair. Other associated features include general malaise, polyarthralgias, polymyalgias, fever, and unilateral or bilateral loss of vision. This type of headache usually occurs in patients older than 55 years but has been reported in patients in their thirties. The diagnosis is suggested by a high sedimentation rate (often >100 mm/hour) and confirmed by temporal artery biopsy. Corticosteroid treatment usually produces a dramatic and rapid improvement in headache.

Migraine headaches usually start in adolescence or early adulthood. There is often a positive family history. The headaches are intermittent, sometimes preceded by 15- to 30-minute prodromes such as scintillating scotomata, usually unilateral, throbbing, and associated with nausea, vomiting, or photophobia. The pain usually builds to a peak in less than 1 hour and persists for hours to 1 or 2 days and is exacerbated by noise and bright light. In some patients, the headaches are precipitated by stress, fasting, menses, and certain foods such as alcohol, chocolate, cured meats, and monosodium glutamate (often used in Chinese food). Often, the headache is relieved with sleep.

Cluster headaches are characterized by recurrent, nocturnal, unilateral, usually retro-orbital searing pains, lasting 20 to 60 minutes and typically accompanied by unilateral lacrimation and nasal and conjunctival congestion. These headaches normally occur in men older than 20 years and often include an ipsilateral Horner's syndrome and rhinorrhea during the headache. Episodes are characteristically precipitated by alcohol.

Vascular headaches (Table 2-1) should be distinguished from nonvascular headaches, such as those associated with (1) cerebral trauma (subdural hematoma, posttraumatic headache); (2) infections or tumors of the central nervous system; (3) contraction, inflammation, or trauma related to cranial or cervical muscles (tension and muscle contraction headache); (4) paranasal sinus disease; (5) glaucoma; (6) benign intracranial hypertension; and (7) nonspecific headaches related to use of various drugs (for example, bromides and indomethacin).

Headache is a very common symptom of subacute (2–14 days) or chronic (>14 days) **traumatic subdural hematoma.** The headache often fluctuates in severity, with a deep-seated, steady, unilateral, or, less commonly, generalized presentation, often proceeding to involve alterations of consciousness and focal neurologic dysfunction. The diagnosis is established by computed tomography or magnetic resonance imaging of the head. **Posttraumatic headaches** may be intermittent, continuous, or chronic (bilateral or, less commonly, unilateral) and are often associated with giddiness, vertigo, or tinnitus. Posttraumatic dysautonomic cephalalgia is characterized by severe, episodic, throbbing, unilateral headaches accompanied by ipsilateral mydriasis and excessive facial sweating.

Meningitis or encephalitis often produces intense, deep, constant, and increasing headache that is usually generalized and associated with stiff neck, Kernig or Brudzinski signs, and fever. The diagnosis is established by lumbar puncture. Acute persistent headache over a period of hours or days may also occur in systemic infections, such as influenza, without definite central nervous system involvement.

Headaches associated with brain tumors are usually unilateral, slowly progressive in frequency and severity, and have a tendency to occur when the patient awakens in the morning. As the tumor grows, the pain is frequently associated with focal neurologic signs or signs of increased intracranial pressure. As with other lesions causing mass effect, the headaches may be brought on by bending over with the head downward or engaging in Valsalva maneuvers (coughing, sneezing, straining to defecate).

Tension-type headache (muscle contraction headache) is usually steady, deep, generalized, bilateral, and occipital, frontal, or in a bandlike distribution around the head with associated tightness and tenderness of the neck muscles. It may persist unremittingly for

Table 2-1.   Classification of headache

Major cause of headache	Clinical forms of headache
Migraine	Migraine without aura, migraine with aura, hemiplegic migraine, basilar migraine, ophthalmoplegic migraine, retinal migraine
Tension-type	Tension headache, episodic or chronic, caused by excessive stress, anxiety, depression, cervical osteoarthritis, cranial or cervical myalgias
Cluster/chronic paroxysmal hemicrania	Cluster headache, chronic paroxysmal hemicrania
Vascular disorders	Ischemic cerebrovascular disease (transient ischemic attack, ischemic stroke), intracranial hemorrhage (intracerebral, subdural, epidural, subarachnoid), unruptured aneurysm or arteriovenous malformation, vasculitis, carotidynia, dissection
Nonvascular intracranial disorders	High cerebrospinal fluid pressure (primary or metastatic tumor, intracranial hemorrhage, ischemic stroke with edema, abscess, hydrocephalus, pseudotumor cerebri) Low cerebrospinal fluid pressure (after lumbar puncture, other cerebrospinal fluid leak) Infection (bacterial, viral, fungal, other) Chemical meningitis
Substance use or withdrawal	Acute substance exposure (nitrates, carbon monoxide, alcohol, monosodium glutamate) Chronic substance exposure (ergotamine, analgesic overuse, birth control pills, estrogens) Withdrawal (alcohol, ergotamine, caffeine, narcotics)
Noncephalic infection	Viral, bacterial
Metabolic disorders	Hypoxia, hypercapnia, hypoglycemia, dialysis, other
Trauma	Acute and chronic posttraumatic headache
Facial/cranial structures	Eye (including glaucoma, inflammatory disorders, refractive errors), ears, nose, and sinuses, temporomandibular joint, teeth, cranial bone, neck
Neuralgia/nerve trunk	Compression of upper cranial nerve, demyelination or infarction of cranial nerve, inflammation (herpes zoster, postherpetic neuralgia), Tolosa-Hunt trigeminal neuralgia, glossopharyngeal neuralgia, occipital neuralgia
Other	Benign cough or exertion headache, headache with sexual activity, cold stimulus headache, idiopathic stabbing headache

Adapted from Headache Classification Committee of the International Headache Society: Classification and diagnostic criteria for headache disorders, cranial neuralgias and facial pain. Cephalalgia 8(Suppl 7):1–96, 1988. By permission of Scandinavian University Press.

days or weeks and is usually associated with excessive stress or tension, anxiety, insomnia, or depression.

Headache caused by **paranasal sinus disease** is usually localized over the affected sinuses, often with associated purulent nasal discharge and fever. The diagnosis is established by tomography of the sinus or by computed tomography or magnetic resonance imaging of the head.

Headache of ocular origin (ocular muscle imbalance, hyperopia, astigmatism, impaired convergence/accommodation, narrowangle glaucoma, iridocyclitis) is usually located in the ipsilateral orbit, forehead, or temple and has a steady, aching quality that may follow prolonged, intensive use of the eyes for close work (with glaucoma, the pain is often associated with loss of vision). A careful description of the type of headache and a history of its onset, relationship to use of the eyes, duration, and associated symptoms often suggests the diagnosis, which is established from other eye signs. For example, long-lasting, mild-to-moderate headache that occurs toward the end of a day and is relieved by a few hours of rest or sleep is more likely to be related to an ocular disorder.

Benign intracranial hypertension usually produces intermittent mild or severe headache that may be brought on by Valsalva maneuvers or by bending with the head down and is associated with papilledema. Criteria for this diagnosis include evidence of increased intracranial pressure and absence of clinical or laboratory evidence of a focal brain lesion, infection, or hydrocephalus.

Low cerebrospinal fluid pressure headache, sometimes called **spinal headache** (usually occurring after lumbar puncture), is usually generalized and characteristically worsens substantially when the person is sitting or standing. Characteristically, the headache is relieved entirely when the person lies down.

Dizziness

It is important to determine whether the patient is describing a sensation of self or environmental movement or spinning (that is, vertigo), a sensation of light-headedness with or without visual graying or postural swaying (that is, faintness or near syncope), or something else (such as an unusual head sensation or gait unsteadiness).

VERTIGO

Vertigo indicates dysfunction in the peripheral or central components of the vestibular system. Central vertigo results from disorders affecting brain stem or vestibulocerebellar pathways; peripheral vertigo indicates involvement either of the vestibular end organ (for example, semicircular canals) or of their peripheral neurons, including the vestibular portion of the eighth cranial nerve. A method for categorizing the causes of vertigo is presented in Table 2-2.

Central vertigo is a common part of posterior circulation disturbances such as cerebellar or brain stem infarction, hemorrhage, or vertebrobasilar transient ischemic attack. In the context of vascular disease, vertigo is almost always associated with other symptoms of brain stem or cerebellar dysfunction. Central vertigo also may be

Table 2-2.   Causes of vertigo

Degenerative	**Toxic**	**Neoplastic**
Cerebellar degeneration	Phenytoin	Acoustic neuroma, other cerebellopontine angle tumors
Syringobulbia	Aminoglycosides	
Arnold-Chiari malformation	Alcohol	Meningioma
	Quinine	Cholesteatoma
Platybasia	**Metabolic**	Cerebellar astrocytoma, other cerebellar neoplasms
Infectious or inflammatory	Beriberi	
	Pellagra	Glomus jugulare tumor
Labyrinthitis	Hypothyroidism	
Otitis media	Hypoglycemia	**Vascular**
Viral illness	**Traumatic**	Brain stem ischemia
Cerebellar abscess	Petrous bone fracture	Cerebellar hemorrhage
Syphilis of CNS	Concussion	Inferior auditory artery occlusion
Arachnoiditis	Other head trauma	
Meningitis		Migraine
Multiple sclerosis		**Other**
		Ménière's disease
		Seizure

CNS = central nervous system.

caused by neoplasms of the posterior fossa (often associated with headache, gait or limb ataxia), demyelinating disease, arteriovenous malformation, brain stem encephalitis, and vertiginous epilepsy (tornado epilepsy) originating in the temporal lobe. Medications, such as analgesics, antiarrhythmics, anticonvulsants, antibiotics, loop diuretics, and sedatives also may lead to vertigo.

Peripheral vertigo may be caused by unilateral or bilateral labyrinthine dysfunction (infection, trauma, ischemia, or toxins), vestibular neuronitis, lesions of the cerebellopontine angle impinging on the eighth cranial nerve (such as acoustic neuroma), Ménière's disease (recurrent attacks of vertigo associated with hearing loss, tinnitus, and a sensation of ear fullness, which may improve after the attack subsides), or benign positional vertigo (episodic vertigo occurring after changes of head position, which diminishes with repeated attempts to elicit vertigo with the same movement).

Positional vertigo resulting from peripheral and central causes may be differentiated on the basis of clinical features, nystagmus characteristics, and findings with Nylen's maneuver (Table 2-3). Nylen's maneuver is performed by having the patient abruptly lie down from a sitting position and orient the head approximately 30 degrees below the horizontal plane. The test is repeated with the head positioned to the left, straight, and to the right, with observation for nystagmus and notation of any clinical symptoms.

LIGHT-HEADEDNESS (FAINTNESS)

Light-headedness is analogous to feelings that precede syncope (near syncope) caused by generalized cerebral ischemia. True vertigo almost never occurs during the presyncopal state. Presyncopal, stereotyped faintness may be associated with visual graying, heavi-

Table 2-3. Differentiating features of peripheral and central vertigo

Feature	Peripheral vertigo	Central vertigo
Clinical		
Onset	Sudden	Insidious, less often sudden
Pattern	Paroxysmal	Continuous, occasionally paroxysmal
Severity	Intense	Mild
Tinnitus	Common	Rare
Fall on Romberg's test	To side of lesion, away from fast component of nystagmus	To side of lesion, to fast component of nystagmus
Caloric stimulation	Nonreactive	Normal
Nystagmus		
Spontaneous	May be present	May be present
Types	Horizontal or rotatory, no vertical	Horizontal, rotatory, or vertical
Fast component direction	Consistent direction in all directions of gaze	Varies with direction of gaze
Nylen's maneuver		
Latency	3–45 sec	None
Fatigability	Yes	No
Visual fixation	Inhibits vertigo	No change
Nystagmus direction	Fixed	Independent
Reproducibility	Inconsistent	Consistent
Intensity	Severe vertigo, nausea	Mild vertigo, rarely nausea

ness in the lower limbs, and postural swaying. The causes of light-headedness relate to generalized cerebral hypoperfusion and include various causes of postural hypotension, orthostatic hypotension, decreased cardiac output (for example, cardiac arrhythmias), anemia, or other vasovagal disorders.

OTHER CAUSES OF NONVERTIGINOUS DIZZINESS

Other causes include hyperventilation syndrome (often associated with shortness of breath, rapid heartbeat, and a feeling of fear), diabetes mellitus (related to hypoglycemia, autonomic neuropathy, or postural hypotension), and various drugs, such as tricyclic antidepressants, antihypertensives, and tranquilizers.

Visual Disturbances

Visual disturbances most often involve **visual loss** (including blurriness) or **diplopia.** It is very important to determine whether these symptoms are a result of cerebrovascular disease, a nonvascular neurologic disorder, a primary ocular disturbance, or something else (for example, a psychogenic disorder). Visual disturbances can be caused by defects in the retina, optic nerve, chiasm, optic tract, lateral geniculate nucleus, geniculocalcarine tract (optic radiation), and striate cortex of the occipital lobes.

Many disturbances of vision are caused by primary ocular disease (Table 2-4). For example, astigmatism or macular lesions may produce distortion of the normal shapes of objects **(metamorphopsia).** **Photophobia** is usually caused by corneal inflammation, aphakia, iritis, ocular albinism, or certain drugs, such as chloroquine or acetazolamide. Color change **(chromatopsia)** may result from systemic disturbances (for example, yellow vision accompanying jaundice), drug use (such as yellow and white vision in digitalis toxicity), chorioretinal lesions, or lenticular changes. **Rings** seen when viewing lights or bright objects may be caused by lens changes, incipient cataract, glaucoma, or corneal edema. **Spots** or **dots** before the eyes, which move with movement of the eye, are commonly caused by benign vitreous opacities (floaters). Difficulty seeing in the dark **(nyctalopia)** may result from congenital retinitis pigmentosa, hereditary optic atrophy, vitamin A deficiency, glaucoma, optic atrophy, cataract, or retinal degeneration.

VISUAL FIELD DEFECTS

Symptoms of visual loss include loss of visual acuity, various types of visual field defects (Table 2-5), and unilateral or bilateral visual loss (the clinical approach to evaluating visual acuity and fields is discussed in Chapter 5).

Vascular retinal lesions may cause **arcuate, central, or cecocentral scotomata** corresponding to the area of vascular supply of the arteriole involved (the patient sees them as wedge-shaped dark spots) (Fig. 2-1). **Arcuate scotomata** may also be caused by compressive or vascular lesions of the optic disk as a result of glaucoma or by hyaline bodies (drusen) of the disk. Optic neuritis and retrobulbar optic nerve lesions (demyelinating disease; infiltrative, neoplastic or infectious diseases; degenerative diseases; aneurysm; tumor) often produce **cecocentral scotomata.** Small, **central scotomata** in macular disease often cause distorted vision for straight lines (metamorphopsia), a trait that aids in the distinction between macular and optic nerve lesions. Toxic states or nutritional disorders

Table 2-4.   Visual disturbances caused by primary ocular disorders

Effect on vision	Ocular disease
Metamorphopsia	Astigmatism, macular lesion
Photophobia	Corneal inflammation, aphakia, iritis, ocular albinism, drugs
Chromatopsia	Systemic disturbance, drug use, chorioretinal lesions, lenticular changes
Rings seen	Lens changes, incipient cataract, glaucoma, corneal edema
Spots, dots	Vitreous opacities
Nyctalopia	Congenital retinitis pigmentosa, hereditary optic atrophy, vitamin A deficiency, glaucoma, optic atrophy, cataract, retinal degeneration

Table 2-5.   Causes of visual field defects

Defect	Cause
Scotomata	
Arcuate	Compressive or vascular lesions of optic disk
Cecocentral	Optic neuritis, retrobulbar optic nerve lesions
Symmetric central, cecocentral	Toxic states, nutritional disorders
Scintillating	Migraine, epilepsy
Peripheral constriction of visual field	Papilledema, perioptic sheath meningioma, psychogenic
Hemianopia	
Bitemporal	Lesions of optic chiasm
Incongruous (less often congruous) homonymous	Lesions of lateral geniculate nucleus, optic tract, optic radiation
Congruous homonymous	Lesions of calcarine cortex

(tobacco-alcohol amblyopia) may produce relatively symmetric **central or cecocentral scotomata. Scintillating scotoma** (the patient sees bright, colorless or colored lights in the field of vision) usually occurs as a part of migraine or epilepsy with occipital lobe involvement. Progressive **peripheral constriction of the visual field** may be caused by papilledema or perioptic sheath meningioma or may be psychogenic (tunnel vision).

Lesions of the optic chiasm (pituitary tumor, craniopharyngioma, sellar meningioma, suprasellar aneurysm of the circle of Willis) produce **bitemporal hemianopias** (blindness in the temporal half of the visual fields). Pregeniculate optic tract lesions (infection, tumor) produce **homonymous hemianopia** associated with optic atrophy and afferent pupillary defects. Lesions of the lateral geniculate nucleus (infection, tumor, circle of Willis aneurysm) or postgeniculate lesions in the optic radiation (ischemic or hemorrhagic stroke, arteriovenous malformation, glioma) produce **incongruous homonymous hemianopias** (field defects in the two eyes are not identical) with normal pupillary reflexes. **Congruous homonymous hemianopia** (field defects in the two eyes are identical) with normal pupillary reflexes signifies a lesion in the calcarine cortex, usually the result of a cerebrovascular or neoplastic disorder, such as ischemic stroke or glioma.

UNILATERAL LOSS OF VISION

Unilateral visual loss may be caused by opticoretinal ischemia, occlusion of the central retinal artery or vein, anterior ischemic optic neuropathy, optic or retrobulbar neuritis, or optic nerve dysfunction resulting from mechanical compression (Table 2-6).

Transient monocular blindness from episodic opticoretinal ischemia (**amaurosis fugax**) is frequently caused by ipsilateral carotid system occlusive disease and results in hemodynamic ocular blood flow disturbances or in retinal emboli (cholesterol, fibrin platelet) originating from proximal carotid system plaque. Alternatively, emboli may reach the eye from the heart in circumstances of valvular

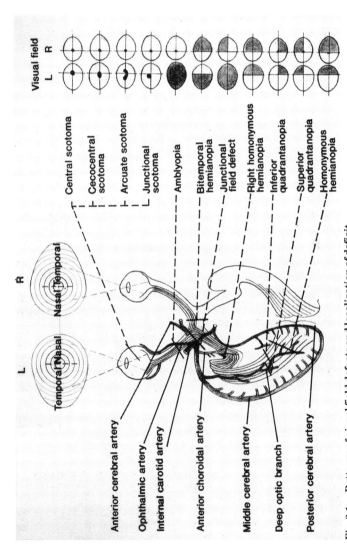

Fig. 2-1.   Patterns of visual field defects and localization of deficit.

Table 2-6. Causes of unilateral loss of vision

Type of vision loss	Cause
Sudden	Ipsilateral carotid system occlusive disease, cardiac valvular abnormalities, blood stasis, cardiac shunts, cranial arteritis, occlusion of central retinal artery or vein, ischemic optic neuropathy
Subacute	Optic neuritis, retrobulbar neuritis, papilledema, migraine
Gradual	Optic nerve dysfunction caused by mechanical compression

abnormalities, blood stasis (arrhythmias, myocardial infarction, congestive heart failure), or right-to-left cardiac shunts with systemic venous thrombosis.

The patient with amaurosis fugax often describes the episode as an acute, transient loss of vision (a perception of a shade being pulled from above downward or from below upward over one eye, or occasionally, proceeding in a circular pattern peripherally to centrally in one eye) that usually lasts seconds or minutes. The clinician must carefully question the patient to determine whether the patient is describing loss of vision in one eye or a homonymous field defect (to localize this field defect some patients may have alternately closed one eye and then the other at the time of the attack).

The clinical picture of amaurosis fugax may infrequently occur with (1) cranial arteritis (often in patients with associated new-onset, severe, persistent headache; enlarged, beaded, or pulseless temporal arteries; pain or cramping in the jaw during chewing [jaw claudication]; polyarthralgias and polymyalgias), (2) papilledema (rarely, producing transient unilateral blindness in the form of very brief blurring of vision in one or both eyes, usually during sudden changes of posture), and (3) migraine (although bilateral scotomata are much more common in migraine than are unilateral blindness and visual loss).

Sudden unilateral blindness may also be caused by occlusion of the central retinal artery (typically, complete, long-lasting or permanent visual loss), occlusion of the central retinal vein (usually causing a milder visual loss), ischemic optic neuropathy (sudden mild-to-moderate visual loss that usually gradually worsens), or optic neuritis (generally in young adults with diminished visual acuity, central or paracentral scotomata, and sometimes painful eye movements, all of which develop subacutely and worsen over a few days). These diagnoses are usually established from characteristic ophthalmoscopic findings.

Gradual onset of unilateral blindness is usually caused by optic nerve dysfunction resulting from mechanical compression that is generally associated with neoplasms or inflammatory lesions within the orbit or in the retro-orbital-parasellar areas, such as optic gliomas, meningiomas, hamartomas, hemangiomas, lymphomas, multiple myeloma, sarcoid, paranasal sinus infections or inflammatory disease, pituitary adenomas, and medial sphenoid wing meningiomas. As the compression progresses, acuity becomes further impaired, along with impaired color vision, afferent pupil reflex abnormalities, and, eventually, optic atrophy. The diagnosis is often established with computed tomography or magnetic resonance imaging of orbital, retro-orbital, and sellar areas.

BILATERAL COMPLETE LOSS OF VISION

Diseases affecting both **optic nerve**s (bilateral optic neuritis, toxic and nutritional optic neuropathies, demyelinating or degenerative disease, cranial arteritis, ischemic optic neuropathy), the **optic chiasm** (usually large lesions, including pituitary adenomas with or without pituitary apoplexy, craniopharyngiomas, meningiomas, suprasellar aneurysms of the circle of Willis), or, rarely, both **optic tracts** (multiple infarcts, intracerebral hemorrhages, or tumors), both **optic radiations** (multiple infarcts, intracerebral hemorrhages, or tumors), or both **calcarine cortices** (hypertensive encephalopathy, tumors, bilateral infarcts, or intracerebral hemorrhages) may produce bilateral complete visual loss (Table 2-7). Often, a partial bilateral visual loss progresses over time before becoming complete. Characteristic visual field defects (see above) and visual acuity or pupillary reflex abnormalities help to establish the diagnosis.

Occasionally, brief episodes of bilateral darkening of vision lasting seconds to a few minutes may precede a basilar territory infarction. Demyelinating or degenerative diseases usually produce intermittent bilateral loss of vision associated with bitemporal optic atrophy and early impairment of color vision. Tumors (for example, meningiomas) or aneurysms affecting the above-mentioned structures often lead to gradual, progressive (usually asymmetric) losses of vision.

Simultaneous bilateral impairment of vision with relatively symmetric central or cecocentral scotomata, developing during a period of days to weeks, may occur with toxic or nutritional optic neuropathy associated with such agents as methyl alcohol, isoniazid, ethambutol, penicillamine, chloroquine, or phenylbutazone, with tobacco-alcohol abuse, or with deficiencies of thiamine, riboflavin, pyridoxine, niacin, vitamin B_{12}, or folic acid. Drug-induced alterations in color vision may be caused by trimethadione, sulfonamides, streptomycin, methaqualone, barbiturates, digitalis, or thiazides.

Nonorganic (functional) bitemporal sudden visual loss is characterized by no objective evidence of ocular pathology or disease of the

Table 2-7.   Causes of bilateral complete loss of vision

Type of vision loss	Cause
Complete	Diseases or lesions of both optic nerves, optic chiasm, both optic tracts, both calcarine cortices
Episodic, bilateral darkening	Basilar territory transient ischemia
Intermittent	Demyelinating or degenerative
Gradual, progressive	Tumors, aneurysms
Impairment simultaneous with scotomata	Toxic or nutritional optic neuropathy

optic pathways (including negative results of computed tomography or magnetic resonance imaging of the head). Some patients may have tunnel vision (the remaining tunnel of vision does not change, regardless of the size of the target or the testing distance) or variable visual field defects with anatomic inconsistencies.

DIPLOPIA

Diplopia may be caused by a wide variety of disorders. A careful history is very helpful for determining the diagnosis and origin of diplopia and may even provide information about the most likely location of the lesion. The clinician should clarify several issues (Table 2-8). **Did the diplopia develop suddenly or gradually?** Sudden onset is typical for acute brain stem ischemia or hemorrhage, and gradual onset with slow progression is typical for growing aneurysms or tumors. **Has the diplopia been associated with orbital or periorbital pain?** Pain around the eye and frontal area may be caused by cavernous sinus thrombosis, by aneurysms of the internal carotid artery at the infraclinoid-intracavernous or middle cranial fossa levels, or by inflammatory disease of the orbit. Bleeding from the aneurysms usually causes generalized severe headache. **Does closing one eye change the diplopia in any way?** If the diplopia is caused by misalignment of the eyes, closing either eye will correct it; if not (monocular diplopia), either an ocular problem (such as a dislocated lens, cataract, retinal or macular lesion) or a functional disorder should be suspected. **Are the two objects seen horizontally, vertically, or as a combination of both?** Horizontal displacement of the objects may be a sign of dysfunction of the

Table 2-8.   Questions to answer in evaluation of diplopia

Question	Significance
Was onset sudden or gradual?	Sudden: brain stem ischemia or hemorrhage
	Gradual: aneurysm, tumor
Is diplopia associated with orbital or periorbital pain?	Pain may be caused by cavernous sinus thrombosis, aneurysm of ICA, inflammatory orbital disease
Does diplopia change with eye closing?	If corrected with closing: misalignment
	If not corrected: ocular problem or functional disorder
Are the objects horizontal, vertical, or both?	Horizontal: possible dysfunction of abducens nerve or lateral rectus muscle
	Vertical: possible involvement of oculomotor nerve or trochlear nerve
	Horizontal and vertical: possible dysfunction of oculomotor nerve or trochlear nerve
Does a direction of gaze widen or narrow distance between images?	Images farthest apart when looking in direction of action of weak muscle: dysfunction of cranial nerves III, IV, VI
Is the diplopia intermittent or constant?	Constant: tumor, inflammation, infarction, infection
	Intermittent: transient ischemic attack, aneurysm, neuromuscular junction defect, extraocular muscle dysfunction

ICA = internal carotid artery.

abducens nerve or lateral rectus muscle, vertical displacement of the images may indicate involvement of the oculomotor nerve or trochlear nerve, and combined horizontal/vertical diplopia also may occur with dysfunction of the oculomotor nerve or trochlear nerve.

Is there a direction of gaze that widens or narrows the distance between the images? The images are displaced farthest apart when the patient is looking maximally in the direction of action of the weak muscle in cases of dysfunction of the third, fourth, or sixth cranial nerve, but this test cannot be used easily in assessing weakness of multiple extraocular muscles, such as in myasthenia gravis or ocular myopathies. Also, the eye may be displaced forward (exophthalmos) or in other directions as a result of an orbital mass lesion with or without diplopia.

Is the diplopia intermittent or constant? It is important to know the time and mode of onset of the diplopia and whether it is constant or intermittent. Constant or slowly changing diplopia may result from tumor, inflammation, infarction, or infection; intermittent diplopia is more suggestive of transient ischemic attack, aneurysms, and disorders of the neuromuscular junction or ocular muscles.

Lesions of the third, fourth, and sixth cranial nerves may occur at the level of their nuclei, along their course from the brain stem through the subarachnoid space, cavernous sinus, or superior orbital fissure. Isolated horizontal or vertical diplopia resulting from oculomotor nerve palsy is commonly caused by head trauma, diabetic vasculopathy, intracranial aneurysm of the internal carotid or posterior communicating artery, herniation of the uncus, or other rare conditions such as a tumor at the base of the brain, infarction of the nerve, inflammation, mass lesions or thrombosis of the cavernous sinus, syphilis, vasculitis, demyelinating disease, or complicated migraine (ophthalmoplegic migraine).

Common causes of vertical or vertical/horizontal diplopia resulting from trochlear nerve palsy include brain stem ischemic stroke, entrapment against the tentorium in herniation and trauma, cavernous sinus thrombosis, and inflammation or mass lesion. Isolated trochlear nerve palsy may be caused by aneurysms or neoplasms of the posterior fossa, trauma, sphenoid sinusitis, diabetic angiopathy, complicated migraine, nerve infarction, and syphilitic or tuberculous meningitis.

Isolated, unilateral, horizontal diplopia resulting from abducens nerve palsy may be caused by diabetic angiopathy, aneurysms of the circle of Willis, increased intracranial pressure with or without downward herniation, or, less commonly, sixth cranial nerve infarction, mass lesions in the orbit, and pontine glioma in children or metastatic nasopharyngeal tumor in adults.

Muscle Weakness

When a patient experiences weakness, heaviness, or difficulty in performing some activity, several historical features must be considered. The clinician should clarify the precise area of the body that is involved: Is the process focal, multifocal, or generalized? One must also inquire about onset: Was the problem acute or insidious in onset,

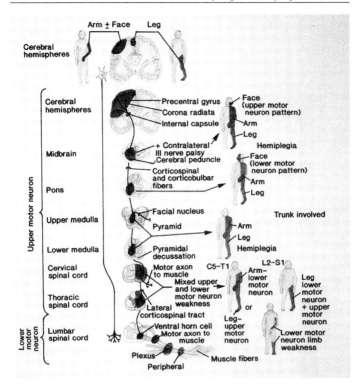

Fig. 2-2. Clinical features of motor system lesions at different levels.

and was there progression after the symptoms started? Are the symptoms episodic or continuous? Does anything seem to bring on the symptoms, and what leads to worsening? What is the pattern of weakness? Are there any symptoms other than weakness? After these questions are answered and a comprehensive examination is performed, the location of the neurologic abnormality leading to the weakness may be determined and a differential diagnosis outlined.

Important aspects of the neurologic examination are the pattern of muscle weakness, the appearance of the muscles, and the presence of fasciculations, atrophy, or hypertrophy. Deep tendon reflexes and muscle tone also should be evaluated. Other aspects of the neurologic examination should delineate the presence of abnormalities in other areas of the nervous system. Symptoms and signs associated with muscle weakness caused by lesions at various sites are reviewed in Table 2-9 and Figure 2-2.

Sensory Disturbances

When patients with ischemic or hemorrhagic cerebrovascular events have a sensory abnormality, it is usually in the form of numbness. It is important to clarify that the numbness nearly always reflects

Table 2-9. Localization of muscle weakness

Location	Symptoms	Signs (side, relevant to lesion site)
Cortical/hemispheric	Weakness: in a single limb or in the face, may involve combinations of weakness on single side Other: associated sensory loss ipsilateral to weakness, visual loss, speech difficulty	Contralateral limb, face, or tongue weakness Spasticity Increased reflexes Extensor plantar response Aphasia Apraxia Hemianopia
Subcortical/internal capsule	Weakness: more likely to involve entire side, including face, arm, and leg Other: sensory loss may involve same areas as weakness; no aphasia, apraxia, hemianopia	Contralateral limb, face, or tongue weakness Spasticity Increased reflexes Extensor plantar response Sensory loss
Brain stem	Weakness: in arm and leg, may involve only face or tongue, may be bilateral Other: diplopia, vertigo, dysphagia, hoarseness, numbness in face or limbs	Same as for subcortical site Ipsilateral cranial nerve deficits, including face or tongue weakness Ipsilateral (mid to low brain stem) or contralateral (high brain stem) facial pain and temperature loss Contralateral limb pain, trunk pain, and temperature loss
Spinal cord (segment)	Weakness: in arm and leg, often bilateral Other: bowel and bladder problems, numbness	Limb weakness Spasticity Increased reflexes below lesion Decreased reflexes at level of lesion Extensor plantar response Contralateral pain and temperature loss Ipsilateral proprioception loss

	History	Signs
Anterior horn cell	Weakness: confined to involved segment(s) Other: cramps, fasciculations	Weakness: confined to involved segment(s) Atrophy Fasciculations Decreased reflexes No extensor plantar response
Nerve root	Weakness: in nerve root distribution Other: local pain, paresthesias, numbness	Weakness in nerve root distribution Decreased reflexes in root distribution Segmental atrophy Segmental sensory loss Segmental fasciculations (uncommon)
Plexus	Weakness: in single limb Other: local pain, paresthesias, numbness	All signs may incompletely involve plexus Weakness in single limb Decreased reflexes in single limb Limb atrophy Sensory loss in single limb Fasciculations in single limb
Peripheral nerve	Distal weakness: footdrop, clumsy gait Other: distal numbness, distal paresthesias	Distal weakness Distal sensory loss Distal atrophy Distal fasciculations (uncommon) Decreased reflexes
Muscle	Weakness: proximal greater than distal, with difficulty arising from chair or elevating arms over head	Proximal weakness Normal sensation and tone Reflexes may be affected late
Neuromuscular junction	Weakness: fluctuating Other: fluctuating ptosis, dysarthria, dysphagia, diplopia	Worsening weakness with repetitive or persistent effort Normal sensation and tone Reflexes usually normal

deadness or a loss of sensation (negative phenomenon), in contrast, for example, to sensory seizures, which characteristically involve a tingling or too much feeling (positive phenomenon). Occasionally, the patient with a thalamic or spinothalamic tract lesion may have a burning discomfort or pain after hemianesthesia or subjective numb feelings in the contralateral limbs. Lacunar stroke affecting the thalamus may also cause **pure sensory stroke,** manifested by loss of sensation over the contralateral side of the body and face, without motor deficit.

In a patient with isolated unilateral or bilateral facial numbness, it is important to carefully analyze the distribution of the numbness. An "onionskin" distribution is diagnostic for a lesion in the descending trigeminal nucleus at the level of the lower pons, medulla, or upper cervical cord, which may be caused by infarction (such as Wallenberg's syndrome of lateral medullary infarction), demyelinating disease, or syringobulbia. Mandibular, maxillary, ophthalmic, or hemifacial numbness may result from lesions involving the extramedullary part of the trigeminal nerve, often a result of tumor or trigeminal sensory neuropathy.

Information should also be sought about the **type of onset, temporal pattern** (intermittent numbness, especially with sudden onset, may occur with a vascular lesion or as a part of epilepsy; gradual onset is more typical of neoplastic lesions), and **association with other neurologic signs** (isolated facial numbness is seldom caused by a cerebrovascular lesion). As mentioned above, a sensory seizure originating in or near the sensory cortex may produce transient, unilateral numbness (tingling or positive phenomenon) of the face, arm, or leg, which usually advances quickly (within a few minutes) from one area to another and may be accompanied by clonic jerks of the involved extremity. Migraine may also produce a sensory spell and involve deadness or tingling, characteristically beginning in one hand and marching up the arm before involving the ipsilateral face and, sometimes, the ipsilateral leg. This type of spell usually lasts 15 to 30 minutes and is often followed by a unilateral, throbbing headache.

Speech and Swallowing Disturbances

Dysarthria, as defined neurologically, is a specific difficulty with articulation caused by a cortical (associated contralateral limb weakness or dysphasia), corticobulbar (accompanying other signs of pseudobulbar palsy), subcortical extrapyramidal (associated with bradykinesia, rigidity, and rest tremor in the extremities), cerebellar (other signs of gait or appendicular ataxia may be noted), or brain stem (often with associated cranial nerve deficits) lesion.

Dysphonia is an impaired ability to produce sound because of respiratory disease or vocal cord paralysis (medullary involvement or a result of a carotid or thyroid surgical procedure, bronchial neoplasm, or aortic aneurysm). In middle-aged or elderly patients, spastic dysphonia may occur. This disorder of unknown nature is characterized by nonprogressive, isolated spasm of all the throat muscles on attempted speech. **Dysphasia** is a loss of production or comprehension of spoken or written language, often as a result of a cortical lesion, such as an ischemic or hemorrhagic stroke.

In a patient with speech and swallowing abnormalities, the physician must determine whether the symptoms are caused by pseudobulbar palsy (bilateral corticobulbar tract involvement) or by true bulbar palsy (including the nuclei of cranial nerves IX, X, and XII, the neuromuscular junction, or muscle involvement) (Table 2-10).

In a patient with acute bulbar palsy, the differential diagnosis should include stroke (often associated with other symptoms of a brain stem lesion), myasthenia gravis (usually with accompanying weakness of extraocular, pharyngeal, or extremity muscles), botulism (often with accompanying dilated, sluggishly reactive pupils and extraocular muscle weakness), Guillain-Barré syndrome (often preceded by ascending symmetric limb weakness), tick paralysis (commonly preceded by tick bite, muscle pain, and fever), and bulbar poliomyelitis (often with asymmetric limb weakness and fever).

Movement and Gait Abnormalities

In a patient with movement or gait disturbances, a carefully obtained history may indicate the likely origin and site of the causative lesion. The physician should ask the patient whether the disturbance occurs more in the dark than in the light, whether there is any accompanying vertigo (brain stem involvement) or other symptoms, whether there is difficulty in the initiation or termination of walking, and whether there is a family history of movement or gait abnormalities.

A patient with unsteadiness and gait disturbances that do not change much in the dark from what they are in the light usually has cerebellar (or cerebellar connection) dysfunction involving either the anterior lobe or the midline vermis. The acute onset of such disturbances suggests a cerebrovascular lesion, most commonly a cerebellar infarct. More gradual onset of isolated gait ataxia is most often caused by aging or chronic alcohol consumption. Other causes of cerebellar gait ataxia include cerebellar hemorrhage, tumor, infection, developmental lesions (agenesis, Dandy-Walker deformity, Arnold-Chiari malformation, von Hippel-Lindau disease), degenerative disorders (ataxia-telangiectasia, Friedreich's ataxia), metabolic, drug, paraneoplastic, or toxic disorders (myxedema, malignancy, inborn disorders of metabolism, use of alcohol, phenytoin), or hydrocephalus.

Unsteadiness on standing, walking, or sitting that markedly increases in the dark or when the patient's eyes are closed, but without substantial impairment of limb coordination or nystagmus, is suspicious for sensory ataxia caused by peripheral nerve or spinal cord posterior column lesions (tabes dorsalis, vitamin B_{12} deficiency, pernicious anemia, paraneoplastic disorders, Sjögren's syndrome, excess vitamin B_6). In contrast, diseases of the cerebellar hemisphere (infarction, hemorrhage, neoplastic or demyelinating disease) often cause prominent impairment of ipsilateral limb coordination.

Table 2-10.   Differentiating features of bulbar and pseudobulbar palsies

Syndrome	Structures involved	Major causes	Characteristic clinical features
Bulbar palsy	Nuclei of cranial nerves IX, X, XII Neuromuscular junction or muscles	Brain stem infarction, demyelinating disease, syringobulbia, botulism, Guillain-Barré syndrome, tick paralysis, bulbar poliomyelitis, diphtheria, myasthenia gravis	Nasal regurgitation of fluids is common; speech tends to be nasal and breathy; flaccid weakness (atrophy may also be present) of the muscles associated with talking, chewing, swallowing, and movement of the tongue and lips
Pseudobulbar palsy	Bilateral corticobulbar tract	Bilateral hemispheric stroke, bilateral lacunar infarction, encephalopathy, demyelinating disease, encephalitis, trauma, amyotrophic lateral sclerosis	Speech tends to be slow, strangulated, low-pitched, and harsh; nasal regurgitation of fluids is rare; emotional incontinence, dementia, bilateral pyramidal tract signs, an active jaw jerk, snout reflex, or grasp reflex

Transient Loss of Consciousness and Seizures

Because the physician usually has not witnessed these disorders, a detailed history, including the time just preceding a spell and the time after it, is very important in the evaluation. The clinician should inquire whether the disturbances occurred with prodromal features (pallor, nausea, and sweating often precede vasovagal **syncopal or presyncopal attacks;** palpitation, sweating, behavioral disturbances, or seizures may precede **hypoglycemic syncope;** vertigo and scintillating scotomata often precede transient loss of consciousness caused by **basilar migraine;** abnormal stereotyped movements, sensations, or experiences just before the loss of consciousness may suggest **seizure**); whether the disturbances occurred suddenly or gradually when the patient was standing (disturbances with standing associated with gradual onset of loss of consciousness are typical of **syncope** or of **functional disturbances**), sitting, or lying (disturbances with lying associated with abrupt onset of loss of consciousness are more suggestive of **seizure**); whether the patient had been using alcohol or other drugs **(drug-induced syncope or seizure);** whether the patient had been ill or febrile at the time the incident occurred (suggestive of **syncope or febrile seizure**); whether there were any focal motor or sensory manifestations such as speech disturbances, localized sensory abnormalities, hemiparesis or monoparesis preceding or following the event (suggestive of a **localized structural cerebral lesion**); and whether there was tongue laceration, bruising, or urinary or fecal incontinence noted after the loss of consciousness (suggestive of **seizure** rather than simple syncope).

The stereotyped and uncontrollable nature of the focal (partial seizures with or without loss of consciousness and secondary generalization) or generalized (absence, myoclonic, clonic, tonic, tonic-clonic, or atonic) seizures is characteristic of epilepsy. Differentiating features of seizures and syncope are reviewed in Table 2-11.

TRANSIENT LOSS OF CONSCIOUSNESS

Transient loss of consciousness most often results from syncope caused by reduced cardiac output or mechanical reduction of venous return or from concussion caused by trauma (Table 2-12). Metabolic disorders, such as hypoglycemia, may cause transient loss of consciousness, and basilar migraine may cause such loss of consciousness, particularly in young women. Primary cerebrovascular insufficiency almost never causes transient loss of consciousness.

Reduced cardiac output (cardiac syncope) most often results from cardiac arrhythmias (especially atrioventricular block with Stokes-Adams attacks, ventricular asystole, sinus bradycardia, episodic ventricular fibrillation, ventricular tachycardia, and supraventricular tachycardia without atrioventricular block), massive myocardial infarction with pump failure, obstruction of left ventricular outflow (aortic stenosis, hypertrophic subaortic stenosis), obstruction of pulmonary flow (pulmonic stenosis, primary pulmonary hypertension, pulmonary embolism), and cardiac tamponade. For patients with suspected cardiac syncope, electrocardiography is mandatory (in many cases, prolonged monitoring,

Table 2-11.   Transient loss of consciousness: seizure compared with syncope

Symptoms	Seizure	Syncope

Prodromal	None: sudden LOC
	Aura
	  Epigastric discomfort
	  Déjà vu
	  Sensation of fear
	  Focal sensory or motor
	    phenomena
		Nausea
		Diaphoresis
		Light-headedness
		Visual darkening

During the spell	Convulsive
	  Tonic-clonic movements
	  Bowel or bladder inconti-
	    nence
	  Tongue biting
	Nonconvulsive
	  Stare
	  Automatistic movements
	    of limbs
		Unresponsive
		Flaccidity
		Occasional stiffness with
		  jerking movements
		Occasional bladder incon-
		  tinence

After the spell	Confusion lasting minutes Agitation lasting minutes	Prompt recovery
Activity	Sleep Standing, sitting, or lying Alcohol use	Standing or sitting Lying (less common) Exertion Alcohol use
Cause	See Table 2-13	See Table 2-12

LOC = loss of consciousness.

tilt-table testing, or cardiac electrophysiology studies are also needed).

Vasovagal (vasodepressor) syncope is characterized by a generalized weakness with loss of postural tone, inability to stand upright, and a loss of consciousness caused by global reduction of cerebral blood flow. A short prodromal phase usually includes various combinations of pallor, nausea, yawning, epigastric distress, hyperpnea or tachypnea, weakness, confusion, tachycardia, pupillary dilatation, and sweating. The patient is pale and has bradycardia and hypotension. This syncope may be experienced by people without significant medical or neurologic disease and tends to take place during emotional stress (especially in a warm, crowded room), and often when the patient is standing (sitting may alleviate or minimize the spell). Circumstances that precipitate this type of syncope include Valsalva maneuver, cough, or micturition. Occasionally, paroxysms of coughing in patients (especially men) with chronic bronchitis produce a **tussive syncope.** After hard coughing, the patient suddenly becomes weak and loses consciousness momentarily. The mechanism is thought to be decreased cardiac venous return associated with the Valsalva maneuver. Defecation syncope has a similar underlying mechanism. In all vasovagal syncope subtypes, loss of consciousness is generally short-lived, but tonic or clonic movements may develop if impaired cerebral blood flow is prolonged (anoxic seizures).

Postural (orthostatic) hypotension with syncope is a fairly common cause of loss of consciousness in middle-aged or elderly

Table 2-12. Classification of causes of syncope

Category	Causes
Cardiopulmonary	
Dysrhythmias	
Tachycardia	Supraventricular
	Atrial fibrillation
	Atrial flutter
	Other
	Ventricular
	Ventricular tachycardia
	Ventricular fibrillation
Bradycardia	Sinus bradycardia
	Second- or third-degree heart block
	Pacemaker failure
Sick sinus syndrome	
Drug toxicity	
Outflow obstruction/	Pulmonary stenosis
cardiac failure	Aortic stenosis
	Pulmonary embolus
	Myocardial infarction
	Hypertrophic obstructive cardiomyopathy
Inflow obstruction	Pericardial tamponade
	Mitral stenosis
	Atrial myxoma
	Cardiomyopathies (restrictive)
Cerebrovascular (unusual cause)	
Stenosis/occlusion of bilateral carotid and/or vertebrobasilar arteries	Multiple causes (see Table 8-1, large vessel diseases)
Other neurologic	
Neurologically mediated	Vasovagal syncope
	Cardiac sinus syncope
	Glossopharyngeal neuralgia
	Micturition syncope
Orthostatic hypotension	Autonomic neuropathy
	Multisystem atrophy
	Prolonged recumbency
Metabolic/hematologic	Hypoglycemia, hypoxia, anemia
Psychological	Anxiety

patients who have instability of vasomotor reflexes. The blood pressure should be measured when the patient is supine, immediately on standing, and 1 to 2 minutes after standing. A decrease in systolic blood pressure of more than 25 mm Hg on standing and associated with near syncope or syncope is highly suggestive of the diagnosis. This syndrome may be caused by medications (antihypertensive agents, beta-adrenergic blockers, tricyclic antidepressants, nitrates, dopaminergics, or dopamine agonists) or concomitant disease (Addison's disease, parainfectious or paraneoplastic autonomic neuropathy, amyloidosis with associated neuropathy, Shy-Drager syndrome, familial dysautonomia), or it may be idiopathic with no evident cause. Although the character of the syncopal attack differs little from that of the vasovagal type, the effect of posture (occurring when the patient arises suddenly from a recumbent position) is its cardinal feature.

Carotid sinus syncope may be initiated by direct palpation over the carotid bifurcation area, by turning of the head to one side, by a tight collar, or by shaving over the region of the sinus, particularly in elderly persons. Carotid sinus palpation and massage should be avoided in patients in whom this diagnosis is suspected. Auscultation of the carotid arteries should be performed carefully and, in selected patients, neurovascular noninvasive investigations may be useful to look for evidence of carotid occlusive disease.

SEIZURES

Seizure is a generic term that can be defined as a transient disturbance in neurologic function related to an abnormal and excessive electrical discharge of a population of neurons in the brain. The clinical manifestations of seizures are many and varied. Spells are generally categorized as generalized (convulsive or nonconvulsive, primary or secondary) or partial (simple or complex) seizures and may be isolated, cyclic, prolonged, or repetitive.

A **jacksonian clonic convulsion** or transient hemiparesis or monoparesis after a motor seizure (**Todd's paralysis**) is indicative of a frontal motor cortex lesion. **Simple sensory seizures** (paresthesia or tingling in a limb or on the face, with or without sensation of body image distortion, or other strange, localized, or stereotyped feelings such as olfactory or visual hallucinations, feeling of familiarity or strangeness, ecstasy, fear, dreamy states, or illusions) are suggestive of a contralateral sensory cortex lesion. The clinical picture of **complex partial seizures** or psychomotor epilepsy (originating usually in the temporal or frontal lobe) usually includes complex aura (stereotyped visceral, memory, movement, or affective disturbances) and loss of consciousness in the form of loss of responsiveness without falling, with or without automatisms (involuntary, often repetitive, and seemingly forced complex motor activity), commonly followed by a confusional state lasting a few minutes or longer. The type of aura before secondary **generalized tonic-clonic seizures** (grand mal) provides information about the site of the lesion.

Once a seizure disorder has been diagnosed, the physician should establish its cause (Table 2-13). Idiopathic epilepsy usually develops when a person is young and is commonly characterized by generalized seizures. The most common causes of seizures in early adulthood include trauma (with or without subdural hematoma), withdrawal from drugs or alcohol (usually within 48 hours after cessation of heavy drinking), central nervous system infection, tumor, and arteriovenous malformation.

The onset of seizures in late adulthood may be associated with cerebrovascular disease (previous cerebral infarction, acute cerebral infarction [especially embolic], arteriovenous malformation, acute subarachnoid hemorrhage, intracerebral hemorrhage), trauma, drug or alcohol withdrawal, tumor, degenerative disease, central nervous system infection, toxic or metabolic encephalopathy (tricyclic antidepressants, phenothiazines, theophylline, hyponatremia, hypoglycemia, nonketotic hyperglycemia, magnesium deficiency, hypocalcemia, hepatic or renal failure), and collagen vascular disorders.

Table 2-13. Classification of causes of seizures

Hereditary/ degenerative	Infectious/ inflammatory	Toxic/metabolic	Neoplastic	Vascular	Other
von Recklinghausen's disease	Meningitis and encephalitis	Severe electrolyte disturbances, hypocalcemia, hyponatremia, vitamin B_6 deficiency, phenylketonuria	Primary brain tumor, brain metastasis	Cerebral infarction	Traumatic hematoma
Tuberous sclerosis	Bacterial			Intracerebral hemorrhage	Subdural
Sturge-Weber syndrome	Fungal			Subarachnoid hemorrhage	Epidural
Inborn errors of metabolism	Viral			Sinus thrombosis	Penetrating brain injury
	Syphilitic	Hypoglycemia		Hypertensive encephalopathy	Fever
	HIV	Hypothyroidism		Cerebral vasculitis	Infantile spasms
	Lyme disease	Drug-induced		Arteriovenous malformation	Idiopathic
	Tuberculosis	Alcohol or other drug withdrawal		Cavernous malformation	Global hypoxia/anoxia
	Parasitic	Liver or kidney failure		Large unruptured intracranial aneurysm	
	Brain abscess				
	Collagen vascular diseases				

HIV = human immunodeficiency virus.

Cognitive Abnormalities

When cognitive function is impaired, the clinician needs to distinguish **dementia** (progressive deterioration of intellect, behavior, and personality caused by diffuse disease processes affecting the cerebral hemispheres) from several **pseudodementias,** including

1. psychiatric illnesses
2. isolated dominant hemisphere lesions
3. isolated nondominant hemisphere lesions
4. isolated memory disturbances
5. acute confusional state (delirium)

Depressed patients and patients with psychosis and other **psychiatric disorders** (such as anxiety) that cause reduced concentration often complain of memory difficulties. In these situations, a careful search for an organic cause should be undertaken.

Dominant hemisphere lesions are often accompanied by abnormalities of language function (aphasia or dysphasia). Gerstmann's syndrome, agraphia, acalculia, right-left confusion, and finger agnosia can all occur with left hemisphere lesions. Apraxia of speech may also occur in patients with dominant hemisphere lesions.

Most patients with **lesions of the nondominant hemisphere** show more dramatic constructional impairment, such as constructional apraxia and dressing apraxia, than do patients with dominant hemisphere lesions. Prosopagnosia (difficulty in recognizing faces), impairment of spatial orientation, anosognosia (ignorance of the presence of disease), motor impersistence, and aprosody may also occur in these patients.

Isolated memory disturbances include **transient global amnesia,** a syndrome usually occurring as a single event in middle-aged to elderly individuals and characterized by the inability to form new memories. The condition usually resolves during a period of minutes to hours and the person has complete recovery. Approximately 10% of patients have recurrent events. The cause of transient global amnesia is probably multifactorial, but, in at least some cases, it appears to involve posterior circulation cerebral ischemia.

Patients with **acute confusional state** (acute brain syndrome, toxic encephalopathy, organic brain syndrome with psychosis) are inattentive, incoherent, agitated, and inconsistent in reporting recent events. In addition, they often demonstrate hallucinations (visual hallucinations are more typical in patients with neurologic disorders, whereas auditory hallucinations are more common in patients with primary psychiatric disease) and fluctuation in their level of consciousness. At night, when environmental stimuli are reduced, the confusion and agitation become accentuated. The most common causes of acute confusional state are (1) toxic-metabolic disturbances, including drug and drug withdrawal reactions; (2) sepsis; and (3) increased intracranial pressure.

When obtaining a history from a patient with **dementia** and from the patient's relative or friend, the physician should obtain details of the **patient's previous mental status** and of the **onset and rapidity of mental deterioration** (acute or stepwise deterioration of the intellectual function may be associated with multi-infarct dementia; subacute progression during a period of days or weeks may be caused by encephalitis; progression during a period of months may result from Jakob-Creutzfeldt disease; chronic progression during several months to years may be associated with Alzheimer's disease, normal-pressure hydrocephalus, or metabolic encephalopathies). Evaluation of the patient's **drug history** enables one to determine dementia caused by taking barbiturates, bromides, tranquilizers, tricyclic antidepressants, lithium, anticonvulsants, steroids, anticholinergic drugs, dopaminergic agents, methyldopa, clonidine, or propranolol.

Questions about **nutritional status** may reveal dementia resulting from thiamine deficiency (chronic alcoholic dementia or Wernicke-Korsakoff syndrome), vitamin B_{12} or folate deficiency, pellagra, alcohol abuse, or toxicity of heavy metals such as arsenic, lead, thallium, or mercury. Questions about **general health and relevant disorders** help to determine the probable cause of a dementing process (Table 2-14).

The physician should also inquire about a **family history of dementia** (suggestive of Huntington's disease and, possibly, Alzheimer's disease). Alzheimer's disease causes about 60% of all dementias; cerebrovascular diseases (multi-infarct dementia, progressive subcortical encephalopathy, or Binswanger's disease) cause 20% of dementias.

Table 2-14.   Classification of common causes of dementia

Hereditary/ degenerative	Infectious/ inflammatory	Toxic/metabolic	Neoplastic	Vascular	Other
Alzheimer's disease	Meningitis and encephalitis	Uremia	Bilateral tumors	Multi-infarct	Multiple head injuries
Pick's disease	Bacterial	Liver failure	Primary	Binswanger's disease	Chronic SDH
Huntington's disease	Fungal	Hypopituitarism	Metastatic	Vasculitis	Hydrocephalus
Parkinson's disease	Viral	Hypothyroidism	Meningeal carcinomatosis		Communicating
Progressive supra-nuclear palsy	Syphilitic	Parathyroid disease	Paraneoplastic syndromes (e.g., limbic encephalitis)		Noncommu-nicating
Wilson's disease	HIV	Hyponatremia			
	Lyme disease	Vitamin deficiencies			
	Brain abscess	Pernicious anemia			
	Jakob-Creutzfeldt disease	B_{12}			
	Collagen vascular diseases	Folate			
		Toxins			
		Medication			
		Heavy metals			

HIV = human immunodeficiency virus; SDH = subdural hematoma.

General Medical Review

The patient's family history, past medical history, and social and environmental history may provide information that clarifies the cause of an ischemic or hemorrhagic cerebrovascular event (Table 3-1). Familial risk factors for ischemic stroke have been difficult to define with certainty, although hypertension, atherosclerosis, diabetes mellitus, and hyperlipidemia appear to have at least some hereditary predisposition in many patients. A family history of ischemic stroke and formation of arterial or venous thromboses should be noted. In persons with subarachnoid hemorrhage or intracerebral hemorrhage, one should ask about a family history of intracranial hemorrhage, saccular aneurysm, arteriovenous malformation, polycystic kidney disease, and bleeding disorders.

A comprehensive medical history also should be obtained. Previous cerebrovascular events of either ischemic or hemorrhagic types should be recorded. Because the presence of systemic atherosclerosis is a risk factor for cerebrovascular atherosclerosis, one should ask about previous myocardial infarction, angina, and claudication of extremities. A history of hypertension, diabetes mellitus, or hyperlipidemia is also an important risk factor for atherosclerosis. Other medical disorders that may be relevant for ischemic stroke are cardiac arrhythmias, valvular heart disease, connective tissue disorders, and coagulopathy of both thrombotic and hemorrhagic subtypes. Previous head or neck trauma or radiation therapy also should be noted. For ischemic or hemorrhagic strokes, use of antiplatelet agents, anticoagulants, fibrinolytic therapies, and estrogen supplements should be recorded.

The social and environmental history should include clarification of the quantity and duration of tobacco use, alcohol consumption, and recreational drug use.

Table 3-1.   General medical history for persons with stroke

Risk factors for cerebral ischemia	Risk factors for cerebral hemorrhage	Risk factors for subarachnoid hemorrhage
Family history		
Ischemic stroke, arterial or venous thromboses	Intracerebral hemorrhage, saccular aneurysm, AVM, bleeding disorders	Subarachnoid hemorrhage, saccular aneurysm, AVM, polycystic kidney disease, Ehlers-Danlos syndrome, Marfan's syndrome, neurofibromatosis, pseudoxanthoma elasticum, bleeding disorders
Previous diseases		
Ischemic stroke(s) or TIA; ischemic cardiac disease; hypertension; diabetes mellitus; hyperlipidemia; systemic atherosclerosis; cardiac arrhythmias; valvular heart disease; hematologic or venous thromboses; hematologic disorders such as lupus anticoagulant positivity (history of multiple miscarriages), anticardiolipin antibody positivity (history of livedo reticularis), polycythemia, thrombocythemia, thrombocytopenic purpura, sickle-cell disease, leukemia; connective tissue diseases; recent operation; head or neck trauma; head or neck radiation therapy	Intracerebral hemorrhage; head trauma; hypertension (particularly severe or poorly treated); intracranial aneurysm or AVM; embolic stroke; CNS infection; SBE; systemic vasculitides, primary CNS angiitis; intracranial neoplasm; hematologic disorders such as thrombocytopenic purpura, sickle cell anemia, leukemia, hyperocoagulable states (venous thrombosis); moyamoya disease	Subarachnoid hemorrhage(s), head trauma, unruptured aneurysm(s), unruptured AVM(s), other disorders listed under "family history" (above), coarctation of the aorta, tuberous sclerosis, fibromuscular disease, bleeding disorders, SBE, primary CNS angiitis, head trauma
Social and environmental history		
Cigarette smoking, use of oral contraceptives or recreational drugs	Anticoagulant or fibrinolytic therapy, heavy alcohol consumption, recreational drug use	Anticoagulant or fibrinolytic therapy, heavy alcohol consumption, recreational drug use

AVM = arteriovenous malformation; CNS = central nervous system; SBE = subacute bacterial endocarditis; TIA = transient ischemic attack.

General Examination

A systematic general examination of the patient with cerebrovascular disease is directed at finding evidence of disease of the cardiovascular system and at evaluation of the functional status of other vital internal organs (lungs, kidneys, liver). The examination of a patient with neurologic symptoms should begin with brief observation and proceed with comprehensive general and neurologic examinations.

Observation

BODY AND LIMB POSITION AND SPONTANEOUS MOVEMENTS

Patients with acute monoparesis or hemiparesis have variable spontaneous movements of the affected limb(s). Often, comatose patients with acute hemiplegia lie with the affected leg externally rotated and occasionally have unilateral twitching, unilateral myoclonic jerks, or spontaneous unilateral or asymmetric bilateral decerebrate or decorticate movements (see Chapter 6). Various metabolic disturbances may produce bilateral myoclonic jerks (seen with uremia) and asterixis (irregular flapping movements of the hands with the arms out straight and the wrists extended) in association with tremor and diffuse twitching (seen with hepatic failure, hypoglycemia, or hyponatremia).

GENERAL APPEARANCE AND HYGIENE

These traits usually reflect the patient's self-image and may provide information about underlying preexisting medical or neurologic conditions.

SPECIFIC SIGNS OF CHRONIC ILLNESS

Observation of some specific signs of chronic illness may provide information about the underlying pathophysiology for various neurologic signs and symptoms, including altered levels of consciousness. Although the odor of alcohol on a patient's breath usually indicates alcohol intoxication, one must also consider superimposed subdural hematoma, other intracranial hemorrhage, trauma, seizure, Wernicke's encephalopathy, or infection. Other examples are the smell of ketones, which often indicates diabetic ketoacidosis, and fetor hepaticus, which suggests liver failure. Gingival hypertrophy is common in patients who are taking phenytoin for epilepsy. Lacerations on the lateral borders of the tongue (recent seizure), needle marks on the arms (drug intoxication), and skin ecchymoses and petechiae (recent trauma or bleeding disorder) may also be very helpful signs.

DERMATOLOGIC EXAMINATION

Among patients with trauma, "raccoon's eyes" may indicate the presence of orbital fracture, Battle's sign may signify underlying mastoid fracture, and other **bruises or abrasions** on the head or body may indicate trauma as the underlying cause. One should also characterize skin color changes by the nature of the pigmentation (hypo- or hyperpigmentation), localization (focal or generalized), presence of erythema, and specific pattern of the changes. The features may allow consideration of the presence of an underlying medical or neurologic disorder (Table 4-1).

Cyanosis in the distal extremities associated with cool skin may indicate vasoconstriction in patients with severe heart failure. Venous obstruction or venous hypertension usually results in localized or generalized cyanosis. Arterial obstruction in an extremity caused by embolism, arteriolar constriction, or cold-induced vasospasm usually results in localized pallor and coldness.

Various conditions may be associated with **localized** or **generalized edema**. Possible causes of localized edema include deep venous thrombosis, lymphatic obstruction caused by tumor, primary lymphedema, stasis edema of a paralyzed leg, and facial edema caused by obstruction of the superior vena cava or limited effect from an allergic reaction. Bilateral leg swelling is seen in cardiac failure, inferior vena cava obstructions, or cirrhosis. Hypothyroidism may be associated with periorbital puffiness. Drugs, such as steroids, estrogens, and vasodilators, and pregnancy and refeeding after starvation may also cause edema.

Varicose veins may indicate increased intra-abdominal pressure or, in rare instances, arteriovenous fistulas. **Thrombophlebitis** that leads to deep venous thrombosis may result in pulmonary thromboembolism.

Table 4-1.   Differentiating features of some abnormalities of skin color

Skin color abnormality	Most common cause(s)
"Butterfly" rash on the face	Systemic lupus erythematosus
Erythematous rash on the elbows and knees	Dermatomyositis
Livedo reticularis	Idiopathic, collagen vascular diseases, hematologic disorders, Sneddon's syndrome, drug ingestion, cholesterol emboli, prolonged immobility
White macules on the trunk or limbs	Diabetes mellitus, vitiligo, hypothyroidism, thyrotoxicosis, pernicious anemia, adrenal insufficiency, sarcoidosis, leprosy, tuberous sclerosis
Generalized diffuse brown hypermelanosis	Addison's disease, ACTH-producing tumors, hemochromatosis, systemic scleroderma, porphyria cutanea tarda
Circumscribed brown macules	von Recklinghausen's neurofibromatosis, malignant melanoma, Peutz-Jeghers syndrome
Localized pallor or coldness	Arterial obstruction (embolism, arteriolar constriction, cold-induced vasospasm)
Cyanosis of the nailbeds, lips, or mucous membranes	Chronic pulmonary insufficiency, pulmonary arteriovenous fistula, congenital heart disease with right-to-left shunting, severe heart failure, venous obstruction, or venous hypertension

ACTH = adrenocorticotropic hormone.

Cardiac Evaluation

During the general examination, special attention should be given to the patient's heart, including cardiac auscultation, precordial palpation, and evaluation of heart rate and rhythm. **Cardiac auscultation** may reveal abnormalities of the cardiac valves, the presence of pulmonary hypertension, ventricular septal or atrial septal defect, cardiac wall abnormalities, or constrictive pericarditis (Table 4-2). Precordial palpation will clarify cardiac size and may also suggest the presence of valvular disease (Table 4-3).

Table 4-2.   Cardiac evaluation: auscultation

Auscultation feature	Common cause
Accentuated first heart sound	Mitral stenosis, hyperkinetic heart, thin chest wall
Diminished first heart sound	Heart failure, mitral regurgitation, thick chest wall, pulmonary emphysema
Abnormal splitting of second heart sound	Pulmonary hypertension, pulmonic stenosis, right bundle-branch block, mitral regurgitation, atrial septal defect, aortic stenosis
Low-pitched third heart sound	Left ventricular failure or volume overload
High-pitched third heart sound	Constrictive pericarditis
Low-pitched fourth heart sound	Aortic stenosis, systemic hypertension, hypertrophic cardiomyopathy, coronary artery disease
High-pitched opening snap after second heart sound	Mitral stenosis
High-pitched ejection clicks after first heart sound	Dilatation of aortic root or pulmonary artery, congenital aortic stenosis or pulmonary stenosis
Systolic murmurs	Mitral or tricuspid regurgitation, ventricular septal defect, aortic stenosis, aortopulmonary shunt
Diastolic murmurs	Aortic or pulmonary regurgitation, mitral stenosis, patent ductus arteriosus, coarctation of aorta, pulmonary arteriovenous fistula

Table 4-3.   Cardiac evaluation: precordial palpation

Examination finding	Common cause
Exaggerated amplitude, duration, and lateral displacement of left ventricular apex impulse	Left ventricular hypertrophy
Presystolic distention of left ventricle	Excess left ventricular pressure, myocardial ischemia
Double systolic impulse	Hypertrophic cardiomyopathy
Low-frequency vibrations	Mitral or aortic valve disease
Pulsation of right sternoclavicular joint	Aneurysmal dilatation of ascending aorta, right-sided aortic arch

Peripheral Vascular Examination

Absence or reduction of the peripheral arterial pulses in the upper and lower limbs is indicative of primary arterial stenotic or occlusive lesions or lesions resulting from proximal emboli. The **time of arrival** of the radial pulse at the wrist may also be helpful. A tardy radial pulse may result from an occlusive lesion in a proximal vessel, usually the subclavian artery. Simultaneous palpation of the radial and femoral arterial pulses, which normally are virtually coincident, allows one to detect the **weaker and delayed pulse,** which is suggestive of aortic coarctation. A **decreased or thready pulse** may occur in patients with myocardial infarction, restrictive pericardial disease, and other conditions associated with decreased cardiac output or in patients with increased peripheral vascular resistance. An **increased, bounding pulse** occurs characteristically in patients with anemia, fever, mitral regurgitation, aortic regurgitation, or peripheral arteriovenous fistula. **Alterations of the pulse amplitude** may result from severe left ventricular decompensation, paroxysmal tachycardia, premature ventricular contraction, pericardial tamponade, airway obstruction, or obstruction of the superior vena cava.

Blood pressure should be measured in both arms with the patient supine, and, if possible, sitting and standing to detect significant asymmetry in blood pressure and to document postural hypotension. One must be certain that the cuff size is appropriate for the arm size of the patient. A difference of 20 mm Hg or more in either systolic or diastolic pressure between two arms may be caused by occlusive disease in or distal to the subclavian artery on the side of the lower systolic or diastolic blood pressure or more proximally in the innominate artery or aorta between the innominate and left subclavian arteries. A significant decrease in the brachial blood pressure when the patient assumes the upright position indicates postural hypotension, which may be symptomatic. The absence of compensatory tachycardia may signify central (such as Shy-Drager syndrome) or peripheral (such as autonomic neuropathy) autonomic dysfunction. A diastolic pressure that is consistently 95 mm Hg or more or a systolic pressure that is 160 mm Hg or more is considered to be definite hypertension (a blood pressure of 140–159/90–94 mm Hg is considered borderline hypertension).

Although as much as 90% of all patients with hypertension have so-called idiopathic or essential hypertension, the physician should try to determine a specific cause for the elevated blood pressure (Table 4-4). The essential components of evaluation are (1) the past medical history (including salt intake, use of oral contraceptives or hormones, presence of diabetes mellitus, smoking history, lipid abnormalities, and cardiac or renal disease) and family history of hypertension; (2) physical examination—ophthalmoscopy, assessment of thyroid size, auscultation for neck and abdominal bruits, palpation of peripheral pulses, determination of heart and kidney size, auscultation of the heart and lungs; and (3) laboratory evaluation—determination of hematocrit, blood urea nitrogen or creatinine, serum potassium, leukocyte count, blood glucose, cholesterol, triglycerides, serum calcium, phosphate, and uric acid; urinalysis; electrocardiography; and chest radiography. In certain circum-

Table 4-4. Common clinical forms of arterial hypertension

Form of hypertension	Clinical feature	Common causes
Essential (primary) hypertension	Varies	Unknown
Secondary hypertension	Primarily systolic hypertension	Aortic atherosclerosis, aortic regurgitation, thyrotoxicosis, hyperkinetic heart syndrome, fever, arteriovenous fistula, patent ductus arteriosus
	Systolic and diastolic hypertension	Renal causes: stenosis of a main or branch renal artery, renal infarction, arteriolar nephrosclerosis, pre-eclampsia, eclampsia, chronic pyelonephritis, acute or chronic glomerulonephritis, polycystic renal disease, diabetic nephropathy, renin-producing tumors
		Endocrine causes: primary hyperaldosteronism, Cushing's syndrome, pheochromocytoma, congenital adrenogenital syndromes, acromegaly, hypercalcemia, myxedema, oral contraceptives
		Neurogenic causes: diencephalic syndrome, familial dysautonomia (Riley-Day), bulbar poliomyelitis, acute increased intracranial pressure, acute spinal cord transection
		Other causes: coarctation of aorta, toxemia of pregnancy, acute intermittent porphyria, and excessive transfusion

stances, special studies, such as determination of creatinine clearance, renal ultrasonography, renal angiography, and 24-hour urine study for metanephrine, catecholamine, or cortisol levels, may be indicated.

Head, Chest, and Abdomen Examination

The clinical examination of the head (scalp and face), chest (lungs), and abdomen (liver, spleen, gastroenteric and urogenital systems) may provide additional important findings.

Palpation and examination of the patient's **scalp, mastoid area, and zygomatic arches** may reveal a depressed fracture or laceration. Examination of the **auditory meatus and nose** to detect the presence of a cerebrospinal fluid leak or hemorrhage may indicate fracture of the cribriform plate or of the petrous portion of the temporal bone. The ocular sclerae also should be examined for hemorrhage because a hemorrhage of the lateral aspect of the eye, which is not bordered posteriorly by normal sclera, is somewhat characteristic of fracture of the anterior cranial fossa.

The neck (cervical vertebral bodies), **chest** (clavicles, ribs, trunk, vertebral bodies), and **limbs** (long bones) must be examined for the presence of fracture, particularly in comatose patients who have uncertain histories or evidence of possible injury. **Lymph node enlargement** is most frequently indicative of infectious, immunologic, or malignant disease.

Pulmonary examination may reveal unsuspected lung or heart disease, including pneumonia, chronic obstructive pulmonary disease, and congestive heart failure.

The patient's abdomen should be palpated for the presence of muscle rigidity as evidence of possible abdominal hemorrhage or infection. **Hepatomegaly** may indicate tumor, hepatitis, cirrhosis, right-sided heart failure, Budd-Chiari syndrome, or hepatic infiltrative disorders. **Splenomegaly** occurs in a wide variety of hematologic, infectious, hepatic, and connective tissue disorders, such as sickle-cell disease, thalassemia, hemolytic anemias, thrombocytopenias, neutropenias, infectious mononucleosis, septicemia, endocarditis, tuberculosis, parasitic infection, acquired immunodeficiency syndrome (AIDS), histoplasmosis, and rheumatoid arthritis. Splenomegaly may also be associated with various forms of portal or splenic venous hypertension or with primary splenic tumor or abscess.

Neurologic Examination

Neurologic examination of the patient with cerebrovascular disease is similar to any other formal neurologic examination. However, certain combinations of neurologic signs may establish the location of the disease. A complete neurologic examination is necessary to determine current neurologic status, and serial assessments are often desirable to determine whether there is any improvement or worsening of the condition. Some elements of the neurologic examination relating to preliminary evaluation of the level of consciousness, mental status, speech, vision, and focal weakness of the limbs are completed when the history is taken and also during the general examination.

Other elements of the neurologic examination provide further detail about whether the patient's current illness is caused by cerebrovascular disease and, if so, the location and sometimes the type and origin of the lesion(s). With the data from the history and the general and neurologic examinations, a logical differential diagnosis and evaluation strategy can be proposed. Further evaluation of laboratory study results usually helps to clarify the diagnosis and define an appropriate treatment plan.

Neurovascular Examination

AUSCULTATION

Auscultation of the proximal great vessels (Fig. 5-1) arising from the aortic arch (over the supraclavicular fossa), the carotid arteries (particularly over the carotid bifurcation below the angle of the mandible), the orbits (while closing the eye being auscultated), and the cranial vault is performed to listen for bruits. With the patient lying or sitting, the bell of the stethoscope should be applied over the area examined without using pressure, which may produce artificial noise. First, the cardiac sounds should be auscultated over the base of the heart, and then the stethoscope should be moved superiorly to distinguish transmitted cardiac sounds from sounds arising in brachiocephalic, subclavian, vertebral, or carotid arteries. Bruits heard proximally over the aortic arch vessels may be associated with transmitted cardiac murmurs, underlying large vessel stenosis or tortuosity, or no identifiable underlying abnormality.

All bruits should be graded on a scale of 1 to 6 according to their intensity (1, barely audible with stethoscope; 6, audible without a stethoscope). The quality of a carotid bruit is a poor predictor of the severity of the underlying stenosis, although high-pitched bruits may be more predictive of an underlying significant stenosis. A bruit is a reflection of turbulence in the underlying artery. A carotid bruit, without regard to its quality or duration, is a relatively poor predictor of stenosis of the internal carotid artery in asymptomatic patients. It is noted in about 40% of patients with stenosis of more than 90% of the diameter of the artery, but 10% of patients with

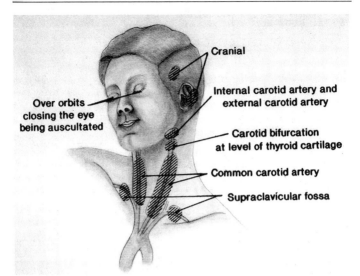

Fig. 5-1.   Sites for neurovascular auscultation.

stenosis of less than 50% of the artery's diameter may have an audible bruit. In patients with symptoms of cerebral ischemia, however, a diffuse or localized bruit is 85% predictive of a moderate or high-grade stenosis. Soft, continuous cervical bruits that vary with changes in neck position or that can be obliterated by jugular compression are suggestive of a benign venous hum.

Most **arterial bruits** begin in systole, but **systolic-diastolic bruits** strongly suggest high-grade arterial stenosis (>90% cross-sectional area stenosis). While listening over the carotid arteries, the physician should distinguish **diffuse** bruits (relatively constant magnitude and pitch along the carotid arteries in the neck or mildly decreasing distal intensity) from **localized** carotid bruits, although either may or may not be associated with underlying carotid stenosis. Diffuse bruits, especially if bilateral, often reflect a transmitted heart murmur, aortic arch lesion, or a condition of diffuse, increased flow and turbulence without an underlying structural lesion. It may be difficult or impossible to distinguish lesions of the internal carotid artery from stenoses of the common carotid or external carotid arteries or to distinguish lesions of the vertebral artery from those of the subclavian or brachiocephalic arteries on the basis of the location or sound characteristics of a bruit.

Orbital bruits, particularly continuous, machinery-like bruits, are encountered with occlusive lesions of the carotid siphon, ipsilateral internal carotid artery occlusion with increased ophthalmic collateral backflow in the external carotid system, and other lesions producing intracranial turbulent flow, such as arteriovenous malformations. **Cephalic bruits** are commonly found in otherwise normal children but may also be found in 10% to 25% of patients with intracranial arteriovenous malformations (often associated with the symptom of a rhythmic, localized head noise).

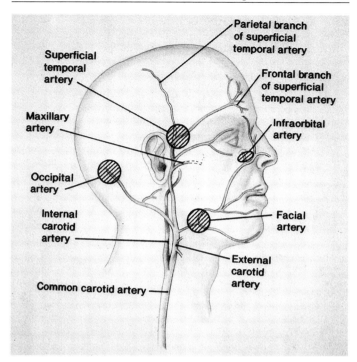

Fig. 5-2. Common sites for palpation of the external carotid artery system.

PALPATION

Palpation of the carotid pulses in the neck is generally unreliable (minor differences in the pulses of the left and right carotid arteries are unlikely to be important) and may even be dangerous, particularly at the level of the carotid bifurcation or over carotid arteries with associated bruit. Material from atheromatous plaques may be dislodged and cause cerebral infarction distally in the carotid system. Direct pressure applied to the carotid sinus may also cause cardiac arrhythmias.

Palpation of the superficial temporal, facial, infraorbital, and occipital arteries provides an estimate of flow in the external carotid system (Fig. 5-2). This flow may be reduced in the cranial arteries or with an ipsilateral common carotid or external carotid artery occlusion. Increased external carotid flow may reflect an occlusive lesion of the internal carotid artery with increased compensatory collateral flow. In addition, palpation of the superficial temporal arteries may be helpful in the diagnosis of cranial arteritis, which is indicated by a decreased pulse, increased arterial tenderness or beading, and erythema of the overlying skin. Palpation of the radial arteries may provide information about the status of the subclavian systems: A weaker pulse in one radial artery or one pulse that follows the other asynchronously (delayed) suggests proximal stenosis in the subclavian system on that side.

OPHTHALMIC OCULAR EXAMINATION

Ophthalmic examination consists of a careful evaluation of the patient's history (see Chapter 2, Visual Disturbances), a general ocular examination, and special ophthalmic examinations.

General Ocular Examination

General examination includes inspection of external ocular structures (lids, conjunctivae, corneas, sclerae, and lacrimal apparatus), irides, pupils, and position of the eyes, determination of visual acuity, and confrontational visual field testing.

Inspection of the **external ocular structures** allows detection of various disturbances, such as pupillary abnormalities, ptosis, exophthalmos, foreign bodies, inflammation, dryness, corneal clouding, and iridic color abnormalities. Both upper eyelids normally cover 1 to 2 mm of the irides. Unilateral ptosis of 1 to 2 mm associated with miosis is usually caused by Horner's syndrome. Ptosis also may be caused by a lesion of the third cranial nerve (accompanied by convergent strabismus and pupillary dilatation) or by muscle (such as muscular dystrophy) or neuromuscular junction abnormalities (such as myasthenia gravis—often fluctuating, gradually worsening, unilateral or bilateral ptosis with fatigability and associated diplopia). Other varieties are congenital ptosis, ptosis associated with aging (usually with redundant eyelid[s]), and ptosis associated with other mechanical factors (lid swelling, tumor, or xanthelasma). Erythema or congestion of the lids, conjunctivae, or sclerae may be caused by infection, trauma, allergy, or acute glaucoma.

Unilateral subconjunctival hemorrhage is commonly caused by trauma or rupture of a small conjunctival vessel; bilateral and recurrent subconjunctival hemorrhages may be caused by blood dyscrasias. The corneal reflex is tested by touching the lateral edge of the cornea with a wisp of cotton. The normal response is a bilateral equal and prompt blink and may be diminished or lost as a result of abnormality in the afferent portion of the fifth cranial nerve, the efferent portion of the seventh cranial nerve, or damage to their reflex connections within the pons.

Both **irides** are normally the same color (a lack of melanin pigment within the iris may cause a unilateral blue iris resulting from Horner's syndrome occurring congenitally or during the first 2 years of life; differences in iris color may also be inherited without Horner's syndrome). Holes on the iris usually indicate atrophy; capillaries on the surface (rubeosis) usually indicate anterior segment ischemia.

Extraocular Muscle Movements

Movement of the eyes is normally smooth, in the same direction, and at the same speed, except for convergence, when both eyes move mediad. Ocular movements are normally tested by having the patient direct gaze to follow the examiner's finger to the extreme right and left in the horizontal plane, upward and downward in the vertical plane, and within a few inches of the face in the midline to test convergence.

Reflex ("doll's eyes") ocular movements are occasionally tested to differentiate supranuclear from nuclear palsies; the patient fixes gaze on a central point straight ahead and the examiner then moves the patient's head from side to side and up and down. Gaze palsies

Table 5-1.   Localization of eye movement disorders

Localization of lesion	Clinical features
Supranuclear palsies	
Activating lesions in frontal lobe	Jerk-like conjugate deviation of the eyes toward the affected limbs away from the lesion
Destructive lesions in frontal lobe	Conjugate deviation of the eyes toward the side of the lesion away from the hemiparetic limb(s); voluntary eye movement to command away from the side of the lesion is lost
Destructive lesions in occipital lobe	Conjugate deviation of the eyes toward the side of the lesion away from the hemiparetic limb(s); voluntary eye movement to command away from the side of the lesion is spared
Destructive lesions in midbrain, pineal gland tumors	Parinaud's syndrome: loss of voluntary upward and convergence gaze, pupils are sluggish in response to light but constrict briskly to near vision or accommodation, convergence-retraction nystagmus, lid retraction
Nuclear palsies	
Destructive lesions in pons	Conjugate or dysconjugate ocular deviation away from the side of the lesion toward the hemiparetic limb(s), diplopia is common
	Skew deviation (the higher eye ipsilateral to the side of the lesion)
Rostral midbrain lesions	Impairment or paralysis of convergence, diplopia for near vision, with absence of any individual extraocular muscle palsy
Lesions of uncertain localization (multiple lesions)	Spasm of the near reflex: convergent strabismus, diplopia, miotic pupils, and spasm accommodation

may result from supratentorial and infratentorial lesions. **Destructive cerebral lesions,** such as cerebral infarcts, often cause conjugate ocular deviations toward the side of the lesion, with the head turned in the direction of deviation, whereas **activating lesions,** such as seizures, cause deviation of the eyes and head away from the lesion. **Destructive cerebral lesions** typically cause a contralateral hemiparesis in which the eyes look **at** the lesion and **away** from the hemiparesis. Lesions in the **brain stem** may also cause lateral gaze palsies. **Destructive lesions** may cause conjugate or dysconjugate ocular deviation, usually away from the side of the lesion. These brain stem lesions are often accompanied by diplopia and also may produce a contralateral hemiparesis. A lateral gaze deviation with a **lesion at a brain stem site** has the eyes looking **away** from the lesion and **at** the hemiparesis. Supratentorial gaze palsies may occur with both frontal and occipital lobe lesions. In **frontal lobe lesions,** voluntary eye movement to command (without following the examiner's finger) away from the side of the lesion is lost; in **occipital lobe lesions,** however, such eye movement to command is spared (Table 5-1).

Vertical gaze palsy affecting downgaze may be caused by infarcts in the territory of the paramedian thalamomesencephalic or posterior cerebral arteries. **Ocular apraxia,** inability to move the eyes voluntarily to command, with a full range of random eye movements, occurs with bilateral prefrontal motor cortex damage. In **internuclear ophthalmoplegia,** weakness of adduction on the side of a lesion of the medial longitudinal fasciculus occurs with monocular, horizontal nystagmus of the abducting eye. Typical causes include various disorders involving the brain stem, such as multiple sclerosis, infarction, trauma, encephalitis, and syringobulbia.

Tectal or pretectal lesions in the midbrain, caused by pineal region tumors, infiltrating gliomas, infarction, hemorrhage, trauma, or multiple sclerosis, may produce **Parinaud's syndrome.** This syndrome is characterized by loss of voluntary upward gaze, light-near reflex dissociation of the pupils (sluggish in response to light but brisk constriction to neargaze or accommodation), and, occasionally, retraction nystagmus, paralysis of convergence, ptosis, papilledema, or third cranial nerve palsy. **Spasm of the near reflex** (convergent strabismus, diplopia, miotic pupils, and spasm of accommodation) is usually caused by encephalitis, tabes dorsalis, meningitis, or functional disturbances. **Skew deviation** (a vertical misalignment of the eyes) usually signifies a structural brain stem lesion with the higher eye ipsilateral to the side of the lesion. **Impairment or paralysis of convergence** (sudden onset of diplopia for near vision, with absence of any individual extraocular muscle palsy) may be caused by rostral midbrain lesions (such as infarction, multiple sclerosis, encephalitis, tabes dorsalis, tumors, or Parkinson's disease) or may be functional. Limitation of ocular movements may also result from paresis of the third, fourth, or sixth cranial nerve (see Oculomotor [III], Trochlear [IV], and Abducens [VI] Nerves, page 59).

Nystagmus

Nystagmus is an involuntary, rapid to-and-fro eye movement that may be either pendular in type, with smooth movements, or jerk nystagmus, with a slow drift and quick corrective movement. When classifying nystagmus, one must consider the type of movement (horizontal, vertical, rotatory, mixed), whether it is pendular or has quick-and-slow components, the direction of the fast component, whether the nystagmus direction changes with gaze direction, and whether the nystagmus is similar in both eyes. Nystagmus subtypes are classified in Table 5-2.

Pupils

The **pupils** should be inspected for (1) size, (2) shape (they should be approximately equal in size and round), (3) reaction to light (bright light directed into the pupil of one eye normally causes equal and quick constriction of both pupils; the contralateral response is called the consensual response), and (4) accommodation/convergence (the pupils normally constrict equally under the stimuli of accommodation and convergence). Pupillary constriction on neargaze is tested by asking the patient to look first at a distant object and then at a close object.

The pupils may be markedly **constricted** from the effect of narcotics, parasympathomimetic drugs, central nervous system syphilis, or pontine disorders such as pontine hemorrhage, in which the reaction to light is difficult to observe but should be present. **Argyll**

Table 5-2. Classification of nystagmus

Subtype	Characteristic
Voluntary or functional	Horizontal, rapid movements, nonsustained
End-position	Nonsustained, at end of horizontal gaze; normal; not noted with vertical gaze
Retinal disease	Conjugate and horizontal, persisting throughout life, caused by congenital macular defect or albinism
Congenital defects	Conjugate, horizontal jerk; occurs from birth, often with impairment of vision or strabismus
Labyrinthine disease (Ménière's disease labyrinthitis, vascular lesions of vestibular apparatus or vestibular nerve)	Jerk nystagmus, fast component toward lesion in all directions of gaze; generally has rotatory component
Cerebellar-brain stem (vascular disease, multiple sclerosis, tumor, alcohol intoxication, Wernicke's encephalopathy, phenytoin toxicity)	Multidirectional nystagmus with fast component in direction of gaze; other nuclear or tract involvement; may be pendular, jerky horizontal, or vertical nystagmus in brain stem lesions
Retraction nystagmus (midbrain tectum, pretectal lesions, pineal lesions)	Best seen with optokinetic testing in downgoing direction; convergence and retraction movements, especially with convergence or upgaze
Down-beating (cervicomedullary junction)	Fast component down-beating nystagmus in primary or lateral gaze
Up-beating (medulla, cerebellum)	Fast component up-beating nystagmus in primary or lateral gaze
Cyclic rotatory or seesaw (lesions in region of optic chiasm and diencephalon)	Regular reciprocating oscillations in which one eye rises and the other falls; bitemporal hemianopia may be associated
Dissociated nystagmus (posterior fossa disease)	Direction of nystagmus differs when eyes are compared
Periodic alternating (cerebellum)	Primary gaze nystagmus with 60- to 120-sec episodes of jerk nystagmus, then brief period with no nystagmus, followed by similar episode of nystagmus in contralateral direction

Robertson pupils caused by central nervous system syphilis are commonly irregular, eccentric, and small (less than 3 mm in diameter). They react promptly on convergence and accommodation for near objects but do not contract to light and dilate poorly with mydriatics. This type of light-near dissociation of pupillary response, with greater response to convergence than to light, may also occur in patients with tumors of the midbrain, diabetes mellitus, encephalitis, multiple sclerosis, central nervous system degenerative disease, meningitis, and chronic alcoholism. The pupils may be relatively fixed and equally **dilated** as a result of diffuse cerebral swelling or sympathomimetic or anticholinergic drugs (epinephrine, ephedrine, amphetamine, cocaine, atropine, homatropine, scopolamine, pilocarpine, acetylcholine).

Adie's pupil is typically a unilaterally dilated pupil with slow reaction to light, which may respond to accommodation. This is a benign condition that usually affects young women and may be related to dysfunction of the ciliary ganglion or postganglionic neuron. The pupil characteristically promptly constricts with administration of low-dose pilocarpine. When the pupil is completely unreactive to both light and accommodation, with depressed or absent deep tendon reflexes, the condition is called **Holmes-Adie syndrome.**

Nonreactive pupils 3 to 5 mm in diameter may accompany a midbrain lesion. A unilaterally dilated, fixed, and unreactive pupil may be a sign of third cranial nerve compression caused by temporal lobe herniation. **Unequal pupils (anisocoria)** may be a normal finding, especially when associated with a normal reaction to light. However, if one or both pupils do not react well to light, a pathologic process is strongly suggested. For example, pathologic anisocoria may result from third cranial nerve involvement at the level of the midbrain (infarction, basilar aneurysm, demyelination, tumor), interpeduncular cistern (aneurysm of the posterior communicating or basilar artery, transtentorial herniation, basal meningitis, or oculomotor nerve trunk infarction), cavernous sinus (intracavernous aneurysm, cavernous sinus thrombosis, pituitary adenoma, meningioma, metastasis, nasopharyngeal carcinoma), or orbit or orbital fissure (tumor, periostitis, sphenocavernous lesion).

Horner's syndrome, with unilateral miosis, ptosis, lower eyelid elevation, and loss of sweating on the same side of the face, may result from an ipsilateral lesion causing sympathetic nervous system damage at various levels: **hypothalamus** (tumor, vascular lesion), **brain stem** (tumor, vascular lesion, syringobulbia), **middle fossa** (tumor, granuloma), **carotid artery in the neck** (dissection, occlusion, aneurysm, trauma), **cervical sympathetic chain** (enlarged cervical lymph node, goiter, aneurysm of the subclavian artery, carcinoma of the lung apex, apical tuberculosis, or mediastinal tumor), **anterior C-8, T-1, T-2, or T-3 roots** (neurofibroma, lower brachial plexus palsy, Pancoast tumor), or **other cervical lesions** (vertebral fractures, tabes dorsalis, syringomyelia, tumor).

Visual Acuity

Visual acuity is usually tested for each eye separately at a near point (approximately 14 cm) with a handheld card (patients who wear glasses for reading should wear them during the test). To overcome hypermetropia or myopia refractory errors without glasses, the patient may look at the card through a pinhole to restrict vision to the central beam of light, which is undisturbed by abnormal ocular distances or transparent media. Once refractory defects have been excluded, **acute impairment of visual acuity** in one eye usually suggests a vascular lesion such as acute occlusion of the ophthalmic or central retinal artery, a lesion affecting the macular region of the retina (for instance, a hemorrhage in the macular area), or ischemic optic neuropathy. **Gradual impairment of vision** may be caused by optic atrophy resulting from compression, toxins, ischemia, neuritis, retinitis pigmentosa, macular degeneration, choroiditis, diabetic retinopathy, or retinoblastoma (Table 5-3). Unilateral lesions of the optic tract, lateral geniculate body, optic radiation, or striate cortex usually do not impair optic acuity, but bilateral occipital cortex lesions can cause complete blindness.

Table 5-3. Causes of unilateral visual loss

Acute unilateral visual loss	Subacute or chronic unilateral visual loss

Central retinal artery occlusion (embolism, vasospasm, hypercoagulable state, vasculitis)
Papillitis (retrobulbar neuritis)
Retinal detachment (traumatic or spontaneous)
Optic nerve trauma
	Primary optic atrophy caused by:
	  Compression resulting from orbital lesions (tumor, granuloma); lesions within optic canal (meningioma, granuloma, hyperostosis); intracranial lesions (aneurysms of internal carotid, anterior cerebral, or anterior communicating artery, prechiasmal neoplasms such as meningioma of sphenoid wing or olfactory groove, granuloma, optic nerve glioma, craniopharyngioma, neoplasm of frontal lobe or pituitary, osteosarcoma, prechiasmal arachnoiditis, third ventricle dilatation). Central scotoma is common early in the course of the compression.
	  Toxins (alcohol or tobacco amblyopia). Centrocecal scotoma is common.
	  Ischemia (often associated with diabetes mellitus, hypertension, glaucoma, or vasculitis, such as temporal arteritis, or syphilis)
	  Optic neuritis (viral, parasitic, fungal, postinoculation syphilis, polyneuritis, bacterial or tuberculous meningitis)
	  Metabolic (Addison's disease, uremia, pernicious anemia, hyperthyroidism, toxemia)
	  Degenerative (multiple sclerosis, vitamin deficiency or starvation, Paget's disease of bone, Hand-Schüller-Christian disease, Tay-Sachs disease, Niemann-Pick disease, Laurence-Moon-Biedl syndrome, fibrous dysplasia)
	  Congenital/hereditary (Leber's hereditary optic atrophy, oxycephaly)
	Secondary optic atrophy after papilledema (enlarged blind spot is common with or without contraction of the fields)
	Retinitis pigmentosa
	Glaucoma or choroiditis (toxoplasmosis, cytomegalovirus infection). Arcuate scotoma is common.
	Diabetic or hypertensive retinopathy
	Malignant melanoma, macular degeneration
	Cataract

Visual Fields

Visual fields are assessed clinically to detect areas of partial or complete loss of vision by confrontation testing. The examiner covers one of the patient's eyes at a time. The examiner then holds up one or two fingers in the six primary visual quadrants, and the patient identifies whether the examiner is holding up one or two fingers while looking straight ahead at the examiner's nose. Alternatively, the examiner may move his or her finger or, for a more precise determination, move a red 5-mm pin from the extreme periphery toward the center. The patient reports when he or she first sees the object while looking straight ahead at the examiner's nose. Repeated testing from multiple directions provides a record of affected or spared visual fields.

For detection of **visual neglect** (in which the patient ignores one-half the visual field), both eyes are uncovered, and the patient looks at the examiner's nose. The examiner then asks the patient to identify which finger(s) is wiggling while wiggling fingers in one of the primary peripheral quadrants, either unilaterally or bilaterally. Patients with neglect often ignore fingers to one side when the examiner is wiggling fingers simultaneously on each side. In addition, the patient with left visual neglect, when drawing a clock face, will write all the numbers on the right-hand side of the clock or, when trying to mark the center of a line, will place the mark far to the right of the real midpoint of the line.

Monocular visual field defects are usually caused by retinal or optic nerve lesions; binocular defects usually reflect a lesion localized at or behind the optic chiasm. The precise determination of visual field defects has an important role in the localization of vascular lesions. Some of the most common variants of visual-spatial disorders are depicted in Figure 2-1. **Central scotoma** may result from retrobulbar neuritis (sometimes as the first sign of multiple sclerosis) or optic nerve compression (anterior communicating artery aneurysm, meningioma, granuloma, or hyperostosis of the optic canal from Paget's disease). **Cecocentral scotoma** is characteristic of toxic (alcohol, tobacco) amblyopia. An **arcuate scotoma** often reflects underlying glaucoma, and a **junctional scotoma** indicates the presence of an optic nerve lesion immediately anterior to the optic chiasm.

Bitemporal hemianopia with involvement of the upper quadrants first indicates compression of the optic chiasm from below by lesions such as a pituitary adenoma, nasopharyngeal carcinoma, or sphenoid sinus mucocele; involvement of the lower quadrants first indicates compression of the optic chiasm from above, such as a craniopharyngioma or third ventricular tumor. **Homonymous hemianopia** may have sudden onset, typically of vascular cause, or gradual onset, caused by neoplastic, infectious, or inflammatory conditions. Lesions may involve the contralateral geniculate body (homonymous defect in the upper and lower quadrants with sparing of a horizontal sector), optic radiations, or occipital lobe. **Inferior quadrantanopia** is more often caused by lesions of the optic radiations deep in the parietal lobe or cuneus of the occipital lobe; **superior quadrantanopia** arises from lesions involving the temporal loop of the optic radiations or inferior bank of the calcarine fissure.

Bilateral homonymous hemianopia results in complete visual loss **(cortical blindness)** with or without sparing of a small central visual field (macular sparing) and the pupillary response. In **Anton's syndrome,** the patient denies the visual defect and confabulates about what is being seen because of bilateral visual association cortex damage resulting from occlusion of either the basilar or both posterior cerebral arteries.

Ophthalmoscopy

Use of ophthalmoscopy is important in evaluating patients with suspected cerebrovascular disease. The normal optic disk is a yellowish red, round or oval, platelike structure, is typically flat with a white central depression (physiologic cup), and has an average diameter about one-third the disk diameter. Margins are clearly defined, although the nasal edge is often slightly less distinct than the temporal edge. The arterioles of the retina diverge from, and the veins converge toward, the disk; in 80% of normal patients, venous pulsations may be seen, an indication that the intracranial pressure is less than 200 mm Hg.

The ophthalmoscopic examination may help define the underlying mechanism through direct visualization of parenchymal and vascular retinal changes. Ophthalmoscopy allows detection of diabetic, ischemic, or hypertensive retinopathy; retinal hemorrhage; and various types of emboli. The arteriolar and venous caliber and appearance should be examined. Disappearance of spontaneous venous pulsations may be the earliest sign of venous congestion, which may be associated with increased intracranial pressure. The retina should be inspected for microaneurysms, papilledema, papillitis, optic atrophy or disk pallor, areas of exudates, abnormal pigmentation, and subhyaloid hemorrhages.

Retinal emboli may be associated with central retinal artery or branch occlusion. The three most common types of retinal emboli are cholesterol, fibrin-platelet, and calcium emboli. **Cholesterol emboli** are composed of cholesterol crystals, generally originating from an ulcerated atheromatous intimal lesion of the ipsilateral internal carotid artery, appearing as shiny orange-yellow lesions, and they are often situated at the bifurcation of retinal arterioles. **Fibrin-platelet emboli** are grayish white lesions, usually indicative of an underlying atheromatous lesion of the ipsilateral carotid system, and they tend to cause arteriolar occlusions much more commonly than do cholesterol emboli. **Calcium emboli** are less common and consist of white particles of calcium, generally originating from calcific aortic stenosis. Septic, talc, polytef (Teflon), cornstarch, and some other emboli may also be seen in the retina but are very uncommon.

Atherosclerosis may manifest ophthalmoscopically in the retinal arterial walls. **Hypertension** may be associated with various changes, including retinal arteriolar narrowing, sclerosis, or even occlusion. Hypertensive retinopathy usually involves retinal edema, cotton-wool patches, hemorrhages, and papilledema. In addition to hypertension, retinal hemorrhages and exudates also may be caused by other systemic disorders, such as diabetes mellitus, systemic lupus erythematosus, and blood dyscrasias. Retinal changes associated with **diabetes mellitus** may be similar to the changes associated with hypertension, but microaneurysms, dilated veins, and neurovascularization are often present.

Other ophthalmoscopic findings ipsilateral to carotid occlusive lesions include venous stasis (low-flow) retinopathy and asymmetric (lesser) hypertensive arteriolar changes. Venous stasis (low-flow) retinopathy resembles diabetic retinopathy but tends to be located more peripherally (microaneurysm formation, venous engorgement, retinal hemorrhages, neovascularization) and may be associated with secondary glaucoma.

In **papillitis** caused by passive congestion, the disk becomes abnormally vascular (hyperemic) and slightly elevated (edema), and small hemorrhages may be seen (cecocentral scotoma may be present). In **retrobulbar** neuritis, however, because of the location of the inflammatory lesion in the posterior portion of the optic nerve, the disk is not swollen. Papillitis is typically unilateral, and the disk appears similar to that seen in papilledema. Visual acuity is usually severely affected early, in comparison with papilledema, which may be associated with more chronic changes in visual acuity.

Papilledema is indicative of increased intracranial pressure and in its early stage is characterized by hyperemia of the rim of the disk. Later, the vessels on the surface of the disk are engorged, and disk swelling, hemorrhages, and nerve fiber infarctions (cotton-wool spots) may occur. In massive papilledema, large areas of the nerve fiber layer may become infarcted. Papilledema developing within 12 to 24 hours of a neurologic event frequently indicates increased intracranial pressure from intracranial mass lesions, such as brain trauma or hemorrhage; pronounced papilledema at the onset of symptoms usually indicates lesions of longer duration, such as brain tumor or abscess.

Subhyaloid hemorrhage is a preretinal hemorrhage commonly associated with intracranial hemorrhage, particularly aneurysmal subarachnoid hemorrhage, but may be seen with severe brain trauma or any condition producing suddenly increased intracranial pressure.

In **anterior ischemic optic neuropathy,** altitudinal or segmental disk swelling, hyperemia, disk margin hemorrhages, and other signs of disk infarction are often noted after the sudden or subacute onset of an altitudinal or segmental visual field loss. Potential causes include diabetes mellitus, hypertension, inflammatory vasculitis, hypercoagulable state, and unknown cause (idiopathic). **Occlusion of the central retinal vein** often produces extensive hemorrhage in the region of the optic disk, disk swelling, dilated veins, and partial visual loss. **Central retinal artery occlusion** causes sudden visual field loss associated with a pale disk and retina. Weeks to months later, the disk whitens as a result of optic atrophy.

Special Ophthalmic Examinations

Special examinations include **perimetry** to assess the peripheral and central visual fields with manual or automated methods; **ophthalmodynamometry** to measure relative pressures in the central retinal arteries, used as an indirect means of assessing the pressure of the carotid arterial system (see Chapter 7, Ophthalmodynamometry); **Schiøtz tonometry** to measure intraocular pressure, in which a pressure of 20 mm Hg or more is considered above average and most often reflects underlying glaucoma; and **fluorescein angiography** to detail the choroidal and retinal vasculature.

Cranial Nerves

Cranial nerve functions, symptoms of cranial nerve deficits, and some of the syndromes affecting the cranial nerves are reviewed in Tables 5-4 and 5-5.

Table 5-4. Location and general function of the cranial nerves and major signs and symptoms of impaired function

Cranial nerve	Major anatomic structures and relationships	General function	Major signs and symptoms of impaired function
Olfactory (I)	Orbital surfaces of the frontal lobe (olfactory nerve, bulb, tract, lateral olfactory gyrus, amygdaloid nucleus, septal nuclei, hypothalamus)	Smell	Anosmia; parosmia, cacosmia
Optic (II)	Retina; optic nerve; optic chiasm; optic tract; lateral geniculate bodies; optic radiation; visual cortex of occipital lobe	Vision	Impaired visual acuity and visual fields (scotoma)
Oculomotor (III)	Midbrain (nucleus or fascicular portion); subarachnoid space; cavernous sinus; superior orbital fissure; orbit	Eye movement (levator palpebrae muscle); pupillary constriction	Downward and outward deviation of affected eye; horizontal and vertical diplopia; ptosis; pupil dilatation
Trochlear (IV)	Dorsal midbrain (nucleus and fascicles); undersurface of tentorial edge; cavernous sinus; superior orbital fissure; orbit	Eye movement (superior oblique muscle)	Vertical diplopia with tilt greatest on downward gaze to the side opposite the lesion. Corrects with tilting head toward the lesion
Trigeminal (V)	Pons (motor portion); semilunar ganglion in middle cranial fossa (sensory portion); brain stem nuclei; gasserian ganglion (ophthalmic, maxillary, mandibular divisions)	Facial sensation; jaw movement	Trigeminal neuralgia or ipsilateral dissociated (nucleus) or total (nerve roots or ganglion) hemianesthesia of face; weakness, atrophy of masticatory muscles; loss of corneal reflex
Abducens (VI)	Lower pons; sulcus between pons and medulla; prepontine cistern; cavernous sinus; superior orbital fissure; orbit	Eye movement (lateral rectus muscle)	Inward deviation of affected eye; ipsilateral gaze palsy with horizontal diplopia worse when looking toward paralyzed side

Table 5-4. (continued)

Cranial nerve	Major anatomic structures and relationships	General function	Major signs and symptoms of impaired function
Facial (VII)	Caudal pons; cerebellopontine angle; internal auditory meatus; facial canal in petrous bone; tympanic and mastoid segments	Facial movement; taste on anterior two-thirds of tongue	Peripheral type of facial nerve palsy (Bell's palsy) with or without ipsilateral loss of taste on anterior two-thirds of tongue; impairment of lacrimation, salivation, and hyperacusis
Vestibulocochlear (VIII)	Pons; upper medulla; internal auditory meatus; vestibular and cochlear nerves; cochlea (organ of Corti); ampullae and semicircular canals; utricle; saccule	Hearing and balance	Sensorineural deafness or vertigo; nausea or vomiting; horizontal or rotatory nystagmus
Glossopharyngeal (IX)	Medulla; jugular foramen; cerebello-pontine angle; space between internal carotid artery and internal jugular vein; pharynx; base of tongue	Palatal and pharyngeal movement; taste to posterior one-third of tongue	Mild dysphagia; homolateral loss of taste over posterior one-third of tongue; depressed pharyngeal or gag reflex
Vagus (X)	Medulla; jugular foramen; auricular, meningeal, pharyngeal, and cardiac rami; recurrent laryngeal nerve	Palatal, pharyngeal, and laryngeal movement; control of visceral organs	Ipsilateral palatal, pharyngeal, and laryngeal paresis (dysphagia and dysphonia) associated with unilateral laryngeal anesthesia and depressed gag reflex
Spinal accessory (XI)	Medulla (cranial part); spinal cord (spinal part); foramen magnum; jugular foramen	Sternocleidomastoid, trapezius muscles	Paresis and atrophy of sternocleidomastoid and trapezius muscles
Hypoglossal (XII)	Medulla (hypoglossal trigone of floor of fourth ventricle); medullary-pontine junction; hypoglossal canal	Tongue movement	Ipsilateral paresis and atrophy with or without fasciculations in one-half of tongue; dysarthria

Table 5-5.   Syndromes involving cranial nerves

Eponym (syndrome)	Structures involved	Symptoms / signs	Usual cause
Foster Kennedy	Frontal lobe, olfactory (I) nerve	Ipsilateral anosmia, optic atrophy with contralateral papilledema	Tumors, saccular aneurysms of anterior portion of circle of Willis
Claude	Tegmentum of midbrain, oculomotor (III) nerve nucleus and red nucleus, brachium conjunctivum	Oculomotor palsy, horizontal diplopia with contralateral ataxia and cerebellar tremor	Infarction, hemorrhage, basilar aneurysm compression, tumor
Benedikt	Tegmentum of midbrain, subthalamic region, corticospinal tract, oculomotor (III) nerve nucleus, red nucleus, brachium conjunctivum	Oculomotor palsy with contralateral ataxia, cerebellar tremor, corticospinal signs	Infarction, hemorrhage, basilar aneurysm compression, tumor
Nothnagel	Tectum of midbrain (brachium conjunctivum below the decussation), oculomotor (III) nerve	Oculomotor palsy with ipsilateral cerebellar disturbance	Infarction, hemorrhage, basilar aneurysm compression, tumor
Weber	Tectum of midbrain and cerebral peduncle, oculomotor (III) nerve	Oculomotor palsy with contralateral hemiparesis	Infarction, hemorrhage, basilar aneurysm compression, tumor
Parinaud	Dorsal midbrain (periaqueductal gray matter)	Paralysis of upward gaze and accommodation; light-near dissociation, retraction nystagmus	Tumor, hydrocephalus, infarction, hemorrhage
Millard-Gubler	Base of pons, abducens (VI) and facial (VII) nerves	Facial and abducens palsy with contralateral hemiplegia	Infarction, tumor
Foville	Base of pons, nerve VII	Facial and conjugate gaze palsies, contralateral hemiplegia	Infarction, tumor
Gradenigo	Ophthalmic division of trigeminal (V) and abducens (VI) nerves	Retro-orbital pain, palsy of nerve VI, deafness, excessive lacrimation	Inflammation at level of petrous apex, infection; tumor, trauma, aneurysm

Table 5-5. (continued)

Eponym (syndrome)	Structures involved	Symptoms/signs	Usual cause
Raeder	Ophthalmic division of nerve V (sometimes IV, VI)	Miosis and ptosis (no facial anhidrosis), facial or retro-orbital pain	Tumor at level of petrous apex, infection, trauma, aneurysm
Tolosa-Hunt	Cranial nerves III, IV, V, VI	Retro-orbital pain with multiple ophthalmoplegia	Inflammation in cavernous sinus
Wallenberg	Lateral tegmentum of medulla, spinal nerves V, IX, XI	Dysphagia, dysarthria, gait and limb ataxia, ipsilateral dissociated hemianesthesia of face, contralateral hemisensory loss in limbs and trunk, Horner's syndrome	Occlusion of ipsilateral vertebral artery or posterior-inferior cerebellar artery
Vernet	Glossopharyngeal (IX) and vagus (X) nerve roots	Dysphagia, dysphonia, depressed gag reflex, homolateral vocal cord paralysis, loss of taste or pain on posterior one-third of tongue, soft palate with ipsilateral paresis of nerve XI	Tumors, aneurysms, abscess, basal skull fracture at jugular foramen
Collet-Sicard	Cranial nerves IX, X, XI, XII	Unilateral paralysis of trapezius, sternocleidomastoid muscles, vocal cord, half of tongue, loss of taste on posterior one-third of tongue, hemianesthesia of palate, pharynx, and larynx	Tumors of parotid gland, carotid body, secondary and lymph node tumors, tuberculous adenitis
Villaret	Cranial nerves IX, X, XI, XII, sympathetic chain, sometimes cranial nerve VII	Same as for Collet-Sicard syndrome, ipsilateral Horner's syndrome, sometimes facial nerve palsy	Same as for Collet-Sicard syndrome at retroparotid or retropharyngeal space
Schmidt	Cranial nerves X, XI	Paralysis of vocal cord (cranial nerve X) and sternocleidomastoid muscle (cranial nerve XI)	Tumor, aneurysm, abscess (before nerve fibers leave skull)
Jackson	Cranial nerves X, XI, XII	Same as for Schmidt's syndrome, hemiparalysis of tongue (cranial nerve XII)	Same as for Schmidt's syndrome, perhaps intraparenchymal

OLFACTORY NERVE (I)

The olfactory nerve is seldom damaged in cerebrovascular disease but may be affected by large intracranial aneurysms. Each of the patient's nostrils should be tested individually with an aromatic material such as camphor or wintergreen. An impaired sense of smell is most commonly associated with rhinitis, head injury, heavy cigarette smoking, or nasal obstruction, but sometimes may be caused by space-occupying lesions of the frontal lobe (tumors of the sphenoid or frontal bone, meningiomas, pituitary tumors, and saccular aneurysms of the anterior portion of the circle of Willis), producing the so-called **Foster Kennedy syndrome** characterized by ipsilateral anosmia and optic atrophy with contralateral papilledema (see Table 5-5).

OPTIC NERVE (II)

The optic nerve is tested by measuring visual acuity, color vision, and peripheral vision (visual fields) and by inspecting the retina and optic disk with an ophthalmoscope.

OCULOMOTOR (III), TROCHLEAR (IV), AND ABDUCENS (VI) NERVES

The oculomotor, trochlear, and abducens nerves subserve ocular movements (III, IV, and VI), lid elevation (III), and pupillary constriction (III). To evaluate the function of these nerves, the physician should assess each of the patient's eyes separately for the completeness of ocular movements, lid retraction, the presence of ptosis, pupillary abnormalities, abnormal spontaneous eye movements, and abnormal convergence.

An **oculomotor nerve (III) palsy** (Fig. 5-3) results in lateral deviation (divergent strabismus) of the affected eye in association with absence or limitation of convergence, horizontal and vertical diplopia, ipsilateral ptosis, and pupillary dilatation caused by lesions in the midbrain, interpeduncular cistern, cavernous sinus, or orbit.

Lesions in the **midbrain,** which may result from infarction, hemorrhage, basilar aneurysm, demyelination, or tumor, may produce the syndromes outlined in Table 5-5.

Lesions in the **interpeduncular cistern** include aneurysmal compression of the posterior communicating or basilar arteries (oculomotor paresis may be incomplete) and basal meningitis. More distally, the third cranial nerve rests on the tentorial edge and may be compressed by uncal herniation. The dilated and fixed pupil may be affected before the extraocular muscle function in this type of compressive syndrome because the pupillomotor fibers predominantly travel in the outer portions of the nerve. Nerve trunk infarction may occur anywhere along its course as a result of hypertension, diabetes, or inflammatory arteriopathy; the pupil is typically spared.

In the **cavernous sinus,** lesions affecting the third cranial nerve may also affect the fourth, fifth, and sixth cranial nerves, the optic nerve, and oculosympathetic fibers as a result of intracavernous aneurysm, cavernous sinus thrombosis, pituitary adenoma, meningioma, metastasis, and nasopharyngeal carcinoma. The combination of third cranial nerve paresis and small, poorly reactive pupils is highly suggestive of a cavernous sinus lesion.

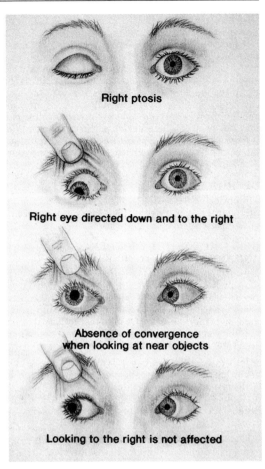

Right ptosis

Right eye directed down and to the right

Absence of convergence when looking at near objects

Looking to the right is not affected

Fig. 5-3.   **Right oculomotor (III) nerve dysfunction.**

Lesions in the **orbit or orbital fissure** include tumor, periostitis, or sphenocavernous lesion associated with fourth, fifth, and sixth cranial nerve dysfunction.

Trochlear (IV) and abducens (VI) nerve palsies result in mild convergent strabismus associated with limited movement of the affected eye to the paralyzed side, vertical diplopia when the person looks downward **(fourth nerve palsy)** (Fig. 5-4), and horizontal diplopia when the person looks toward the side of the lesion **(sixth nerve palsy)** (Fig. 5-5). The palsies may be caused by the same lesions that cause palsy of the third cranial nerve. However, lesions of the fourth cranial nerve in the midbrain are usually associated with other midbrain syndromes, such as hemiparesis and hemisensory loss, predominantly involving the leg. Nuclear or intramedullary lesions of the sixth cranial nerve are usually associated with

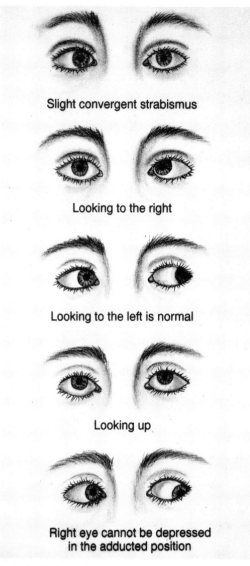

Slight convergent strabismus

Looking to the right

Looking to the left is normal

Looking up

Right eye cannot be depressed
in the adducted position

Fig. 5-4. Right trochlear (IV) nerve dysfunction.

ipsilateral gaze palsy to the same side, contralateral hemiparesis, hemisensory loss, and ipsilateral lower motor neuron facial weakness; upper and lower face weakness is caused by palsy of the seventh cranial nerve. Pontine lesions, typically of vascular origin, may produce various syndromes, as outlined in Table 5-5.

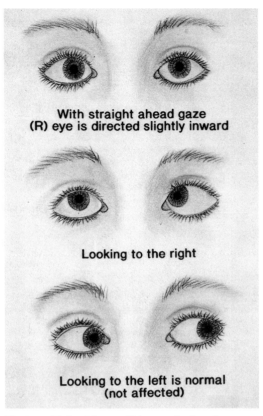

**With straight ahead gaze
(R) eye is directed slightly inward**

Looking to the right

**Looking to the left is normal
(not affected)**

Fig. 5-5.   Right abducens (VI) nerve dysfunction.

TRIGEMINAL NERVE (V)

The trigeminal nerve may be damaged by many conditions, including cerebrovascular disorders (supranuclear or nuclear infarct or hemorrhage, basilar aneurysm), tumor, infection, or trauma. The sensory portion of the trigeminal nerve is evaluated by testing pain, temperature, and light touch sensation (including corneal reflex) over the whole face. The motor portion of the fifth cranial nerve is tested by having the patient clench the jaw and move the jaw from side to side against resistance and by checking the jaw jerk.

Unilateral **supranuclear lesions** (such as a thalamic lesion) may result in anesthesia of the contralateral face; bilateral supranuclear lesions produce an exaggerated jaw reflex. **Nuclear lesions affecting the dorsal midpons** may produce ipsilateral trigeminal paresis, atrophy, and fasciculations of the muscles of mastication with associated contralateral hemiplegia, ipsilateral dissociated (loss of pain or temperature sensation, touch retained) hemianesthesia of the face, contralateral hemisensory loss of the limbs and trunk, and ipsilateral tremor.

Lesions affecting the spinal tract of the fifth cranial nerve include brain stem infarction, syringobulbia, demyelination, and tumor. The best-known vascular syndrome affecting this tract is the **lateral medullary (Wallenberg) syndrome,** caused by a posterior-inferior cerebellar artery infarct and most often a result of occlusion of the ipsilateral vertebral artery; symptoms include dysphagia, dysarthria, gait unsteadiness, ipsilateral limb ataxia, vertigo, and hoarseness. Examination shows ipsilateral Horner's syndrome, ipsilateral dissociated hemianesthesia of the face, contralateral hemianesthesia in the limbs and trunk, gait ataxia, and ipsilateral limb ataxia.

Trigeminal nerve lesions may result from various pathologic processes, such as tumor, acute infection, chronic meningitis, trauma, or aneurysm located in the **preganglionic cisternal course** of the nerve, at the cerebellopontine angle, and in the petrous apex, orbital fissure, and cavernous sinus. Some syndromes affecting the trigeminal nerve are reviewed in Table 5-5.

FACIAL NERVE (VII)

Evaluation of facial nerve function begins with watching the patient talk and smile. The physician should be alert for asymmetric eye closure, elevation of one corner of the mouth, and flattening of the nasolabial fold. The patient is instructed to wrinkle the forehead, close the eyes while the physician attempts to open them, purse the lips while the physician presses the cheeks, and show the teeth (Fig. 5-6). Corneal reflexes should be tested and any asymmetries noted. Facial nerve palsies may be caused by vascular, neoplastic, demyelinating, or infectious processes at different anatomic levels. Vascular damage to the seventh cranial nerve usually occurs at supranuclear, pontine (infarction, hemorrhage), and, rarely, cerebellopontine angle (aneurysm) levels (see Fig. 5-6, Table 5-5).

VESTIBULOCOCHLEAR NERVE (VIII)

Hearing function is tested in several ways, such as tone audiometry, speech threshold testing, and impedance measures. **Pure tone audiometry** measures hearing sensitivity as a function of frequency and can be tested either by air conduction through earphones or by bone conduction through a tuning fork on the skull. Bone conduction tests include the **Weber test,** in which a vibrating tuning fork is placed over the midline of the skull; normally, hearing is equal in both ears without lateralization. In the **Rinne test,** the vibration of the tuning fork is applied to the mastoid bone until vibration disappears; the tuning fork is then placed next to the ear, 1 inch from the external auditory meatus. The test is normal if the vibrations are still perceived in the ear. In **conductive deafness,** bone conduction is better than air conduction; thus, the Weber test lateralizes to the affected ear, and the Rinne test is abnormal. In **nerve deafness,** both bone and air conduction are impaired but air conduction remains greater than bone conduction; thus, the Weber test lateralizes to the normal ear, and the Rinne test is normal. Beyond these neurologic examination techniques, other special studies, such as speech discrimination tests and impedance measures made with a tympanogram and acoustic reflex, may be performed.

The **vestibular component** of eighth cranial nerve function may be evaluated with the **Romberg test.** The patient, standing with

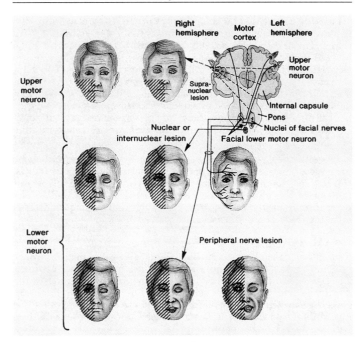

Fig. 5-6.   Facial paralysis—upper and lower motor neuron.

eyes closed and feet together, will fall or veer to the side that has vestibular dysfunction.

Vascular causes of central vestibular dysfunction include vertebrobasilar ischemia or infarction with symptoms of vertigo or dizziness, typically associated with other brain stem signs such as diplopia, dysarthria, ataxia, unilateral or bilateral homonymous hemianopia, alternating unilateral or bilateral sensory or motor deficits, **labyrinthine ischemic stroke** caused by occlusion of the internal auditory artery and resulting in vertigo, tinnitus or deafness, and nausea or vomiting), and **Wallenberg's syndrome**. Other causes are **cerebellar infarction or hemorrhage** with associated nystagmus, truncal and limb ataxia, and intention tremor and **basilar migraine,** which frequently affects young women and is characterized by occipital throbbing headache, bilateral visual symptoms, unsteadiness, dysarthria, vertigo, and limb paresthesia, with or without loss of consciousness. **Subclavian steal syndrome** is caused by stenosis of the proximal subclavian artery and results in retrograde flow down the vertebral artery with arm exercise and a clinical picture of vertebrobasilar insufficiency, such as vertigo or nystagmus, facial or extremity numbness, double vision, unsteadiness, weakness, and diminution of pulse and blood pressure in the affected arm.

GLOSSOPHARYNGEAL (IX) AND VAGUS (X) NERVES

The glossopharyngeal and vagus nerves should be examined together because their functions (speaking, swallowing, palatal movements, gag reflex) are seldom individually impaired. When the palate is examined, the middle of the palate should rise in the midline when the patient is asked to say "ah." If one side is weak, the midline deviates to the intact side.

Bilateral supranuclear lesions, often of vascular origin because of bilateral infarction, result in pseudobulbar palsy with severe dysphagia, dysarthria, spastic tongue, depressed or exaggerated gag reflex, and emotional lability. **Nuclear or intramedullary lesions** caused by vascular disease, syringobulbia, demyelinating disease, or tumor commonly involve other brain stem structures. **Extramedullary lesions affecting these nerves** include tumor, aneurysm, or abscess and may cause a **cerebellopontine angle syndrome** of dysphagia, dysphonia, depressed gag reflex, tinnitus, deafness, vertigo, and facial sensory loss. Other syndromes affecting the ninth and tenth cranial nerves are reviewed in Table 5-5.

SPINAL ACCESSORY (XI) AND HYPOGLOSSAL (XII) NERVES

The spinal accessory nerve innervates the sternocleidomastoid and trapezius muscles, which are tested by asking the patient to rotate the head against resistance and to shrug the shoulders against resistance. To examine the hypoglossal nerve, the physician asks the patient to open the mouth and protrude the tongue. When the hypoglossal nerve or nucleus is involved, the protruded tongue deviates toward the side of the lesion. The side of involvement also may show atrophy and fasciculations.

Supranuclear lesions (such as cerebral infarction at the level of the internal capsule) usually do not cause weakness of the tongue. However, upper motor neuron lesions affecting corticobulbar fibers going to the hypoglossal nucleus typically lead to slowing of tongue movements and may cause contralateral weakness of half the tongue, resulting in tongue deviation toward the side of the hemiplegia. **Nuclear lesions** (syringomyelia, intraparenchymal tumor, demyelinating disease, vascular insult) of the spinal accessory nerve are unusual but may result in paresis of the trapezius and sternocleidomastoid muscles with atrophy and fasciculations. Nuclear or intramedullary lesions of the hypoglossal nerve may result in **Dejerine's anterior bulbar syndrome** (ipsilateral paresis, atrophy, and fibrillations of the tongue associated with contralateral hemiplegia with facial sparing, contralateral loss of position, tactile and vibratory sensations on the trunk and limbs, and sparing of pain and temperature sensation).

Peripheral lesions of the eleventh and twelfth cranial nerves may be caused by trauma, carotid aneurysms, local infections, or neck surgery (complications may result in **floppy head syndrome** [isolated palsy of the eleventh cranial nerve, weakness of neck extension against gravity]), or they may be associated with one of the syndromes reviewed in Table 5-5.

Motor System

Muscle bulk, muscle tone, muscle power, and reflexes should be examined in each limb. **Muscle wasting** may indicate lower motor neuron disease, **hypertrophy** may suggest some form of myopathy, and prominent **fasciculations or fibrillations** may indicate anterior horn cell disease or nerve root damage. A **decrease in muscle tone** may indicate lower motor neuron disease, and **hypertonicity or spasticity** manifested by the "clasp-knife" phenomenon (initial resistance to passive movement is precipitously overcome) may indicate an upper motor neuron lesion. "Cogwheel" or "lead-pipe" ratchet-like **rigidity** involves a steady increase in resistance throughout the movement and may indicate an extrapyramidal lesion.

Severe weakness or plegia of the limbs is usually easily recognized. Individual muscle testing is typically necessary to detect mild weakness. Examination of alternating motion rates in the patient's fingers, hands, and feet also may clarify more subtle degrees of weakness. The presence of pronator drift also may indicate a subtle pyramidal tract lesion. To examine for drift, the physician may ask the patient to close the eyes and hold the arms outstretched with the hands supinated for as long as 1 minute—subtle drift starts with finger flexion, and the weak arm gradually pronates and drifts downward. In addition, the physician may observe a patient's voluntary movements (for instance, in dressing or walking); the weak limb will be used less than the strong limb.

In addition to examination of muscle power, **deep tendon reflexes** (biceps, brachioradialis, triceps, patellar, and Achilles), plantar reflex, and, in some circumstances, snout, grasp, palmomental, glabellar, and abdominal reflexes should be examined, with attention given to asymmetries between the two sides.

If limb weakness results from damage to the motor system at the upper motor neuron level (corticospinal pyramidal tract), deep tendon reflexes will be exaggerated in the affected limbs compared with the unaffected limbs, and extensor plantar responses and other pathologic reflexes in the affected limbs may be noted. Superficial reflexes will be depressed or absent on the affected side.

In contrast, if limb weakness results from motor system damage at the lower motor neuron level (anterior horn cell level and lower), deep tendon and superficial reflexes will be depressed (all or selectively, depending on the extent of damage and level of damage) in the affected limbs. Examination of power, tone, and reflexes of individual muscles or muscle groups is essential to localize the lesion at the level of the spinal root or nerve. The clinical features differentiating upper motor lesions from lower motor lesions are summarized in Table 5-6.

Posture, Gait, and Coordination

The cerebellar syndromes can be divided into four groups by location. The **rostral vermis syndrome** involving the anterior lobe leads to a wide-based stance and gait, ataxia of gait with proportionally little ataxia on the heel-to-shin maneuver with the patient lying down, normal or slightly impaired arm coordination, and infrequent presence of hypotonia, nystagmus, and dysarthria. The **caudal vermis syndrome** is caused by a flocculonodular and posterior lobe lesion; associated findings include axial dysequilibrium and staggering gait, little or no limb ataxia, and occasional spontaneous nystagmus and

Table 5-6. Clinical features differentiating upper motor lesions from lower motor lesions

Upper motor neuron lesions
General clinical features: Hemiplegia or hemiparesis (predominantly distal weakness); spasticity; hyperactive deep tendon reflexes; clonus; absent abdominal reflexes; Babinski's sign; suck/snout and Hoffmann's reflexes

Lower motor neuron lesions
General clinical features: Weakness with atrophy, hypotonia, decreased deep tendon and superficial reflexes, fasciculations in affected muscles of face, trunk, or extremities; vasomotor disturbances; absent Babinski's sign

Weaker muscles	Stronger muscles	Structure involved	Clinical features
Face (lower face)	Face (forehead)	Nucleus of cranial nerve III	Horizontal diplopia, downward and outward deviation of affected eye, bilateral incomplete ptosis, pupillary dilatation
Upper extremities External rotator Deltoid Triceps Digit extensors Hypothenar Interossei	Upper extremities Pectoralis major Biceps Wrist flexors Digit flexors Thenar	Cranial nerve IV Cranial nerve VI	Vertical diplopia with tilt component Horizontal diplopia, worsens toward the paretic side, often as Foville's syndrome
		Cranial nerve VII	Unilateral weakness of ipsilateral upper and lower facial muscles (often as Millard-Gubler or Foville's syndrome)
Lower extremities Iliopsoas Thigh abductors Hamstrings Peronei Toe flexors	Lower extremities Adductor thigh Gluteus maximus Quadriceps Tibialis anterior Toe extensors Tibialis posterior	Cranial nerves IX, X, XI, XII Anterior horn cells	Bulbar syndrome, Wallenberg, Vernet, Schmidt, Jackson, Collet-Sicard syndrome Weakness, prominent atrophy, fasciculations in affected muscles of trunk and extremities

Table 5-6.   (continued)

Weaker muscles	Stronger muscles	Structure involved	Clinical features
	Gastrocnemius Soleus	Root and radicular	Radicular pain, weakness, atrophy in myotomal distribution of the affected root, sensory loss, paresthesias
		Plexus	Weakness and distal atrophy in affected muscles with or without sensory disturbance
		Peripheral nerve	Weakness and atrophy of specific muscle group(s) involved with or without sensory, vasomotor, and trophic disturbances in distribution of specific nerve(s)

rotated postures of the head. A **hemispheric syndrome** with posterior lobe and variable anterior lobe involvement leads to incoordination of ipsilateral appendicular movements, particularly when they require fine-motor coordination. The **pancerebellar syndrome** affects the cerebellum globally and leads to bilateral signs of cerebellar dysfunction affecting the trunk, limbs, and cranial musculature.

To examine posture and coordination, the physician should ask the patient to stand with heels and toes together, first with eyes open and then with eyes closed **(Romberg test)**. The presence of loss of balance with the eyes open or closed may indicate a cerebellar or cerebellar-spinal pathway deficit. This ataxia is usually associated with other cerebellar symptoms such as **asynergia** (lack of synergy of the various muscles performing complex movements), **dysmetria** (abnormal in movement), **dysdiadochokinesia** (difficulty with rapid alternating movements), **intention tremor, rebound phenomena** (the outstretched arm[s] overcorrects when displaced), **decreased muscle tone, or nystagmus** (the fast component of the nystagmus is usually to the side of the cerebellar damage). Deep tendon reflexes may be normal or decreased.

Gait disorders are detected on examination by instructing the patient to walk normally "as though you are walking down the street," on the toes, on the heels, and in tandem, "one foot in front of the other, heel touching toe." Gait ataxia with uncoordinated steps, falling, or near falling may indicate a cerebellar deficit or spinocerebellar tract impairment. Most persons older than 60 years have some degree of tandem gait ataxia. Gait ataxia alone usually indicates anterior cerebellar lobe dysfunction and is most commonly caused by aging or alcohol intake, although mass lesions (including tumors, arteriovenous malformations, and abscesses) and cerebellar hemorrhage and infarction are occasional causes.

Appendicular ataxia, or incoordination of the arms or legs, is usually ipsilateral to a cerebellar hemispheric lesion or lesion of the cerebellopontine angle (including infarction, hemorrhage, or other mass lesion such as hemangioma, metastasis, and astrocytoma). Such incoordination is manifested by intention tremor and clumsiness independent of weakness on finger-to-nose and heel-to-shin testing.

Truncal ataxia, usually involving both gait ataxia and ataxia when the patient is sitting, may be apparent only when the patient attempts to correct sitting posture after it is slightly displaced. Lesions producing such disturbances are usually located in or near the cerebellar vermis or its brain stem connections. The differential diagnosis of such lesions includes sensory ataxias and cerebellar ataxias. Sensory ataxias, which worsen when the patient has eyes closed, are often the result of separate vestibular or proprioceptive disturbances. Cerebellar ataxias are generally about the same whether the patient has eyes open or closed.

Sensation

The sensory examination is usually conducted with the patient's eyes closed while the physician tests each half of the body (face, trunk, and limbs) separately. Each neurologic examination should include at least one type of testing of the spinothalamic tract system (such as pain or temperature) and function of the dorsal column (such as proprioception or vibration). Lateral spinothalamic system modalities may also reflect thalamic function (as does vibration); the modalities of joint position (proprioception), stereognosis, two-point discriminations, and graphesthesias involve higher cortical functions.

Clinically, **lesions of the parietal cortex** usually produce a contralateral discriminatory type of hemisensory loss (impaired two-point discrimination, astereognosis, sensory ataxia) or, if partial, selective sensory deficit in the face, arm, trunk, or leg.

Lesions of the thalamus or the internal capsule usually result in contralateral hemisensory loss (including the face) of all modalities. In addition, thalamic lesions may also produce other sensory disturbances such as **thalamic pain,** an unpleasant or severe burning, dysesthetic pain on the contralateral side of the body, or **anesthesia dolorosa** (reduction of pinprick sensation in the painful area).

Brain stem lesions may produce ipsilateral loss of pain and temperature or loss of sensation and numbness over the ipsilateral side of the face and contralateral loss of all modalities in the limbs, depending on the size and location of the lesion.

Spinal cord lesions involving only the spinothalamic tract on one side cause loss of pain, temperature, and light touch sensations below and contralateral to the lesion, but in lesions involving half of the spinal cord **(Brown-Séquard syndrome),** the spinothalamic tract signs plus ipsilateral loss of proprioception and discriminatory touch sensation occur as far as the level of the lesion. Complete cord lesions result in bilateral loss of all modalities, and central cord lesions usually lead to bilateral loss of pain and temperature sensation with sparing of proprioception and discriminatory sensation and sacral sparing of pain and temperature.

To determine whether the patient has central or peripheral nervous system damage and at what level, the physician must first systematically evaluate two or more of the above-mentioned sensory modalities in the spared half of the body (face, arm, trunk, leg) and then evaluate the affected side, comparing the normal side with the corresponding area on the opposite side and with contiguous dermatomes. Familiarity with sensory distributions over the various parts of the body is important (Fig. 5-7).

Cognitive Function

An adequate assessment of cognitive function is possible only if the patient is alert and oriented to time, place, and person and if the patient is not aphasic. Evaluation of the patient's intellectual or mental ability includes assessment of language, memory (short-term, recent, and long-term), calculation, abstract reasoning, judgment, perceptual and constructional functions, right-left orientation, and finger gnosia.

LANGUAGE
Language can be defined as the understanding and production of individual words and grouping of words for the communication of

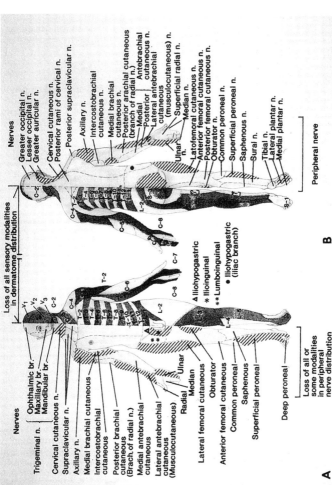

Fig. 5-7. Cutaneous fields of dermatomes and sensory nerves. A. Anterior view. B. Posterior view.

ideas and feelings. Language should be evaluated early in any examination of mental status because the presence of language deficits can influence performance on several parts of the mental status examination. Specific attention must be paid to **spontaneous speech,** including the characteristics such as the nature of speech output, presence of a dysarthria, or specific aphasic errors. Paraphasia is an important aphasic error, with substitution of an incorrect word or sound for the correct one and loss of fluency of speech. **Comprehension** is tested by asking a patient to follow one-, two-, and three-step commands, presented both orally and on paper. A patient is asked to repeat a word or sentence, of increasing difficulty, after the examiner to reveal repetition abnormalities, including possible paraphasias, grammatical errors, omissions, additions, and failures to approximate the examples given.

Naming and word finding are tested by asking the patient to describe a picture or to name various objects. Both reading comprehension and reading aloud should be tested to demonstrate possible alexia (reading deficit). **Writing** is tested by asking the patient to write letters, numbers, names of common objects, and a short sentence from dictation to detect possible agraphia. Aphasic patients are nearly always agraphic and frequently alexic. More than 99% of right-handed persons have a left hemisphere dominance for language, and approximately 60% to 80% of left-handed persons have a left hemisphere dominance or mixed dominance for language.

The common aphasia syndromes may be classified according to four major examination findings, including speech fluency, repetition, comprehension, and naming, as reviewed in Table 5-7. All aphasias are associated with naming difficulties. Transcortical aphasias do not involve lesions in perisylvian locations, and thus they manifest relative sparing of repetition.

Pure alexia without agraphia, in which the patient understands words spelled aloud and can write but is unable to read, may result from lesions of the posterior portion of the corpus callosum and the occipital lobe in the dominant hemisphere. **Alexia with agraphia** indicates inability to read or write and may be caused by lesions in the dominant inferior parietal lobule, in the angular gyrus. **Pure agraphia** occurs rarely and generally with the left hand because of lesions of the anterior corpus callosum; agraphia associated with dyscalculia, right-left confusion, and finger agnosia (**Gerstmann's syndrome**) is more common in patients with lesions in the dominant parietal lobe.

Nonorganic speech and language disorders may occur in some patients with functional disturbances who convert anxiety into a halting, telegraphic speech. Comprehension, repetition, naming, reading, and writing are normal; appropriate psychotherapy alters the abnormal speech patterns. An acute aphonia with total inability to adduct the vocal cord and make audible sounds but normal breathing and no evidence of stridor also responds well to speech therapy. In elective mutism, patients may demonstrate willful reluctance or an outright refusal to speak, but they have no demonstrable language deficit. These patients usually respond to behavior modification.

Table 5-7. Classification of aphasias

| Subtype | Location | Examination findings | | | |
		Fluent	Repetition	Comprehension	Naming
Broca's	Frontal operculum	No	−	+	−*
Wernicke's	Superior temporal	Yes	−	−	−
Conduction	Supramarginal gyrus, arcuate fasciculus	Yes	− −	+	−
Anomic	Angular gyrus, toxic or metabolic encephalopathy; poorly localized	Yes	+	+	−
Global	Middle cerebral artery distribution	No	−	−	−
Transcortical					
Motor	Anterior arterial border zone	No	+	+	−
Sensory	Posterior arterial border zone	Yes	+	−	−
Mixed	Entire border zone	No	+	−	−

+ = normal or relatively unaffected; − = abnormal; − − = markedly abnormal.
*May be good, relative to paucity of spontaneous speech.

Table 5-8.   Short mental status examination

Subtest	Maximal possible score
Orientation	8
Attention	7
Learning	
Number of words learned (maximum of 4)	4
Number of trials (maximum of 4) for acquisition	
Arithmetic calculation	4
Abstraction	3
Information	4
Construction	4
Recall	4
Total score	38

From Kokmen E, Naessens JM, Offord KP: A short test of mental status: Description and preliminary results. Mayo Clinic Proc 62:281–288, 1987. By permission of Mayo Foundation.

MEMORY

To assess short-term (immediate) **memory,** the physician should ask the patient either to recall a sequence of random numbers or to recall the names of items after 5 minutes. To assess recent memory, the physician may ask the patient to recall events of the past few days or to describe the duration of the hospital stay. Long-term (remote) memory may be assessed by asking the patient about his or her date of birth, home address, the years of World War II, or details of other events that have occurred more than 5 years previously.

Memory impairment involves bilateral lesions, and results of the mental status examination may help in differential and topical diagnosis. For instance, **impaired recent memory** is often caused by lesions of the limbic system, whereas **remote memory impairment** is often associated with diffuse cortical lesions. Also, patients with acute cerebrovascular disorders, epilepsy, or recent brain injury may have loss of memory for events that led to the current illness **(retrograde amnesia);** permanent loss of memory of events for a period after a current illness is highly characteristic of brain trauma **(posttraumatic or anterograde amnesia).**

SHORT MENTAL STATUS EXAMINATION

A detailed mental status examination can be very time-consuming. For practical use by physicians and neurologists who do not have special neuropsychological training, the short mental status examination that has been used at the Mayo Clinic provides an efficient and reproducible way of evaluating general cognitive function (Table 5-8). **Orientation** is tested by asking the patient to give his or her (1) full name, (2) address, (3) current location (building), (4) city, (5) state, and (6) the current date—either the day of the week or the day of the month, (7) month, and (8) year. Each correct response is worth 1 point (maximal score is 8). To assess **attention,** the physician tells the patient, "I will give you a series of numbers. Please pay close attention to them, wait until I am finished, and then repeat the numbers to me in the same order as I have given them." Usually, a span of five to seven digits is given to the patient. The number of digits correctly repeated is the patient's score; the maximal score is 7, and the minimal score is 0.

To assess **learning** functions, the patient is told, "I shall now give you four words. I would like you to learn them, keep them in mind, and repeat them to me from time to time when I ask you to do so." The four words are "apple," "Mr. Johnson," "charity," and "tunnel." The patient is asked to repeat the words. If he or she learns the words on the first trial, a score of 4 points is given. If the patient is unable to learn all four words, a point is earned for each word learned. The number of trials (a maximum of four) required to learn the words is recorded separately, but for scoring, the number of trials greater than one is subtracted from the points earned for each word learned.

Arithmetic calculation ability is tested by asking the patient to multiply 5 by 13, to subtract 7 from 65, to divide 58 by 2, and to add 11 and 29. Each correct answer earns 1 point, and the maximal score is 4. Interpretation of similarities by use of word pairs is used as a test of **abstraction.** The word pairs are "orange/banana," "horse/dog," and "table/bookcase." One point for each word pair is given only for definitely abstract interpretations (for example, horse/dog = animal). Concrete interpretations or inability to note a similarity earns 0 points for that word pair. The maximal score is 3. To assess **information,** the patient is asked to name the current president and the first president of the United States, to state the number of weeks per year, and to define an island. Each correct answer earns 1 point, and the maximal score is 4. **Construction** ability is tested by asking the patient to draw the face of a clock showing 11:15 and to copy a three-dimensional cube (impaired constructional functions may result from lesions in the nondominant parietal lobe). The patient is able to view the diagram of the cube while drawing his or her own version. For each construction, an adequate conceptual drawing is scored as 2, a less than complete drawing as 1, and inability to perform the task as 0 (the maximal score for the construction task is 4).

At the end of the short mental status examination, **recall** ability is tested. The patient is asked to recall the four words from the learning subtest: "apple," "Mr. Johnson," "charity," and "tunnel." No cues or reminder is given. The patient earns 1 point for each word recalled, and the maximal score is 4. The total score for each patient is the sum of the scores on the eight subtests. The highest possible score on the test is 38. Any patient who scores less than 29 should have a more detailed evaluation for dementia and related disorders. A single test such as this one **should not be the sole basis** of a diagnosis of dementia or any other cognitive disturbance.

OTHER INTELLECTUAL FUNCTION TESTS

Construction may be tested by having the patient draw a clock, including the numbers, and arrange the hands to indicate a specific time (lesions in the nondominant parietal lobe may result in constructional apraxia). **Right-left orientation** is tested by asking the patient to identify right from left for his or her own body parts (this function may be impaired because of lesions in the dominant angular gyrus). To assess **finger gnosia,** the patient may be asked to name his or her own fingers and to point to and name the appropriate finger of the examiner (impaired finger gnosia may result from focal dominant parietal lesions or, occasionally, from more diffuse lesions).

The differential diagnosis of dementia and other forms of cognitive dysfunction is discussed in Chapter 2.

Approach to the Comatose Patient

Coma is a state of unarousable unresponsiveness (impairment of consciousness) in which the patient is unable to noticeably sense or respond to the environment. When managing a comatose patient, the physician should initiate therapeutic actions aimed at maintaining vital functions to help avoid permanent brain damage from potentially reversible conditions while performing diagnostic procedures to define the cause of the comatose state. Management of specific coma-producing processes (for example, stroke, trauma, infections, tumor) requires careful evaluation of the patient because this state may derive from various systemic and intracranial causes. The following is a general outline for the clinical approach to the comatose patient, including a discussion of how to distinguish among various cerebrovascular and noncerebrovascular causes of coma. Further aspects regarding the management of comatose patients with stroke are discussed in Chapter 11.

Major Types of Coma

Wakefulness is maintained by a diffuse system of upper brain stem and thalamic neurons, the reticular activating system (RAS), and its connections to the cerebral hemispheres. Therefore, depression of either the RAS or generalized hemispheric activity may produce impaired consciousness. Three major types of coma result from various pathophysiologic mechanisms by which consciousness may be impaired (Fig. 6-1): (1) **focal cerebral lesion with mass effect** on deep diencephalic structures caused by intracerebral hematoma, subdural or epidural hematoma, tumor, abscess, large supratentorial infarct (although large hemispheric infarct may not produce coma caused by increasing edema for 1–4 days after stroke); (2) **intrinsic brain stem lesions** affecting the RAS, including infarct, hemorrhage, tumor, abscess, and cerebellar masses causing direct brain stem compression; and (3) **processes causing diffuse bilateral cortical and brain stem dysfunction,** occurring most commonly in cases of **metabolic encephalopathy**, **hypoxic encephalopathies**, and **infectious or inflammatory central nervous system disease**. The differential diagnosis of coma is reviewed in Table 6-1.

Neurologic Examination

Because coma has many causes, a systematic approach is required for the examiner to quickly establish the location and probable nature of the lesion, define appropriate laboratory tests, and outline appropriate intervention. Before the neurologic examination is performed, one must be certain that the patient's airway, breathing, and circulation are evaluated. Emergency treatment of airway compromise or insufficient ventilation may require suction, supplemental

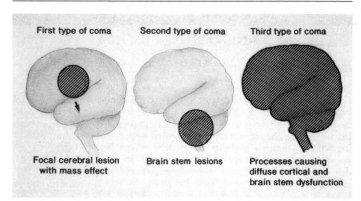

First type of coma   Second type of coma   Third type of coma

Focal cerebral lesion   Brain stem lesions   Processes causing
with mass effect   diffuse cortical and
                                                        brain stem dysfunction

Fig. 6-1.   Three major types of coma.

oxygen, or intubation. Hemodynamic instability also should be treated appropriately before more comprehensive neurologic evaluation. **Neurologic examination should include evaluation of the following five major neurologic functions:**

1. level of consciousness
2. respiratory pattern
3. pupillary size and response to light
4. ocular position at rest and following vestibular stimulation
5. motor and reflex activity

LEVEL OF CONSCIOUSNESS

Level of consciousness can be determined by applying verbal, tactile, visual, and painful stimuli. Initially, the patient should be observed for the presence of spontaneous movement or postures. Spontaneous purposeful movement implies intact brain stem pathways. The degree of stimulus that is necessary to evoke a response should be recorded. One initially attempts verbal stimuli, followed by tactile stimuli, then painful stimuli, which includes sternal rub or fingernail or toenail pressure. The type of movements evoked with these maneuvers also should be noted. Patient movements may include appropriate withdrawal, which indicates intact spinal cord, brain stem, and cortical pathways. One should consider corticospinal tract dysfunction if movement is asymmetric. Decerebrate or decorticate posturing is also of localizing significance (see Motor and Reflex Activity, p. 83).

The **Glasgow coma scale** is an objective scale that may prove useful for measuring the depth of coma or level of consciousness in patients who have had stroke. This scale (see Appendix B) has a score range from 3 (minimum score, deepest coma) to 15 (maximal score, normal consciousness). Assessment of the level of coma alone does not establish the cause, but documentation of progression or regression of the level of coma is vitally important.

RESPIRATION

Generally, normal respiration is characterized by rhythmic breathing with a frequency of approximately 10 to 15 breaths/minute (a

Table 6-1. Major types of coma

Type	Examples
Focal cerebral lesion with mass effect	Intracerebral hematoma, subdural or epidural hematoma, tumor, abscess, large supratentorial infarct
Brain stem lesions	Brain stem infarct, hemorrhage, tumor, abscess, basilar migraine
	Cerebellar masses with brain stem compression, including tumor, hemorrhage, abscess, infarction
Processes causing diffuse cortical and brain stem dysfunction	Metabolic Endogenous Hypoglycemic, hyperosmolar coma; diabetic acidosis Renal or hepatic failure Thyroid, pituitary, adrenal dysfunction Hyponatremia or hypernatremia, hypokalemia or hyperkalemia, acidosis or alkalosis, hypocalcemia or hypercalcemia Wernicke's encephalopathy Exogenous Alcohol, sedatives, narcotics, antidepressants, anticonvulsants, anesthetic agents, carbon monoxide Other Severe hypothermia, hyperthermia Hypoxia or anoxia Cardiac disorders: cardiac arrest, severe congestive heart failure Chronic obstructive pulmonary disease Infectious disorders Meningitis Encephalitis Systemic infections Other diffuse disorders Subarachnoid hemorrhage Postictal state Concussion Hypertensive encephalopathy Hydrocephalus Degenerative neurologic disorders

normal breath is about 500 ml of inspired air). Some respiratory patterns can have a localizing significance and help in the diagnosis of coma (Fig. 6-2).

Cheyne-Stokes respiration is a periodic pattern in which episodes of hyperpnea alternate with apnea and implies bilateral, deep hemispheric lesions or diffuse cortical and brain stem dysfunction. This respiration pattern may be the first sign of transtentorial herniation in patients with a unilateral supratentorial lesion. The pattern may also be seen in normal individuals and in those with metabolic disorders and other causes of diffuse cortical and brain stem dysfunction. **Central neurogenic hyperventilation**, a regular, rapid, deep, machinery-like breathing, usually indicates a lesion of the brain stem tegmentum between the low midbrain and the middle third of the pons or diffuse cortical or brain stem dysfunction. A sys-

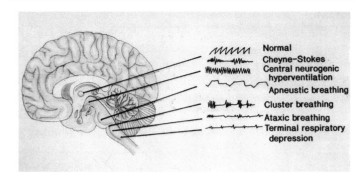

Fig. 6-2.   Respiratory patterns characteristic of lesions at different levels of the brain. (Redrawn from: The localization of lesions causing coma. In: Brazis PW, Masdeu JC, Biller J. Localization in Clinical Neurology (3rd ed). Boston: Little, Brown, 1996, pp 565–595.)

temic, acid-base imbalance also must be considered if hyperventilation is noted. Central neurogenic hyperventilation resulting in metabolic acidosis may be caused by pneumonia (often accompanied by an expiratory grunt, cyanosis, and fever), neurogenic pulmonary edema, or diabetic or uremic acidosis, and may occur in hepatic coma and salicylate poisoning. **Apneustic breathing** consists of a prolonged inspiratory cramp followed by an expiratory pause and usually denotes a lesion (especially infarction or primary hemorrhage) in the pons. **Ataxic breathing,** which is irregular and variable, and **cluster breathing,** with irregular pauses between breaths, are often terminal patterns signifying a high medullary dysfunction. With further depression of the medulla, respiration becomes more erratic and may eventually decrease (**suppression**) and then stop (**apnea**).

PUPILS
Pupillary size, symmetry, and reactivity to light (Fig. 6-3) are all important in the evaluation of the comatose patient. The response of the pupils to light in a comatose patient should be tested with a bright light to be certain of the response. Pupillary light response is relatively resistant to metabolic abnormalities, and the preservation of light response in association with other signs of midbrain dysfunction indicates a probable metabolic cause. Although the presence of the light reflex is the single most important physical sign differentiating diffuse (cortical and brain stem dysfunction) from structural brain disease, metabolic disorders can mimic structural brain disease. Glutethimide, scopolamine, and atropine may cause fixed and dilated pupils; opiates may cause constricted pupils.

Bilateral dilated (6–7 mm) and fixed pupils usually signify brain death but may also occur with barbiturate intoxication or severe hypothermia. Midposition (4–5 mm), equal, and reactive pupils usually occur in patients with diffuse cortical and brain stem dysfunction; midposition pupils that are fixed to light indicate a midbrain lesion. Unilateral pupillary dilatation may indicate uncal herniation through the tentorial notch or a third cranial nerve compressive lesion such as a posterior communicating artery aneurysm. Bilateral

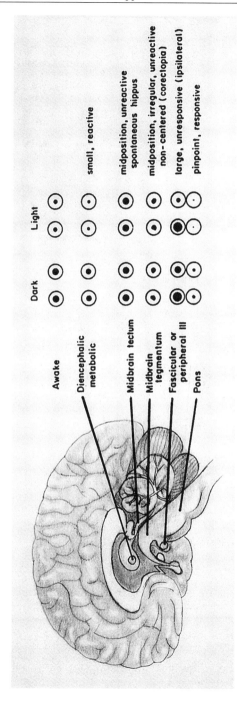

Fig. 6-3.   Pupillary responses characteristic of lesions at different levels of the brain. (Redrawn from: The localization of lesions causing coma. In: Brazis PW, Masdeu JC, Biller J. Localization in Clinical Neurology (3rd ed). Boston: Little, Brown, 1996, pp 565–595.)

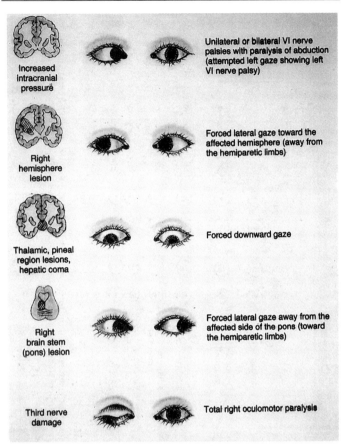

Increased intracranial pressure — Unilateral or bilateral VI nerve palsies with paralysis of abduction (attempted left gaze showing left VI nerve palsy)

Right hemisphere lesion — Forced lateral gaze toward the affected hemisphere (away from the hemiparetic limbs)

Thalamic, pineal region lesions, hepatic coma — Forced downward gaze

Right brain stem (pons) lesion — Forced lateral gaze away from the affected side of the pons (toward the hemiparetic limbs)

Third nerve damage — Total right oculomotor paralysis

Fig. 6-4. Examination of eye position and movements in comatose patients.

very small (pinpoint) and reactive pupils suggest pontine hemorrhage, infarction, or narcotic use.

OCULAR POSITION AND MOVEMENTS

Careful assessment of eye position and movements in comatose patients is often very helpful for localizing the offending lesion(s) (Fig. 6-4). Spontaneous, roving, conjugate eye movements indicate intact brain stem pathways. Dysconjugate ocular movements typically indicate abnormal brain stem function. Lateral gaze deviation is also localizing, as noted below.

Unilateral or bilateral paralysis of abduction may be caused by increased intracranial pressure resulting from a massive hemispheric lesion. Conjugate lateral gaze deviation may be caused by frontal or pontine lesions. In frontal hemispheric destructive lesions, the **eyes deviate toward the damaged hemisphere** and away from the affected limbs; in pontine lesions, the **eyes deviate away from the damaged brain stem** and toward the affected limbs (forced lateral gaze). In irritative lesions, such as a seizure, the eyes deviate away from the frontal seizure and are directed toward the hemiparetic limb. **Absence of eye movements** with reactive pupils suggests a process causing diffuse cortical and brain stem dysfunction. Deviation of one eye laterally and down, complete ptosis, and pupil dilatation are characteristic of damage to the ipsilateral third cranial nerve (see Fig. 6-4).

In a patient with a hemispheric lesion, the eyes are fully deviated but can be brought beyond the midline toward the other side by either cold water caloric stimulation (oculovestibular caloric reflex) or passive head turning (doll's eye maneuver). **Cold water caloric stimulation** (10–20 ml ice-cold water introduced into the ear canal, with the head inclined at 30 degrees) helps to evaluate brain stem function between the upper medulla and midbrain: In a patient with a functioning brain stem, the eyes will slowly deviate toward the stimulated side. In a patient with a pontine lesion, ipsilateral caloric stimulation may bring the eyes only to the midline. In a comatose patient with intact brain stem function, rotation or flexion of the head produces eye movements in a direction opposite to the direction of head movement **(oculocephalic [doll's eye] reflex);** in patients with brain stem dysfunction, this maneuver produces no eye movement or ocular movement may not be conjugate.

Nystagmus (rapid, jerking eye movements) in a comatose patient may be caused by brain stem or cerebellar dysfunction as a result of vascular disease, demyelination, infection, neoplasm, alcohol intoxication, or toxicity from phenytoin (in cases of localized cerebellar damage, the direction of the fast phase of nystagmus tends to occur to the affected side of the cerebellar lesion). In conscious patients with functional coma, nystagmus develops when caloric testing is performed.

Forced downgaze usually occurs with thalamic hemorrhage, a mass lesion in the pineal region, or diffuse cortical and brain stem dysfunction; rapid downgaze followed by slow upgaze is more characteristic of a caudal pontine lesion. Unilateral loss of the **corneal reflex** signifies a pontine lesion (bilateral loss or diminution of the corneal reflexes may be observed in the deep stages of coma, indicating depression of brain stem function).

MOTOR AND REFLEX ACTIVITY

An important component of the neurologic examination of the comatose patient is to determine whether hemiplegia or other focal neurologic signs are present. Because the comatose patient is unable to respond, the face and limbs should be observed to detect subtle asymmetries of neurologic function. When one cheek puffs out with each expiration, one eyelid does not close completely after passive lifting and release (compared with the other side of the face), or there is homolateral absence of the corneal reflex, the affected side of the face is usually paretic or plegic. Absence of **movements** on one side of the body, or asymmetry of movements, is suggestive of hemiparesis. Symmetric limb responses, especially when associated with reactive pupils and full eye movements, suggest diffuse cortical and brain stem dysfunction. Focal **seizures** may point to a localized cerebral lesion. Multifocal seizures, myoclonic jerks, or asterixis are suggestive of diffuse cortical and brain stem dysfunction.

In addition to general observation of the position of the patient's body and limbs, paralysis of the limbs also can be determined through the examination of muscle tone. By lifting each limb and allowing it to fall (the paralyzed limb falls rapidly and heavily, and the spared one falls more gradually) or by flexing the patient's knees so the heels approach the buttocks (with the patient supine, the paralyzed leg falls farther to the side and more rapidly when the knees are released), paralysis may become apparent. Bilateral paratonic rigidity or gegenhalten (plastic-like increase in muscle resistance to passive movements of the extremities) is suggestive of diffuse cortical and brain stem dysfunction.

The predominant posture of the limbs and body should be noted. **Decorticate rigidity** (arm[s] flexed and adducted, and leg[s] extended) usually results from deep hemispheric lesions above the red nucleus (cerebral white matter, internal capsule or thalamus) (Fig. 6-5). Lesions below the level of the vestibular nuclei usually produce flaccidity and absence of all postures and movements. **Decerebrate rigidity** (opisthotonos, jaw clenching, stiff limb extension, internal rotation of the arms, and plantar flexion of the feet) typically suggests a lesion in the upper brain stem between the red nucleus in the midbrain and the upper medulla, but a similar-appearing posture also may be noted in bilateral diencephalic and cortical dysfunction (see Fig. 6-5).

Deep tendon reflexes usually add little to the testing of motor activity and are seldom needed to localize the abnormality causing coma. Deep tendon reflexes may be normal or slightly reduced on the hemiplegic side, and the plantar reflexes may be absent or extensor. Asymmetries of deep tendon reflexes and limb movements, facial grimace in response to painful stimulation, and the presence of **pathologic reflexes** (Babinski's sign) or clonus of the affected limbs all indicate the probable presence of a structural lesion. Occasionally, all deep tendon reflexes may be lost or very depressed in comatose patients immediately after a stroke, but more commonly the reflexes are hyperactive on the side opposite the cerebral lesion. Bilateral Babinski's signs may occur in a patient with a massive unilateral lesion if cerebral edema has caused midbrain compression. However, Babinski's signs and clonus also can be present in some metabolic comas.

SUMMARY
Key findings in the three main types of coma described are summarized in Table 6-2. After brief neurologic examination, one should be able to localize the neurologic abnormality and define a differential diagnosis for the coma (see Table 6-1).

Additional Evaluation: History and General Examination

Although the neurologic examination aids in localizing a lesion, the cause of the coma may still not be clear. Additional historical and

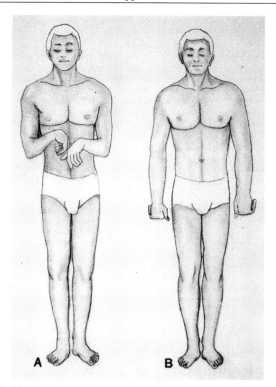

Fig. 6-5. Decorticate and decerebrate posturing. A. Decorticate posture may occur with severe unilateral hemispheric lesion with central hernia-tion, a deep hemispheric lesion, or a high brain stem lesion at or above the level of the red nucleus (midbrain) level. B. Decerebrate posture usually indicates a lesion in the brain stem between the red nucleus in the midbrain and the upper medulla.

general examination findings are useful for narrowing the differen-tial diagnosis and outlining appropriate treatment.

HISTORY
Having determined what type of coma is present, the physician must define the underlying cause of the comatose state. A properly taken **history** is essential in the differential diagnosis. Questioning of friends, relatives, and ambulance personnel should focus on the exact **circumstances** and **mode of onset** of the condition (acute onset of symptoms is typical for intracerebral hemorrhage, sub-arachnoid hemorrhage, or embolic vertebrobasilar infarction; grad-ual development of symptoms is more characteristic of an expanding mass lesion, or various metabolic or infective causes of coma). Ques-tions should elicit information about **previous illnesses** such as transient ischemic attack or stroke, diabetes (may cause hypogly-cemia or, less likely, hyperglycemia), epilepsy (may cause postictal state), drug abuse, previous head injury (may cause diffuse white matter injury, acute intracranial hematoma, chronic subdural

Table 6-2.   Clinical features of major types of coma[a]

Type	Clinical features
I: Focal cerebral lesion with mass effect[b]	Cheyne-Stokes respiration, bilateral paralysis of abduction, eye deviation toward damaged hemisphere and away from affected limbs, eye deviation overcome by cold caloric or oculovestibular testing, forced downgaze, decorticate posture, hemiplegia with unilateral Babinski's sign and reduced tendon reflexes on hemiplegic side, focal seizures ± unilateral third nerve palsy with early pupil dilatation in cases of early herniation
II: Brain stem lesions	Apneustic/ataxic breathing, central neurogenic hyperventilation, ataxic breathing, midposition pupils fixed to light, pinpoint, reactive pupils, eye deviation away from damaged brain stem and toward affected limbs, eye deviation not overcome by cold caloric or oculovestibular testing, rapid downgaze and slow upgaze, nystagmus, skew deviation of eyes, decerebrate posture, hemiplegia (with unilateral Babinski's sign), unilateral loss of corneal reflex
III: Process causing diffuse cortical and brain stem dysfunction[c]	Cheyne-Stokes respiration, central neurogenic hyperventilation or slow or shallow regular breathing, equal and reactive pupils, intact or impaired corneal reflex, brisk ocular response to passive head turning, divergent strabismus, no focal neurologic signs, decerebrate rigidity, asterixis, tremor, multifocal seizures, myoclonic jerks

[a]All forms of coma may produce any of the levels of consciousness.
[b]Other brain stem findings may appear with increasing brain stem compression from mass effect.
[c]The features of this type of coma can be easily remembered with the phrase "nothing works but everything works," referring to the initial appearance of unresponsiveness ("nothing works") but the intact or relatively intact function of respiration, pupils, ocular position and involvement, and motor and reflex activity ("but everything works").

hematoma), or psychiatric disorders (may be associated with drug overdose or functional coma); **previous bacterial or viral infection** (may cause meningitis, encephalitis); **malignancy** (may produce intracranial metastasis); and **previous medications or alcohol intake** (may help to define primary illness, drug overdose, or alcohol abuse).

In patients with **type I coma** (focal cerebral lesion with mass effect), historical features may clarify the cause of the coma. The differential diagnosis includes intracerebral hematoma (history of hypertension, acute onset of deficit with early change in level of consciousness), subdural or epidural hematoma (history of head injury, with a lucid interval in epidural hematoma), large supratentorial infarct (recent onset of a focal neurologic deficit that fits a single arterial territory), tumor (history of malignancy, preceding headache, seizures, mental disturbances, papilledema), and abscess (preceding subacute progression of focal neurologic signs, headache, depressed mental status, evidence of a contiguous or systemic source of infection). In most patients with the first type of coma, a specific diagnosis is established by characteristic findings on computed tomography (CT) of the head.

Brain stem ischemia, hemorrhage, tumor, abscess, or compression should be considered in patients with **type II coma.** Historical features mimic those described for entities causing type I coma.

In patients with **type III coma** caused by diffuse cortical and brain stem dysfunction, the differential diagnosis should include metabolic or hypoxic encephalopathies and infectious or inflammatory central nervous system disorders. Historical features of a previous medical disorder associated with one of the causes reviewed in Table 6-1, history of drug or alcohol use, recent cardiac or respiratory disease, report of previous infection or fever, other history of seizure, hypertension, or head injury may suggest the diagnosis.

GENERAL PHYSICAL EXAMINATION

The differential diagnosis of comatose patients should also be based on the general physical examination, with special attention given to the patient's head, blood pressure, pulse, heart, breathing, skin, chest, abdomen, extremities, temperature, and signs of meningeal irritation.

On examination of the **head,** lacerations, bruising, "raccoon eyes," Battle's sign, localized tenderness, crepitus, and cerebrospinal fluid leakage from the ears or nostrils suggest head injury. Periorbital ecchymosis associated with cerebrospinal fluid leakage from an ear or the nose is an indication of cranial fracture. An enlarged head or tense anterior fontanelle in an infant indicates increased intracranial pressure. Internal auditory meatus pus or an infected sinus may be indicative of cerebral abscess or meningitis.

Hypotension and cardiac arrhythmias may occur in coma as a result of alcohol or barbiturate intoxication, myocardial infarction (decreased cardiac output), internal hemorrhage, septicemia, and addisonian crisis. Hypotension may also occur in diabetic or metabolic coma, dissecting aortic aneurysm, and gram-negative bacillary septicemia. A cardiac murmur may indicate underlying valvular disease with endocarditis. A **slow pulse rate** in combination with hypertension and hyperventilation or periodic breathing may be indicative of an increase in intracranial pressure. An **exceptionally slow pulse rate** suggests primary heart block but may also be caused by medication overdose. **Marked hypertension** usually occurs in patients with hypertensive encephalopathy or intracranial hemorrhage and in those with other causes of greatly increased intracranial pressure.

Respiratory patterns were previously discussed (see Respiration). In addition, the patient's breath may reveal the smell of liquor in cases of alcohol intoxication, fetor hepaticus in cases of liver failure, the spoiled-fruit smell of ketoacidosis in cases of diabetic coma, the uriniferous smell of uremia, or the burnt-almond odor of cyanide poisoning.

Tongue biting suggests epilepsy or a postictal state. **Needle marks** on limbs may indicate drug abuse, and **"snout" rash** indicates solvent abuse. **Emaciation, hepatomegaly, or lymphadenopathy** may be indicative of an underlying malignancy and intracranial metastases. **Generalized cutaneous petechiae** suggest thrombotic thrombocytopenic purpura, a bleeding diathesis causing intracerebral hemorrhage, or systemic infection with meningococcus. Signs of trauma (multiple bruises, especially on the scalp), stigmata of liver disease, skin infection, or embolic phenomena also have diagnostic importance. **Cyanosis of the lips and nailbeds** suggests inadequate oxygenation caused by pulmonary or circulatory insufficiency or methemoglobinemia. **Cherry red coloration** is typical of carbon monoxide poisoning, and **yellow coloration** may indicate underlying liver or kidney disease. **Telangiectases and hyperemia of the face** and conjunctival area are characteristic of alcoholism, **marked pallor** is associated with internal hemorrhage, and a **macular hemorrhagic rash** may be caused by meningococcal infection, staphylococcal endocarditis, typhus, or Rocky Mountain spotted fever. **Excessive sweating** suggests hypoglycemia or shock, but **excessively dry skin** points to diabetic acidosis or uremia. Dehydration results in reduction of **skin turgor. Needle marks** indicate possible narcotic intoxication.

Pyrexia suggests systemic infection, cerebral abscess, meningitis, or subarachnoid, intracerebral, or pontine hemorrhage; if associated with dry skin, it should raise the suspicion of heat stroke. **Hypothermia** may be a complication of exposure during the winter months or may be caused by alcoholic or barbiturate intoxication, peripheral circulatory failure, or myxedema.

The chest and cardiac examinations may reveal evidence for infective lung or valvular disease predisposing to cerebral abscess or meningitis. The presence of abdominal muscle rigidity suggests possible abdominal hemorrhage or infection.

Resistance and pain on neck flexion (the patient's head cannot be completely flexed forward onto the chest or flexion causes pain), **Kernig's sign** (extending the knee with the thigh flexed at the hip causes resistance and pain), and **Brudzinski's sign** (flexion of the knees in response to head flexion) can all be indicative of meningeal irritation caused by subarachnoid bleeding, meningitis, meningoencephalitis, or meningeal carcinomatosis. However, in some patients with subarachnoid hemorrhage, the signs of meningeal irritation may not develop until 12 to 24 hours after the ictus. Resistance to movement of the neck may also be caused by generalized muscle rigidity (as in phenothiazine intoxication) or to disease of the cervical spine. If any signs of meningeal irritation are present, emergency CT should be performed. In the absence of an intracranial mass or other identifiable lesion causative for symptoms, a lumbar puncture should also be undertaken.

LABORATORY STUDIES

Investigations in the acute stage of coma include **routine tests** such as complete blood cell count and determination of electrolyte, creatinine, serum glucose, calcium, aspartate aminotransferase (AST, SGOT), and bilirubin values. Urinalysis, chest radiography, electrocardiography, and arterial blood gas studies also should be done. **Toxin screening,** when clinically indicated (such as patients with type III coma), should be done on blood and urine to screen for opiates, barbiturates, sedatives, antidepressants, cocaine, and alcohol. If routine screening blood tests, arterial blood gas studies, urine and serum toxin screening, and head CT do not reveal an abnormality, additional metabolic screening may be necessary. This screening may include determination of **ammonia, serum magnesium, B$_{12}$, serum amylase, folic acid, and serum cortisol values, thyroid function tests,** and evaluation of **porphyrins**.

In virtually all cases of coma, especially with signs of trauma, focal neurologic signs, or raised intracranial pressure, head **CT or magnetic resonance imaging** is indicated. In patients with types I and II coma and evidence or suspicion of increased intracranial pressure, CT of the head without contrast should be performed as a primary procedure; in other instances, it should be done immediately after the initial laboratory procedures. In patients with type III coma, CT may still be necessary if the cause of the diffuse process is not readily apparent from the laboratory studies. Electroencephalography may provide evidence of subclinical epilepsy, herpes simplex encephalitis, or metabolic encephalopathy.

Lumbar puncture should be performed in patients with a possible diagnosis of meningitis or encephalitis, clinical suspicion of subarachnoid hemorrhage associated with negative findings on CT, and cases with normal findings on CT in which the origin of coma is obscure. **Lumbar puncture is generally contraindicated** if CT reveals an intracranial mass lesion, if there are other signs of increased intracranial pressure, such as papilledema, if clinical findings suggest a focal, probable mass lesion and CT is unavailable, or if the patient has a bleeding disorder.

INITIAL MANAGEMENT

As described earlier, initial management should include stabilization of a patient's airway, breathing, and circulation. Subsequent neurologic and general examinations quickly narrow the differential diagnosis. If the cause of the coma does not become clear after the first few minutes of the evaluation, therapeutic intervention on an empiric basis may be initiated. These initial treatments include 25 ml of 50% dextrose, given immediately after serum glucose determination. One should be certain to give thiamine, 100 mg intravenously, because a patient with heavy alcohol intake or other factors leading to poor nutrition may be thiamine-deficient and glucose intake may precipitate Wernicke's syndrome. Naloxone hydrochloride (Narcan) may be given (0.4 mg intravenously every 5 minutes) if acute narcotic overdose is possible.

The initiation of other interventions should be based on the results of the clinical examination, laboratory studies, and cranial imaging. Other measures that may need to be considered for urgent use include antibiotics for possible meningitis, anticonvulsants for seizures, hyperventilation or osmotic agents for increased intracranial pressure, or neurosurgical consultation for a focal cerebral mass lesion (see Chapter 11).

Coma-Like Syndromes

Several syndromes may mimic comatose states because they produce apparent unresponsiveness. "Waxy flexibility" in a patient without voluntary or responsive movements and with eyes open may suggest a psychiatric state such as **catatonia**. On recovery, patients fully recall events that occurred during their catatonic stupor. Patients with **psychogenic unresponsiveness** voluntarily try to appear comatose and may resist eyelid elevation, blink to threat when the lids are held open, and move the eyes concomitantly with head rotation. Pupils are normal and reactive, and cold caloric testing provokes nystagmus rather than gaze deviation.

Akinetic mutism refers to the appearance of a partially or fully awake patient who is immobile and silent as a result of lesions of both frontal lobes, masses in the region of the third ventricle, or hydrocephalus. In the **locked-in syndrome,** patients are able to communicate by means of blinks or vertical eye movements but otherwise are completely paralyzed. This syndrome results from lesions involving the ventral pons such as infarction, hemorrhage, or central pontine myelinolysis. A similar state may occur in severe cases of acute polyneuritis or myasthenia gravis, but unlike basilar artery stroke, vertical eye movements are not selectively spared in these conditions.

Nonconvulsive status epilepticus is usually characterized by rhythmic blinking of the eyelids or conjugate jerking of the eyes associated with continuous seizure activity on electroencephalography. If this diagnosis is suspected, intravenous administration of benzodiazepine (such as lorazepam, 1–4 mg) should result in improvement.

Persistent Vegetative State and Brain Death

Comatose patients who are chronically unresponsive with preserved brain stem function are said to be in a **persistent vegetative state** (spontaneous pulse, respiration, and blood pressure but no apparent awareness of their environment, no ability to communicate, and only reflex or random motor activity responses to stimuli). This state may follow cardiac arrest, trauma, or drug overdose or be an end stage of a chronic degenerative disease and should be diagnosed only when there are no concomitant medical or toxic conditions. The patient in a persistent vegetative state must be observed for a sufficient time (at least 1 month, even longer in children) to establish the permanence of the syndrome and to look for any signs of neurologic improvement.

Brain death, or irreversible coma, results from total cessation of cerebral function and blood flow at a time when cardiopulmonary functions may remain preserved but depend on ventilatory assistance (no respiratory movements are observed when the ventilator is disconnected). The patient is **fully unresponsive** to external stimuli. **Movements** and **brain stem reflexes** including spontaneous respiration **are absent**; pupils are midposition to fully dilated with no pupil reaction to light, no orbicularis oculi contraction in response to corneal stimulation, no vestibuloocular and oculocephalic reflexes; and no gag reflex is present. An appropriate apnea test should reveal no respiratory movements. Spinal cord reflexes including deep tendon reflexes may persist, but decorticate or full decerebrate posturing precludes the diagnosis of brain death. The **electroencephalogram is flat or isoelectric** and the patient is unresponsive to pain or other stimuli. Transcranial Doppler ultrasonography may also be used to confirm brain death on the basis of a pattern of small systolic peaks in early systole without diastolic flow or reverberating flow. Conventional arteriography reveals no filling at the level of the carotid bifurcation or circle of Willis. **Exogenous and endogenous toxins and hypothermia must be excluded.** Brain death should be diagnosed only if it persists for some period of observation (usually 12–24 hours, but often longer if there is any doubt about the preconditions).

Prognosis of Coma

A definitive prognosis cannot be given for each comatose patient, but the physician can provide some guidance on the basis of existing natural history data. In this respect, examination of the level of consciousness and determination of the duration of coma, pupillary responses, eye movements, age, underlying disease, and general medical condition provide valuable prognostic information. The signs of brain death predict an extremely poor outcome. Unfavorable signs during the first hours after admission of a patient with nontraumatic coma are the absence of any two of the following: pupillary responses, corneal reflexes, or oculovestibular responses.

The survival rate for patients whose pupillary responses or reflex eye movements are absent 24 hours after the onset of coma is about 10%. Nontraumatic coma lasting more than a week; poor motor responses at 3 days despite awakening on day 1; absence of visual, auditory, and somatosensory evoked responses; and persistent coma or vegetative state at 1 week are also unfavorable prognostic signs. In comatose patients, the survival rate decreases with prolonged coma, concurrent medical illness, complications, or advanced age. However, children, young adults, and patients with head trauma, toxic overdose, or metabolic coma are more likely to recover even when ominous signs are present. Patients who have motor responses or spontaneous eye movements with visual fixation at 3 days after onset or obey commands at 7 days after onset have a survival rate of about 75%.

Laboratory Evaluation

Laboratory and radiologic investigations allow anatomical localization of the cerebrovascular event and assist in the determination of its pathogenesis. Techniques available to aid the physician in the diagnosis and management of potential cerebrovascular disease include computed tomography, magnetic resonance imaging, cerebral arteriography, noninvasive neurovascular studies, and other ancillary studies. The proper use of these techniques requires an understanding of the underlying disease process, the principles of the test involved, and the advantages and limitations of each procedure. Specific attention should be focused on how each investigation influences management of a patient.

Computed Tomography

Soon after its introduction in 1973, **computed tomography** (CT) became the preferred method for imaging tissue damage from stroke, and its use was extended to the body and spine. In CT of the head, multiple rotating beams of x-rays pass through the patient's head, and diametrically opposed detectors measure the extent of absorption values for multiple, small blocks of tissue (voxels). Computerized reconstruction of these areas on a two-dimensional, gray-scaled display (pixels) provides the characteristic CT scan appearance. Modern CT scanners have spatial resolution from 1 to 2 mm (for routine scanning, slices are usually 5–10 mm thick). White and gray matter are usually easily differentiated (Fig. 7-1), and the major arteries may be visualized after the infusion of contrast material.

CT FINDINGS IN PATIENTS WITH ISCHEMIC LESIONS

The ability of CT to reveal an ischemic lesion depends on the resolution of the scanner, the size and location of the lesion, and time after onset of symptoms (Table 7-1). After a person has had a transient ischemic attack (TIA), the CT scan may be normal, or it may show an area of decreased density compatible with a small infarction (or rarely, an area of increased density compatible with a small hematoma) in the distribution of the TIA. Therefore, TIA is considered a clinical diagnosis. The main role of CT in patients with TIA is to rule out an unexpected pathologic lesion such as intracranial hemorrhage, vascular tumor, or arteriovenous malformation, which may change the investigative approach and management.

On admission, the CT is negative in approximately one-third of patients in whom ischemic stroke has been diagnosed clinically. However, a negative result does not exclude the diagnosis of ischemic stroke. A CT scan may not detect relatively small infarctions in the vertebrobasilar system, infarcts near the skull base (because of bone-related artifact), infarcts less than 5 mm in diameter, or infarcts with little edema. Furthermore, within the first 24 hours after cerebral infarction, the CT scan may be negative in about 50% of cases. Clinicians should remember that the location of the lesion is important for making the diagnosis of cerebral infarction and helping to identify

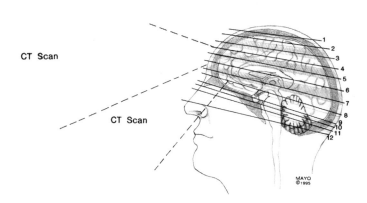

Fig. 7-1.   **Normal CT head scans.**

the underlying pathophysiologic mechanism that produced it. For example, infarcted tissue within a vascular territory of one or more major arteries may suggest large vessel disease or a cardiac source for emboli. In contrast, a tiny lesion in the basal ganglia area may suggest small vessel disease (for example, a lacunar infarct) or a lesion in a border zone between different vascular territories (watershed infarction) may suggest proximal occlusive disease with hemodynamic infarction.

Characteristic CT findings in patients with ischemic stroke include an area of decreased density, which often appears 12 to 48 hours after the stroke. The hypodensity is initially mild and poorly defined, but on the third or fourth day after the stroke the density decreases (in this period, edema is maximal and manifests as decreased density involving both gray and white matter in the area affected by ischemia), the margins of the lesion become better defined, and the lesion is better visualized (Fig. 7-2). Later, the edema and mass effect gradually subside, and the hypodensity becomes less evident. This change sometimes leads to radiologic disappearance of the infarcted area, which may become indistinguishable from the normal surrounding brain. The fogging effect occurs usually during the second or third week after the stroke and corresponds to the period of invasion by macrophages and proliferation of capillaries.

Thus, the peak period for detection of brain infarction by standard CT techniques is between the third and tenth day after stroke. However, small infarcts, particularly lacunes and brain stem infarcts, may not be visible on CT scans even after an appropriate delay. After the third week, phagocytosis of affected tissue ensues, the infarcted area gradually becomes replaced by cystic spaces filled with fluid, and the CT scan again shows a smaller and better-defined area of hypodensity with sharply demarcated margins of the infarct. In this phase, the density of the affected area is closely matched to the density of cerebrospinal fluid (CSF).

Table 7-1. Common CT findings in patients with cerebral infarction and intracranial hemorrhage, by time from event to evaluation

Lesion type	Interval between stroke onset and CT evaluation	CT finding
Infarction[a]	<24 hr	Mass effect with subtle gyral flattening or poorly demarcated zone of slightly reduced density
	24–48 hr	Mild and poorly defined area of decreased density
	3–5 days	Well-defined margins of decreased density; signs of cytotoxic edema (hypodensity involving both gray and white matter in the area affected by ischemia) and mass effect may be noted
	6–13 days	More homogeneous appearance of hypodense lesion, with sharp margination and abnormal contrast enhancement
	14–21 days	Fogging effect (infarcted area may become isodense with normal surrounding brain but may be detected with contrast enhancement as hypodense zone)
	>21 days	Smaller and better-defined area of hypodensity with sharply demarcated margins of infarct (cystic space); ipsilateral ventricular enlargement may occur later
Hemorrhage	First 7–10 days[b]	Well-defined, homogeneous, hyperdense rounded, oval, or more irregular mass lesion, often with surrounding edema appearing as a narrow hypodense margin
	11 days–2 mo	Becomes a hypodense area with peripheral ring enhancement (hemosiderin deposition), an enlarged homolateral ventricle (in small hematomas, hypodense area may become isodense)
	>2 mo	Isodense area (large hematomas can leave a hypodense defect with attenuation values similar to those of cerebrospinal fluid) with decreased intensity of enhancement

[a]Changes of large infarctions may be detected earlier.
[b]In cases of large hematoma, the first 3–4 wk.

The combination of a hyperdense zone and a hypodense adjacent white matter is characteristic of a **hemorrhagic infarction,** which more commonly occurs in embolic vascular occlusions and usually involves the cerebral cortex with sparing of the subcortical white matter. The hyperdense hemorrhagic portion usually appears smaller than a hypodense component representing infarct, and this hemorrhage is usually absorbed within 3 weeks. CT findings in patients

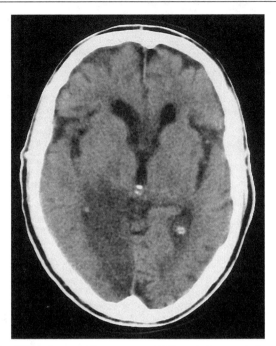

Fig. 7-2.   **CT head scan without contrast, 72 hours after onset of symptoms: area of decreased density in distribution of right posterior cerebral artery, consistent with cerebral infarction.**

with **hypertensive encephalopathy** usually include signs of generalized cerebral edema and mass effect, including compression of lateral ventricles, basal cisterns, and cortical sulcal spaces.

Under normal circumstances, **contrast agents** do not enter the brain, but if the blood-brain barrier is disrupted by a stroke, tumor, abscess, or other process, contrast material leaks into that area and produces better visualization (enhancement). Therefore, the use of a contrast agent (usually iodinated, water-soluble contrast medium administered intravenously) allows visualization of a small percentage of otherwise isodense and undetectable infarcts, particularly in the second to fourth week after stroke, when the fogging effect is present. After 1 month, the area of infarction typically will not enhance with administration of contrast medium. Other indications for contrast enhancement are suspected arteriovenous malformation, intracranial tumor, or intracerebral abscess. Contrast agents (particularly in high doses) may also have neurotoxic effects and cause clinical deterioration.

In patients with **venous infarction** caused by venous sinus or cortical venous thrombosis, CT of the head usually reveals extensive areas of edema with patchy contrast enhancement and multiple small hemorrhages. In the case of sagittal sinus thrombosis, changes tend to occur in a bilateral parasagittal pattern.

CT FINDINGS IN PATIENTS WITH HEMORRHAGIC LESIONS

Immediately after a person has had a hemorrhagic stroke, CT detects freshly extravasated blood (areas of increased density) in virtually all cases of intracerebral hemorrhage and in 80% to 90% of patients with subarachnoid hemorrhage (small amounts of subarachnoid blood may not be detected). **Characteristic CT findings in patients with acute intracerebral hematoma** (the first few days after ictus) include a well-defined, homogeneous, hyperdense mass lesion of a rounded, oval, or more irregular shape. The initial hyperdensity of the hematoma then begins to decline. The average lesion decreases in density by 1.4 Hounsfield units/day as a result of hemoglobin breakdown, progressing through an isodense (subacute) phase to a hypodense (chronic) phase.

Therefore, the differentiation between infarction and intracerebral hematoma is readily made by CT at any time within the first 7 to 10 days after stroke (or as long as 3–4 wk with large hematomas, in which disappearance of the hyperdensity is slower). In the chronic phase, a hematoma is often reduced to a slit-like cavity (with attenuation values similar to those of CSF) or may even disappear. **Subarachnoid hemorrhage** is even more transient, and CSF examination should be considered within 1 day to as long as 6 weeks after the ictus when the clinical history suggests this diagnosis and the CT scan is negative. In patients with **intraventricular hemorrhage,** CT demonstrates a hyperdense cast outlining the ventricular system.

Administration of an intravenous contrast agent is usually unnecessary in the early stages of intracerebral hemorrhage and no significant changes show on CT in the first 7 to 10 days. However, a contrast CT (or magnetic resonance imaging study) is required when the plain CT scan shows white matter abnormalities around the acute hematoma or abnormal densities adjacent to or surrounding the hematoma because these findings may indicate possible underlying arteriovenous malformation, aneurysm, tumor, or abscess. Often, contrast CT or magnetic resonance imaging is delayed a few weeks to provide a better chance for visualizing possible underlying lesions.

Epidural hematomas appear on CT as biconvex to lenticular, hyperdense, homogeneous extracerebral zones adjacent to the inner table of the skull with sharp margins. In cases of subacute epidural hematoma, CT usually shows a biconvex mixed-density lesion (the detached dura can often be seen on plain CT or on contrast CT as a thin, hyperdense stripe between the hematoma and the brain). In patients with **acute subdural hematoma**, the CT scan shows hyperdense, homogeneous, crescent-shaped lesions located between the calvarium and underlying cortex, often accompanied by marked ipsilateral edema and mass effect. **Chronic subdural hematoma** usually appears as a hypodense, lenticular-shaped, extracerebral lesion that is characteristically surrounded by a well-defined capsule.

Magnetic Resonance Imaging

For **magnetic resonance imaging (MRI),** the patient is placed within a uniform, powerful magnetic field. The procedure is based on the resultant interaction within body tissues between pulsed magnetic waves and nuclei of interest. Hydrogen nuclei (such as those in

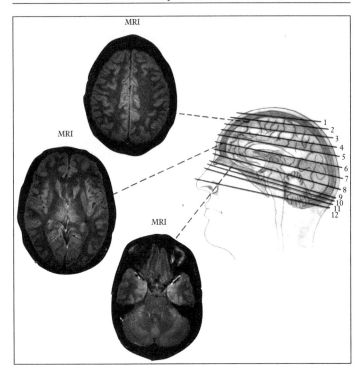

Fig. 7-3.   Normal MRI head scans.

water) absorb energy and are deflected from their alignment. As the nuclei return from a stage of excitation to their rest state, a signal is induced in a receiver, which converts it into a diagnostic image. During the process of energy release en route to tissue relaxation, two tissue-specific relaxation constants (T1, longitudinal or spin-lattice relaxation time, and T2, transverse or spin-spin relaxation time) can be used to reconstruct **T1-weighted images**, in which CSF has decreased signal intensity relative to the brain and fat has increased signal (ventricles appear dark, and gray matter is darker than white matter), and **T2-weighted images**, in which CSF has increased signal relative to the brain (ventricles appear white, and gray matter is lighter than white matter) (Fig. 7-3).

Disease processes such as edema, ischemia, hemorrhage, tumor, abscess, and demyelination typically cause an increase in free water concentration and hence an increase in the observed T1 and T2 relaxation times. An MRI scan can be obtained to accentuate either the T1 or the T2 characteristics of the tissue. The T1 and T2 signal characteristics of cerebral infarction and cerebral hemorrhage are outlined in Table 7-2, and a cerebral infarction is shown in Figure 7-4.

MRI produces images that generally are more detailed than those of CT and that provide more information about tissue characteristics. In many cases of stroke, this technique is not superior to CT, but

Table 7-2. Major MRI signal characteristics of cerebral infarction and cerebral hemorrhage

Type of lesion / hemorrhage composition	MRI signal characteristics	
	T1-weighted image	T2-weighted image
Cerebral infarction	Dark	White
Cerebral hemorrhage, time (days) from stroke to MRI		
1–3 (acute) deoxyhemoglobin formation	Isodense	Dark
3–7 (early subacute) intracellular methemoglobin	White	Isodense
7–14 (late subacute) cell breakdown, free methemoglobin	White	White
>21 (chronic) hemosiderin formation	Isodense, may have dark rim	Very dark rim

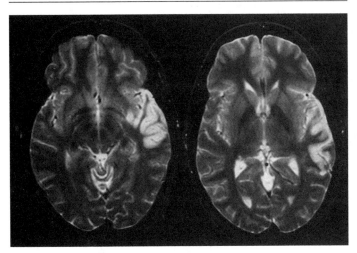

Fig. 7-4.   MRI head scan 72 hours after onset of symptoms: area of increased T2 signal in anterior temporal region consistent with cerebral infarction.

MRI does have some **advantages over CT:** (1) any plane can be selected (coronal, sagittal, oblique); (2) there is no ionizing radiation; (3) it is more sensitive to tissue changes (small infarcts may be detected earlier, within the first few hours, and more precisely); (4) occluded vessels or small arteriovenous malformations may be more easily visible; (5) there are no bone-related artifacts to obscure small infarctions in the vertebrobasilar system and infarcts near the skull base; (6) iodinated contrast agents are not required (paramagnetic contrast agents such as gadolinium allow differentiation of new strokes from old ones on the basis of their enhancement); and (7) cerebral infarction may be differentiated from cerebral hemorrhage even after several weeks have passed.

The **major disadvantages of MRI** compared with CT are (1) slice thickness is limited (3 mm wide); (2) bone imaging is limited to the display of marrow; (3) scanning time is relatively long; (4) claustrophobia occurs in approximately 10% of patients; (5) some patients do not fit into the machine; (6) MRI cannot be done if a pacemaker or other ferromagnetic materials such as shrapnel or certain surgical clips are in the body; and (7) the study may be normal for 24 hours after intracranial hemorrhage.

Since the initial investigations into the use of MRI techniques to demonstrate vascular structures in the mid-1980s, **magnetic resonance angiography (MRA)** has become available on a widespread basis. MRA is a subtype of MRI that can noninvasively visualize extracranial and intracranial arterial and venous circulations. Major advantages over standard x-ray arteriography include imaging without administration of potentially toxic contrast media and without the risks associated with arterial puncture and catheterization. The technique is especially useful for the noninvasive identification of intracranial aneurysms (a three-dimensional image may be obtained, which can be rotated through 360 degrees, a feature that is helpful for differentiating arterial loops from aneurysms). MRA also enables identification of increased intracranial vascularity that may occur with arteriovenous malformations. However, MRA does not clearly distinguish high-grade, cervical vessel stenosis from occlusion, may tend to overestimate the degree of carotid arterial stenosis, cannot clearly detect intimal irregularities, does not provide sequential information on the filling of the cerebral circulation, and generally has limited use in evaluation of the distal intracranial vessels. Overall, for evaluating extracranial carotid arteries, the ability of MRA to detect carotid arterial stenosis is similar to that of color duplex ultrasonography. The sensitivity and specificity of MRA for detection of hemodynamically significant stenoses in the vertebrobasilar system are less well documented.

Magnetic resonance spectroscopy provides information about the biochemical state of the ischemic brain. Its diagnostic and prognostic importance have not yet been clearly delineated. In addition, its clinical use for patients in the acute phase of stroke is limited by long acquisition times and wider slice thickness, precluding sufficient detail to be useful in some stroke syndromes.

Cerebral Arteriography

Cerebral arteriography remains the only method for complete study of both the extracranial and intracranial vasculature. It allows visualization of all phases of the cerebral circulation, including the distal intracranial arteries and venous drainage.

Arteriography is the most reliable method for demonstrating occlusion, recanalization, ulceration, and dissection of large arteries as well as stenosis and irregularity of distal intracranial segments of large and small arteries. It is also used for precisely estimating the degree of extracranial arterial stenosis and for detailed study of aneurysms and arteriovenous malformations. However, arteriography does not reliably image vessels less than 0.5 mm in diameter, is usually not helpful for determining the cause of deep lacunar infarctions, and is seldom used unless specific therapy (such as anticoagulation or a neurosurgical procedure) depends on the study result.

Even in the most skilled hands, neurologic complications occur either during or soon after cerebral arteriography in 2% to 4% of patients with cerebrovascular disease, including transient neurologic deficit in 1.8% to 2.9%, permanent neurologic deficit in 0.1% to 0.6%, and death in 0.1% to 0.5%. These complications may result from embolization of arteriosclerotic plaque or thrombus dislodged by the catheter tip, from the toxic effect of the contrast medium, or from vasospasm after injection of the contrast agent. The risk of complications increases with advanced age or impaired renal function and may be reduced with use of nonionic contrast material (such as iohexol or iopamidol).

Important indications for cerebral arteriography are (1) stroke syndromes in which arterial dissection or arteritis is a diagnostic consideration, (2) subarachnoid hemorrhage, (3) an intracerebral hemorrhage not clearly caused by hypertension or amyloid angiopathy—to define the presence of an arterial aneurysm or arteriovenous malformation, and (4) candidates for carotid endarterectomy—to confirm the degree of stenosis in the extracranial carotid artery and evaluate the intracranial circulation.

Digital subtraction angiography (DSA) uses a computerized technique to subtract or deemphasize unwanted images in order to accentuate intracranial and extracranial vascular structures. It may be performed with intravenous administration of contrast material (IV DSA) or intraarterial injection of contrast material (IA DSA). The major advantages of DSA over standard arteriography are that (1) it is faster and less costly; (2) it requires less contrast material for intraarterial injection, and therefore it has less risk of complications; and (3) IV DSA causes less discomfort and still allows some visualization of extracranial vessels and very good visualization of intracranial veins. DSA also has some disadvantages compared with standard arteriography: (1) IV DSA results in superimposition of vessels, which may mask an abnormality; (2) IV DSA has limited spatial resolution, which may prevent visualization of small intracranial vessels; (3) even a small movement such as swallowing by the patient during DSA can produce artifacts resulting in image blurring; and (4) the quantity of contrast medium used for intravenous injection is much more than that needed for standard arteriography and is more likely to cause renal damage (especially in older patients and those with diabetes mellitus and/or impaired renal function) and allergic reactions.

Electrocardiography and Echocardiography

The heart should be assessed in all patients with cerebrovascular disease. **Electrocardiography** may rapidly reveal evidence of myocardial ischemia or infarction, dysrhythmias (especially atrial fibrillation), or left ventricular hypertrophy as potential causes of ischemic stroke or TIA. Continuous **electrocardiographic** (Holter) **monitoring** for detecting chronic or intermittent cardiac arrhythmia may be used in patients with possible embolic events in whom another source of the event is not defined. Transthoracic and transesophageal **echocardiography** are relatively safe methods of evaluating cardiac anatomy and allow detection of potential cardiogenic sources of cerebral embolism, such as left atrial thrombi, left atrial appendage thrombi, atrial septal aneurysm, and patent foramen ovale with right-to-left shunt (Table 7-3). Other findings, which may be associated with a higher frequency of transient ischemic attack and stroke, may be spontaneous echocardiographic contrast, aortic arch atheromatous debris, and valvular strands.

Echocardiography is used to look for or to confirm valvular abnormality, cardiomyopathy, intracardiac mass (apical thrombi or tumor), and ventricular aneurysm or akinetic segment. Transesophageal echocardiography should be reserved for patients with one or more cerebral ischemic events of unknown or uncertain cause, in whom the detection of a cardiac source would lead to a change in therapy.

Noninvasive Neurovascular Studies

The various noninvasive neurovascular studies can be divided into two major groups: indirect studies such as ophthalmodynamometry,

Table 7-3. Transesophageal and transthoracic
echocardiography for detecting cardiac sources of embolism

Detected better by transesophageal echocardiography	*Detected better or equally well by transthoracic echocardiography*
Atrial septal aneurysm	Left ventricular thrombus
Atrial septal defect	Myxomatous mitral valvulopathy with prolapse
Patent foramen ovale	Mitral annular calcification
Atrial myxoma	Mitral stenosis
Atrial thrombus	Aortic stenosis
Atrial appendage thrombus	Aortic valve vegetations
Aortic arch atheroma/thrombi	
Mitral valve vegetations Infective endocarditis Nonbacterial thrombotic endocarditis	

From Sherman DG, Dyken ML Jr, Fisher M, et al: Antithrombotic therapy for cerebrovascular disorders. Chest 102 (Suppl): 529S–537S, 1992.

ocular pneumoplethysmography, and periorbital directional Doppler
ultrasonography; and direct studies such as real-time B-scan ultrasonic arteriography, duplex scanning, and transcranial Doppler
ultrasonography (see previous discussion of MRA under Magnetic
Resonance Imaging).

Indirect techniques use the ophthalmic and external carotid
arterial systems for indirect assessment of the more proximal carotid
system hemodynamics. All indirect techniques are designed to detect
the presence or absence of lesions that compromise 75% or more of
the luminal area (equivalent to 50% or more reduction in diameter in
all planes) somewhere within the internal carotid system proximal
to and including the ophthalmic artery. None of the techniques can
localize the lesion within the internal carotid system, detect mild
stenosis or ulceration within lesions, or reliably differentiate high-
grade stenosis from occlusion.

Direct techniques provide physiologic or morphologic data about
the external and internal carotid arteries in the neck and some proximal intracranial arteries. The B-mode and duplex scanning techniques are particularly sensitive for detecting mild degrees of stenosis at or near the carotid bifurcation, but the results of these studies
may be adversely affected by calcified plaques that prevent trans-
mission of the Doppler signal and produce acoustic shadowing. Technical difficulties also often occur in patients who have large, short
necks or a very high carotid bifurcation. The differentiation of fresh
thrombus from moving blood with B-scanning is also problematic,
but difficulties can be overcome with the Doppler flow velocity analysis instrumentation incorporated into the duplex scanner.

The clinical application of noninvasive cerebrovascular studies
varies widely. Although arteriography remains the most informative
study regarding the cerebral circulation, noninvasive studies provide useful information without the risks associated with arteriography. Noninvasive studies are often used to select which patients
may be the most likely to benefit from carotid arteriography and

endarterectomy procedures. The studies also may be used repeatedly to follow the condition of the carotid circulation in patients receiving various forms of medical or surgical treatment. The results of all the tests must be interpreted in light of the clinical situation, because patients with symptoms may have test results that are negative.

The indirect and direct tests complement each other and are often used in combination because they provide different types of information. Major principles underlying each of the various noninvasive techniques are outlined in Table 7-4.

OPHTHALMODYNAMOMETRY

Ophthalmodynamometry provides a measure of the central retinal artery pressure and yields information about pressure-significant (75% or more stenosis of the area) ipsilateral lesions of the internal carotid system proximal to and including the central retinal artery. The examiner applies pressure to the side of the globe of the eye with a calibrated, handheld ophthalmodynamometer while observing the patient's central retinal artery with an ophthalmoscope. As the intraocular pressure is increased, the point at which pulsations appear is the diastolic pressure and the point at which pulsations are eliminated is the systolic pressure. Criteria for abnormality include a 15% or more decrease in the systolic pressure of the retinal artery or a 50% or more decrease in the diastolic pressure of the retinal artery in one eye compared with that in the other. Absolute systolic retinal artery pressures less than 40 mm Hg are also considered abnormal in the absence of systolic hypertension. The procedure requires great technical expertise, and results may be subject to wide variation.

OCULAR PNEUMOPLETHYSMOGRAPHY

Ocular pneumoplethysmography provides a simultaneous measure of the systolic pressures of the ophthalmic arteries by an air-filled system. Suction is applied to the anesthetized sclera by eye cups serving as pressure transducers, and the resulting scleral displacement creates an increase in intraocular pressure that can be measured precisely. Recordings are made during continuous release of the applied vacuum (300–500 mm Hg). The point at which the ophthalmic artery pressure overcomes intraocular pressure and produces ocular pulsations represents the systolic pressure of the ophthalmic artery. Asymmetry in ophthalmic artery systolic pressure of 5 mm Hg or more indicates a pressure-significant stenosis of the internal cerebral artery on the side with lower pressure proximal to the central retinal artery.

The systolic pressures of the ophthalmic arteries also are expressed routinely as fractions of the systolic pressures of the brachial arteries. When these ratios decrease below calculated critical values, pressure-significant stenoses can be identified with or without asymmetries in the systolic pressure of the ophthalmic arteries. This technique also may be used for measuring collateral pressure around either carotid system by common carotid artery compression maneuvers performed during ocular pneumoplethysmographic testing. The technique is highly reproducible when performed by trained technicians and is not subject to as much operator-dependent variation as other noninvasive neurovascular studies.

Table 7-4. Major principles underlying indirect and direct noninvasive techniques

Technique	Factor measured	Lesions detected by luminal area stenosis (%)	Accuracy (agreement with arteriogram) (%)	Limitations*
Indirect				
Ophthalmodynamometry	Retinal arterial pulse pressure	75–100	60–76	Do not detect ulceration, do not differentiate high-grade stenosis from occlusion, do not evaluate posterior circulation, do not detect lesions with <75% area of stenosis, do not localize pressure-significant lesions
Ocular pneumoplethysmography	Systolic ophthalmic arterial pressure	75–100	90–95	
Periorbital Doppler ultrasonography	Flow (collateral flow)	75–100	50–90	
Direct				
Real-time B-scan ultrasonic arteriography	Morphology of the arterial wall	<10–100	75–85	Do not detect lesions outside carotid bifurcation area, do not evaluate posterior circulation, affected by calcium in arterial wall
Duplex scanning	Blood velocities and arterial wall morphology	<10–100	85–95	
Transcranial Doppler ultrasonography	Blood velocities	<10–100	75–85	Inadequate bony windows resulting in nondiagnostic transcranial Doppler studies in 4% to 10% of patients

*Limitations of the techniques can be minimized to some extent by using tests in combination, especially direct and indirect tests.

PERIORBITAL DIRECTIONAL DOPPLER ULTRASONOGRAPHY

Periorbital directional Doppler ultrasonography assesses the direction and quality of blood flow in the periorbital arteries and the response of these variables to arterial compression maneuvers about the face and neck. Because the periorbital arteries are terminal branches of the ophthalmic artery, blood flow is normally directed out of the orbit and may be augmented by external compression of carotid artery branches.

After locating one or more periorbital vessels near the orbital rim, the examiner positions the Doppler probe over the vessel to be studied. Reversed flow indicates extracranial collateral flow, usually resulting from a pressure-significant stenosis of the ipsilateral internal carotid system. The source of collateral flow is often better defined by sequentially compressing the superficial temporal, infraorbital, and facial arteries on each side of the head. A diminution or obliteration of periorbital flow indicates that the compressed vessel supplies collateral flow via the external carotid system. Compression of the common carotid artery may detect pressure-significant stenosis of the internal carotid system when intracranial collateral circulation from the circle of Willis maintains periorbital blood flow in the normal direction. In such instances, periorbital blood flow is unchanged or augmented by ipsilateral compression of the common carotid artery.

REAL-TIME B-SCAN ULTRASONIC ARTERIOGRAPHY

A two-dimensional image of the vessel wall is created by sound waves generated and recorded from an **ultrasonic B-mode probe**. Because the sound waves are reflected differently from interfaces of different acoustic impedance, the common and proximal internal and external carotid arteries in the neck can be identified. The blood column is generally sonolucent, but the vessel wall and atherosclerotic deposits are comparatively dense. Both transverse and longitudinal scans are obtained, and the percentage of stenosis in any given area is estimated.

DUPLEX SCANNING

The **duplex scanner** combines real-time B-scan ultrasound with Doppler flow velocity analysis in the same instrument. The B-scan component allows imaging of the walls of the common carotid, internal carotid, and external carotid arteries, and a pulsed Doppler cursor is placed within the lumen of any of the arteries to record flow velocity signals that subsequently can be analyzed by audiofrequency or color-coding methods. The ability of continuous-wave Doppler sonography to reliably identify both obstructive cervical carotid artery disease and subclavian artery obstructions makes it particularly useful in screening patients considered for surgical revascularization.

Color-coded duplex sonography allows characterization of fresh thrombotic material adjacent to the vessel wall and facilitates detection of ulceration within carotid artery lesions. The sensitivity of color-coded duplex sonography compared with that of conventional arteriography for detecting carotid occlusive disease is about 90%; thus, this technique is useful for rapid identification of patients at high risk for stroke from high-grade stenosis of the carotid bifurca-

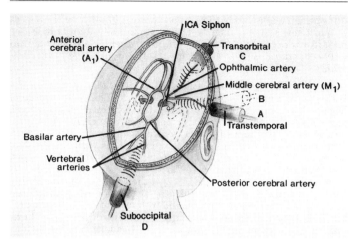

Fig. 7-5. Transcranial Doppler ultrasound windows. Transtemporal approach (A and B) is used to insonate middle cerebral artery stem (M_1); A_1 segment of anterior cerebral artery (A_1); distalmost segment of internal carotid artery siphon (ICA Siphon); and P_1 and P_2 segments of posterior cerebral artery. Transorbital window (C) is used for insonation of ophthalmic artery and immediately supraclinoid and infraclinoid segments of internal carotid artery siphon. Suboccipital transcranial window (D) is used for insonation of distal intracranial segments of both vertebral arteries and basilar artery.

tion area and for studies of the development of atherogenesis and carotid plaques.

TRANSCRANIAL DOPPLER ULTRASONOGRAPHY

Transcranial Doppler ultrasonography was introduced in 1982 as a noninvasive procedure for assessment of the intracranial cerebral circulation. The principle of transcranial Doppler is that a range-gated, low-frequency, pulsed-Doppler ultrasonic beam of 2 megahertz (MHz) crosses the intact skull at points known as windows and allows noninvasive study of the hemodynamic characteristics (blood flow velocity, direction of flow, collateral patterns, state of cerebral vasoreactivity) of the basal cerebral blood vessels (Fig. 7-5). Such criteria as window used, depth of sampling, direction of flow, and velocity measurements allow specific identification of the intracranial arteries. As with other noninvasive techniques, the physician must be familiar with the capabilities and limitations of transcranial Doppler technology to make clinical decisions based on test results. Clinicians will find transcranial Doppler studies most helpful if they have specific questions about the status of the intracranial circulation.

The procedure is safe and can be relatively fast (taking 20–60 minutes), but it requires patience to detect the signal and then to find the best angle for insonation at a given depth because even minor anatomic variations can cause misleading changes in signal strength. Intracranial stenosis is identified by increased blood flow velocities to levels more than 2 standard deviations from normal, and spectrum analysis of the signals allows estimation of the degree of the stenosis. A challenge test of contralateral compression of the carotid artery can be done to determine whether the effects of unilateral extracranial stenosis are compensated or lack anatomic collaterals.

Established clinical indications and potential applications for transcranial Doppler testing are outlined in Table 7-5. Transcranial Doppler ultrasonography is currently used for detection of stenoses of the major intracranial arteries, monitoring and early diagnosis of vasospasm in patients with aneurysmal subarachnoid hemorrhage, assessing intracranial collateral flow in patients with extracranial arterial occlusive disease, detecting intracranial arterial stenosis, identifying the feeding arteries of arteriovenous malformations and monitoring the hemodynamic effects of their treatment, confirming the clinical diagnosis of brain death, monitoring of brain-injured patients in intensive-care units, and intraoperative and postoperative monitoring of patients who have had neurosurgical procedures (including interventional neuroradiology). In addition to the obvious advantage of being noninvasive, transcranial Doppler ultrasonography is performed with lightweight, portable equipment; therefore, bedside assessment of critically ill hospitalized patients and also outpatients is possible. However, approximately 10% of all patients have inadequate bony windows to allow the pulsed-Doppler ultrasonic beam to insonate the intracranial vessels, which precludes completion of the study.

Hematologic Studies

The **clinical and biochemical analysis** of peripheral blood is important in the evaluation of all patients with cerebrovascular diseases, because specific hematologic disorders may be the primary cause of cerebral ischemia or hemorrhage, and other hematologic abnormalities may predispose to cerebrovascular occlusive disorders.

Specific **hematologic disorders** associated with cerebrovascular events are hereditary deficiency of coagulation inhibitors or hereditary abnormalities of fibrinolysis, elevated concentration of coagulation factors, autoantibody syndromes, polycythemia vera, leukemia, other hematologic malignancies, sickle cell disease, platelet disorders, and secondary polycythemias.

Several **tests** are available to aid the physician in the diagnosis and management of these hematologic conditions: determination of platelet count, hemoglobin and hematocrit values, leukocyte count, prothrombin time, partial thromboplastin time, bleeding time, fibrinogen level, lupus anticoagulant, and anticardiolipin antibody levels; hemoglobin electrophoresis; protein C and protein S assay; antithrombin III assay; and evaluation for resistance to activated protein C.

Other blood tests may be needed in patients with cerebrovascular disease. Blood urea nitrogen and serum creatinine analyses help to exclude renal disease, which might be a cause for chronic hypertension. Elevated total cholesterol and low-density lipoprotein cholesterol levels and a low level of high-density lipoprotein cholesterol and

Table 7-5. Established clinical indications and potential applications for transcranial Doppler testing

Established clinical indications	Potential applications
1. Assessment of pattern and extent of intracranial collateral circulation in patients with known regions of severe stenosis or occlusion in the internal carotid arteries, vertebral arteries, or subclavian arteries	1. Preoperative, intraoperative, and postoperative monitoring of neurosurgical patients (such as monitoring of patients during carotid endarterectomy and other revascularization procedures; intraoperative and postoperative study of the hemodynamic behavior of arteriovenous malformations)
2. Detection of hemodynamically significant stenosis in the major intracranial arteries at the base of the brain	2. Monitoring intracranial pressure in patients with head injury, intracranial hemorrhage, brain tumor, or hypoxia
3. Assessment and follow-up of patients with vasoconstriction of any cause, especially vasospasm occurring after subarachnoid hemorrhage	3. Research applications (such as investigation of cerebral hemodynamic changes in response to physiologic and pharmacologic stimuli, investigation of pathophysiologic mechanisms involved in stroke in patients with sickle-cell disease, migraine, cerebral vasculitis, and other conditions)
4. Detection of arteriovenous malformations and study of their feeding arteries and the hemodynamic effects of treatment	
5. Confirmation of clinical diagnosis of brain death	

Adapted from Petty GW, Wiebers DO, Meissner I: Transcranial Doppler ultrasonography: Clinical applications in cerebrovascular disease. Mayo Clin Proc 65:1350–1364, 1990.

lipoprotein (a) often are associated with atheromatous plaques in the cerebral arteries and an increased risk of stroke. A 2-hour postprandial blood glucose test is a reliable screening test for diabetes mellitus, but transient hyperglycemia and glycosuria may also follow hemorrhagic stroke.

Marked elevation of the erythrocyte sedimentation rate occurs in cranial arteritis but also occurs in other conditions such as systemic infection and malignancy. The leukocyte count in the peripheral blood is usually normal in patients with ischemic stroke, but it may be increased after intracerebral hemorrhage or ischemic stroke caused by septic embolus (usually indicating an infection when associated with a polymorphonucleocytosis). Increased platelet aggregability may be associated with TIA or cerebral infarction, particularly in young patients. The treponemal antibody absorption test helps to exclude syphilis.

Lumbar Puncture

Lumbar puncture (LP) is no longer done routinely in cases of stroke but is reserved for circumstances in which CT and MRI are nondiagnostic or unavailable or for specific diagnostic problems, especially in cases of possible subarachnoid hemorrhage, meningitis, or

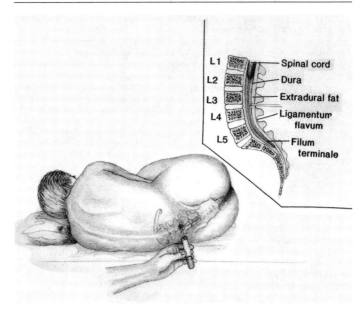

L1 — Spinal cord
L2 — Dura
L3 — Extradural fat
L4 — Ligamentum flavum
L5 — Filum terminale

Fig. 7-6.   Technique of lumbar puncture.

neurosyphilis. In cases of possible subarachnoid hemorrhage, when the patient's clinical history is suggestive but the CT (or MR) scan is negative, LP is usually indicated (often postponed 6–12 hours after the ictus). LP done at least 12 hours after the subarachnoid hemorrhage can reliably detect xanthochromia, but xanthochromia usually disappears by 21 days after the ictus. Relative contraindications to LP include (1) increased intracranial pressure, especially in cases of an intracranial mass lesion (for example, hematoma or tumor), particularly in the posterior fossa; and (2) hypocoagulable states.

When LP is performed, strict aseptic technique is required, and correct positioning of the patient is essential (Fig. 7-6). The patient's back should be perpendicular to the bed, knees drawn up to the chest, the neck flexed, and the patient's head level with the LP needle. The L3–L4 interspace lies directly between the two superior iliac crests and is most easily identified for LP. Local anesthetic should be injected intradermally in the center of the selected interspace and into deeper tissues along the anticipated tract of the spinal puncture needle (but not into the subarachnoid space).

After waiting several minutes, the physician should insert the LP needle with the stylet in place through the patient's skin at a slight angle toward the patient's head, parallel to the spinous processes. As the needle penetrates the ligamentum flavum, there is often a sudden decrease in resistance, after which the stylet is removed, and CSF is collected (if no fluid emerges, the needle may be rotated and withdrawn a few millimeters). After the LP is completed, the patient should be encouraged to remain lying down for the next 6 to 8 hours (preferably supine) and to drink extra fluid. These measures help to avoid spinal headache, which occurs in approximately 10% of patients as a result of persistent leakage of CSF from the subarachnoid space. Spinal headache is usually positional in nature, exacerbated with standing or sitting, and relieved by lying down. The headache can usually be treated with bed rest, analgesics, and hydration. When these measures fail, an epidural patch with autologous blood usually provides relief.

To differentiate whether blood found in CSF is the result of subarachnoid hemorrhage or a traumatic tap (puncture of a blood vessel by the spinal needle), the CSF should be collected in three tubes. A traumatic tap usually results in a diminishing number of erythrocytes in each successive tube. If this change is noted, it is advisable to discard the initial few milliliters and collect only the clear fluid, which should be promptly centrifuged. Clear supernatant fluid characterizes the traumatic puncture, whereas a xanthochromic supernatant indicates that the blood has been in contact with the CSF for at least several hours and, therefore, antedates the LP. However, the supernatant fluid can be clear if a spontaneous subarachnoid hemorrhage has occurred within 1 to 2 hours of collection of the fluid, and xanthochromia may occur in traumatic LP, with erythrocyte counts exceeding 200,000/µl. Differentiation of subarachnoid hemorrhage from traumatic LP may also be possible with the D-dimer assay, although this is still being evaluated.

The opening pressure should be recorded during the procedure, and the CSF should be examined for appearance, cell count, and glucose and protein levels. Some characteristics of normal and abnormal CSF are presented in Table 7-6.

The CSF is bloody in almost all patients with subarachnoid hemorrhage, in 85% of those with intraparenchymal hemorrhage, and in only 10% of those with cerebral infarction. The leukocyte count of the CSF is usually normal in patients with cerebral infarction (a pleocytosis as high as 50 cells/µl is occasionally found). In cases of septic cerebral embolism and rare cases of intracerebral hematoma, a moderate or severe pleocytosis as high as 4000 cells/µl may be found even in the absence of infection, as a result of an aseptic meningeal reaction. The aseptic nature of the reaction can be verified by a normal CSF glucose level and the absence of microorganisms in the fluid. The CSF protein content increases in direct proportion to the amount of blood present in the fluid (1000 erythrocytes/1 mg CSF protein). However, hemolyzed erythrocytes (such as those found in subarachnoid bleeding) may increase the CSF protein to many times this ratio.

In cases of suspected acute infection of the central nervous system, with or without potential cerebrovascular symptoms, an examination of CSF should be performed. Urgent Gram stain, antigen detection, and cultures for bacteria are indicated; and fungal, viral, and mycobacterial cultures are required in selected cases. In patients with positive serum serologic results for syphilis, or other reason to suspect neurosyphilis, a Venereal Disease Research Laboratory study of CSF is needed. Herpes zoster, herpes simplex, and Lyme disease studies may also be performed in certain situations.

Table 7-6. Some characteristics of normal and abnormal CSF

CSF characteristics	Normal CSF	CSF abnormalities and their possible causes
Appearance	Clear and colorless	**Bloody CSF:** traumatic tap, subarachnoid hemorrhage, intraparenchymal hemorrhage, intraventricular hemorrhage **Yellowish color in the CSF (xanthochromia):** recent subarachnoid bleeding, subdural hematoma, intracerebral hematoma, purulent meningitis, Guillain-Barré syndrome, acoustic neuroma, spinal block, hyperbilirubinemia **Turbid to cloudy:** acute purulent meningitis, acute tuberculous or syphilitic meningitis
Opening pressure	60–140 mm Hg	**High pressure:** meningitis, mass lesion (tumor, abscess, hematoma, large infarction), benign intracranial hypertension **Low pressure:** spinal block, intracranial hypotension
Cells	<5 lymphocytes or mononuclear cells	**Lymphocytosis** Infections: bacterial (resolving or partially treated), viral, fungal, mycobacterial, syphilis, Lyme, HIV, parasitic, parameningeal (sinusitis, mastoiditis, subdural empyema, epidural abscess) Vascular: cerebral infarct, cerebral angiitis, cerebral hemorrhage, sinus thrombosis Inflammatory: multiple sclerosis, systemic vaculitides affecting CNS, Guillain-Barré syndrome, sarcoidosis Neoplastic: meningeal carcinomatosis and lymphomatosis, some primary CNS tumors Other: chemical meningitis, drug-related, Mollaret's meningitis, Behçet's disease **Polymorphonuclear leukocytes:** bacterial infections, early in viral, fungal, and mycobacterial infection, brain abscess, subdural empyema, spinal epidural abscess, sphenoid sinusitis/abscess, septic cerebral emboli (infective endocarditis), chemical meningitis, Mollaret's meningitis **Erythrocytes:** traumatic tap, subarachnoid hemorrhage, intraventricular hemorrhage
Malignant cells	No	Meningeal carcinomatosis
Total protein	15–45 mg/dl	**Protein concentration** may be increased in association with various types of infection (see above for lymphocytosis and polymorphonuclear leukocytes), cerebral infarction, intracranial hemorrhage, spinal block, cerebral tumor (benign or malignant), meningeal

IgG index	<8.4 mg/dl	
Newborn's IgM	37–374 ng/ml	
Gamma globulin	6%–13% of total protein	carcinomatosis or lymphomatosis, inflammatory disorders (cerebral angiitis, chemical meningitis, Mollaret's meningitis, Behçet's disease, sarcoidosis) **Gamma globulin, IgG, or IgM value** usually is increased in demyelinating disease of any kind, with neurosyphilis and subacute sclerosing panencephalitis, with other inflammatory diseases of the central nervous system, and with cirrhosis, sarcoidosis, myxedema, multiple myeloma
Oligoclonal bands	0–1 band	**Raised:** in patients with demyelinating diseases, neurosyphilis, subacute sclerosing panencephalitis, fungal meningitis, progressive rubellar panencephalitis
Myelin basic protein	0–4 ng/ml	
Glucose	45–80 mg/dl or 60%–80% plasma glucose	**Reduced:** in various infections including parameningeal infections (purulent, tuberculous, fungal, syphilis, granulomatous, mumps, herpetic meningoencephalitis), subarachnoid hemorrhage (most often in the first week), carcinomatous meningitis, Mollaret's meningitis, Behçet's disease, chemical meningitis, blood hypoglycemia

CSF = cerebrospinal fluid; HIV = human immunodeficiency virus; IgG = immunoglobulin G; IgM = immunoglobulin M.

Ancillary Studies

ELECTROENCEPHALOGRAPHY

The **electroencephalogram (EEG)** records cortical electrical activity. In cases of stroke, the EEG is better for localizing the lesion than it is for identifying which type of stroke is present. For instance, in the case of an intracerebral hemorrhage, focal polymorphic delta activity (with or without bilateral projected dysrhythmia) may be seen on the side of the lesion, but these abnormalities are often similar to those caused by brain tumor or acute cerebral infarction. However, EEG abnormalities caused by acute stroke, in contrast to those caused by a tumor, tend to diminish progressively during the resolution of a cerebrovascular lesion. A subdural hematoma usually produces slowing or reduction in background cerebral voltage over the site of the hematoma, which seldom occurs with cerebral infarction or hemorrhage.

Within a few hours or days after an acute cortical infarction, the EEG sometimes contains periodic lateralized epileptiform discharges (PLEDs), which are frequently associated with clinical focal (partial) seizures, but these discharges are not pathognomonic for cerebral infarction because they may result from many other types of nonvascular lesions. A small, deep cerebrovascular lesion (for instance, in the internal capsule) may produce little or no EEG abnormality, and TIAs almost never produce persistent EEG abnormalities.

The EEG may be helpful diagnostically in comatose patients who have cerebrovascular lesions involving the brain stem (typically showing prominent alpha activity and lacking normal reactivity) and as a supplementary investigation for confirming brain death in stroke patients with irreversible coma (flat or isoelectric EEG).

PLAIN RADIOGRAPHY

Because of the development of advanced radiologic and ultrasound techniques, routine skull radiography has less diagnostic value in the evaluation of patients with cerebrovascular disease, but it still has some potential applications.

Radiographs of the head can show heavily calcified extracranial or intracranial arteries and occasionally calcified arteriovenous malformations, aneurysms, or tumors. Skull fractures (which characteristically accompany epidural hematomas), developmental anomalies (platybasia, basilar impression, occipitalization of the atlas), bony erosion, hyperostosis, signs of increased intracranial pressure (erosion of the posterior clinoid), and shifts of midline structures such as calcified pineal (as may occur with an unsuspected subdural hematoma or vascular tumor posing as a stroke) may also be detected. Cervical spondylosis can cause compression of the vertebral artery in the neck when the head is turned, with resultant obstruction to blood flow and the production of symptoms of vertebrobasilar insufficiency.

Chest radiography provides an estimation of heart size and may reveal the presence of unsuspected pulmonary tumors or other disorders. It is a routine investigation in the evaluation of patients with cerebrovascular disease.

Tests of Undetermined Application

Positron emission tomography (PET) and **single photon emission computed tomography (SPECT)** are methods for imaging various aspects of brain metabolism (functional neuroimaging). However, the clinical usefulness of these methods in the evaluation of patients with cerebrovascular disorders remains uncertain; currently, neither PET nor SPECT is available on a widespread basis.

In the **SPECT** technique, a gamma camera counts (from multiple sites around the head) the density of signals emitted from an injected agent minutes after it is given intravenously. Scanning provides a two-dimensional image depicting the radioactivity emitted from each pixel and detects early regional ischemia in occlusive cerebrovascular disease and regional flow abnormalities in dementia and epilepsy.

PET uses short-lived, positron-emitting isotopes (radionuclides) in a technique similar to that of CT, but because an on-site or nearby cyclotron is needed to supply the isotopes, this study is available in only a few centers. Regional brain biochemical activity is reflected in the emitted metabolic end products of such important substrates as oxygen and glucose. Therefore, PET scanning is of particular value for investigating the relationship between cerebral blood flow and oxygen utilization in focal areas of ischemia.

Suggested Reading for Part I

Akopov S, Grigorian G, Gabrielian E: Noninvasive testing of dynamic component of internal carotid artery stenosis in patients with chronic cerebrovascular disease. Angiology 45:125–130, 1994.

Amarenco P, Hauw JJ: Cerebellar infarction in the territory of the anterior and inferior cerebellar artery: A clinicopathological study of 20 cases. Brain 113:139–155, 1990.

American Academy of Neurology, Therapeutics and Technology Assessment Subcommittee: Assessment: Transcranial Doppler. Neurology 40:680–681, 1990.

Bisese JH: Cranial MRI: A Teaching File Approach. New York: McGraw-Hill, 1991.

Bogousslavsky J, Regli F, Uske A: Thalamic infarcts: Clinical syndromes, etiology, and prognosis. Neurology 38:837–848, 1988.

Bozzao L, Fantozzi LM, Bastianello S: Acute cerebral ischemia: CT and MR findings (letter). AJNR 13:829–831, 1992.

Caplan LR, Wolpert SM: Angiography in patients with occlusive cerebrovascular disease: Views of a stroke neurologist and neuroradiologist. AJNR 12:593–601, 1991.

Comess KA, DeRook FA, Beach KW, et al: Transesophageal echocardiography and carotid ultrasound in patients with cerebral ischemia: Prevalence of findings and recurrent stroke risk. J Am Coll Cardiol 23:1598–1603, 1994.

Department of Neurology, Mayo Clinic and Mayo Foundation: Clinical Examinations in Neurology (6th ed). St. Louis: Mosby–Year Book, 1991.

DeRook FA, Comess KA, Albers GW, et al: Transesophageal echocardiography in the evaluation of stroke. Ann Intern Med 117:922–932, 1992.

Donnan GA: Investigation of patients with stroke and transient ischaemic attacks. Lancet 339:473–477, 1992.

Fisher M, Sotak CH, Minematsu K, et al: New magnetic resonance techniques for evaluating cerebrovascular disease. Ann Neurol 32:115–122, 1992.

Fishman RA: Cerebrospinal Fluid in Diseases of the Nervous System (2nd ed). Philadelphia: WB Saunders, 1992.

Fronek A: Noninvasive Diagnostics in Vascular Disease. New York: McGraw-Hill, 1989, pp 186–268.

Goldstein LB, Matchar DB: Clinical assessment of stroke. JAMA 271:1114–1120, 1994.

Gomes AS: Aortic arch studies and selective arteriography. In: Moore WS, ed. Surgery for Cerebrovascular Disease. New York: Churchill Livingstone, 1987, pp 399–416.

Hanson SK, Grotta JC, Rhoades H, et al: Value of single-photon emission-computed tomography in acute stroke therapeutic trials. Stroke 24:1322–1329, 1993.

Job FP, Ringelstein EB, Grafen Y, et al: Comparison of transcranial contrast Doppler sonography and transesophageal contrast echocardiography for the detection of patent foramen ovale in young stroke patients. Am J Cardiol 74:381–384, 1994.

Jones EF, Donnan GA, Calafiore P, et al: Transoesophageal echocardiography in the investigation of stroke: Experience in 135 patients with cerebral ischaemic events. Aust N Z J Med 23:477–483, 1993.

Kittner SJ, Sharkness CM, Sloan MA, et al: Infarcts with a cardiac source of embolism in the NINDS Stroke Data Bank: Neurologic examination. Neurology 42:299–302, 1992.

Kucharczyk J, Moseley M, Barkovich AJ, eds: Magnetic Resonance Neuroimaging. Boca Raton: CRC, 1994.

Lang DT, Berberian LB, Lee S, et al: Rapid differentiation of subarachnoid hemorrhage from traumatic lumbar puncture using the D-dimer assay. Am J Clin Pathol 93:403–405, 1990.

Latchaw RE, ed: MR and CT Imaging of the Head, Neck, and Spine (2nd ed). St. Louis: Mosby–Year Book, 1991.

Mathews VP, Barker PB, Bryan RN: Magnetic resonance evaluation of stroke. Magn Reson Q 8:245–263, 1992.

Medical Consultants on the Diagnosis of Death to the President's Commission for the Study of Ethical Problems in Medicine and Biomedical and Behavioral Research: Guidelines for the determination of death. JAMA 246:2184–2186, 1981.

Moore WS, ed: Surgery for Cerebrovascular Disease. New York: Churchill Livingstone, 1987, pp 377–381.

Newell DW, Aaslid R, eds: Transcranial Doppler. New York: Raven, 1992.

Niedermeyer E: Cerebrovascular disorders and EEG. In: Niedermeyer E, Lopes da Silva F, eds. Electroencephalography: Basic Principles, Clinical Applications, and Related Fields. Baltimore: Williams & Wilkins, 1993, pp 305–327.

Nuwer MR, Arnadottir G, Martin NA, et al: A comparison of quantitative electroencephalography, computed tomography, and behavioral evaluations to localize impairment in patients with stroke and transient ischemic attacks. J Neuroimaging 4:82–84, 1994.

Peter JB: Use and Interpretation of Laboratory Tests in Neurology (2nd ed). Santa Monica: Specialty Laboratories, 1993–1994.

Petty GW, Wiebers DO, Meissner I: Transcranial Doppler ultrasonography: Clinical applications in cerebrovascular disease. Mayo Clin Proc 65:1350–1364, 1990.

Prichard JW: The ischemic penumbra in stroke: Prospects for analysis by nuclear magnetic resonance spectroscopy. Res Publ Assoc Res Nerv Ment Dis 71:153–174, 1993.

Quast MJ, Huang NC, Hillman GR, et al: The evolution of acute stroke recorded by multimodal magnetic resonance imaging. Magn Reson Imaging 11:465–471, 1993.

Rasmussen D, Kohler O, Worm-Petersen S, et al: Computed tomography in prognostic stroke evaluation. Stroke 23:506–510, 1992.

Riles TS, Eidelman EM, Litt AW, et al: Comparison of magnetic resonance angiography, conventional angiography, and duplex scanning. Stroke 23:341–346, 1992.

Sato A, Takahashi S, Soma Y, et al: Cerebral infarction: Early detection by means of contrast-enhanced cerebral arteries at MR imaging. Radiology 178:433–439, 1991.

Shuaib A, Lee D, Pelz D, et al: The impact of magnetic resonance imaging on the management of acute ischemic stroke. Neurology 42:816–818, 1992.

Taveras JM, Wood EH: Diagnostic Neuroradiology. Baltimore: Williams & Wilkins, 1964.

Tegeler CH, Downes TR: Cardiac imaging in stroke. Stroke 22:1206–1211, 1991.

Turnipseed WD: Digital subtraction angiography: Intravenous and intra-arterial routes. In: Moore WS, ed. Surgery for Cerebrovascular Disease. New York: Churchill Livingstone, 1987, pp 383–397.

Viroslav AB, Hoffman JC Jr: The use of computed tomography in the diagnosis of stroke. Heart Dis Stroke 2:299–307, 1993.

WHO Task Force on Stroke and Other Cerebrovascular Disorders: Stroke—1989: Recommendations on stroke prevention, diagnosis, and therapy. Stroke 20:1407–1431, 1989.

II

Differential Diagnosis and Clinical Features of Cerebrovascular Disease

Differential Diagnosis Made Easy: General Approach

Differential diagnosis in cerebrovascular disease can be divided into ischemic and hemorrhagic disorders. After establishing that a condition is cerebrovascular and determining whether it is ischemic or hemorrhagic (see pages 3–4), the clinician must try to identify the underlying pathophysiologic mechanism for the condition. This step constitutes the bulk of the differential diagnosis in cerebrovascular disease and facilitates optimal treatment. Although the underlying mechanism cannot be identified with certainty in many cases (as much as 40%), the number of such cases can be minimized by following a systematic approach to classification and differential diagnosis.

Ischemic Cerebrovascular Disorders

Ischemic cerebrovascular disorders are often classified according to temporal profile, including transient ischemic attack (resolution of symptoms within the first 24 hours), reversible ischemic neurologic deficit (resolution of symptoms after 24 hours, within 3 weeks), progressive ischemic stroke (progressive deficit, often for as long as 24–72 hours), and completed ischemic stroke (resolution of symptoms after 3 weeks, if ever). However, such classification does not help define pathophysiologic mechanisms because each of the temporal profiles may be associated with any of the various underlying mechanisms for cerebral ischemic events.

An easy method for categorizing all ischemic conditions, which relates to the underlying pathophysiology, is to classify the mechanisms into four main groups, proceeding from proximal to distal in the arterial system: (1) cardiac disease, (2) large vessel disease (craniocervical occlusive disease), (3) small vessel disease (intracranial occlusive disease), and (4) hematologic disease (Table 8-1).

Traditional clinical and radiologic features considered to differentiate cardioembolic events from cerebral ischemic events of other causes have lower predictive value than previously reported. These features may be suggestive of cardioembolic cause, but the clinician must acknowledge that overlap exists. Abrupt onset of maximal neurologic deficit and hemorrhagic transformation, particularly at a subcortical site, may indicate a proximal embolic source. Suggestive clinical syndromes include cortical events, isolated Wernicke's aphasia, posterior cerebral artery ischemia with homonymous hemianopia, and top of the basilar syndrome. The findings of seizures and headache are not useful in differentiating mechanism.

Lacunar infarctions are small infarcts in noncortical cerebral sites and the brain stem and result from penetrating arteriole occlusion. Characteristic symptoms allow clinical characterization as a lacunar syndrome but do not imply a clear localization, although a narrowed differential diagnosis is possible. These infarcts do not typically cause aphasia, hemianopia, significantly altered level of conscious-

Table 8-1.   Four major groups of diseases
associated with ischemic cerebrovascular disorders

Cardiac disorders	**Valve-related emboli:** rheumatic heart disease, calcific aortic stenosis, mitral valve prolapse, cardiac surgery, prosthetic heart valve, infective endocarditis, nonbacterial thrombotic endocarditis
	Intracardiac thrombus or tumor: atrial fibrillation, sick sinus syndrome, other major rhythm disturbances, myocardial infarction, congestive heart failure, cardiomyopathy, atrial myxoma, cardiac fibroelastoma
	Systemic venous thrombi with right-to-left cardiac shunt: interatrial or interventricular septal defect, thrombophlebitis, pulmonary vein thrombosis, pulmonary arteriovenous malformation
Large vessel diseases (craniocervical occlusive diseases)	**Atherosclerosis:** cervical arteries, aortic arch, and major intracranial arteries
	Fibromuscular dysplasia: the internal carotid arteries above the carotid bifurcation
	Carotid artery dissection: traumatic, spontaneous, or caused by fibromuscular dysplasia, aortic dissection
	Takayasu's disease (see also noninfectious arteritis, below)
	Other: vasospasm (migraine), moyamoya disease, homocystinuria, Fabry's disease, pseudoxanthoma elasticum
Small vessel diseases (intracranial occlusive diseases)	**Hypertension**
	Infectious arteritis caused by bacterial, fungal, tuberculous meningitides or other infective processes of central nervous system, such as tertiary syphilis, malaria, Lyme disease, rickettsial diseases, mucormycosis, aspergillosis, trichinosis or schistosomiasis, herpes zoster, basal meningitis (*Cryptococcus, Histoplasma, Coccidioides*)
	Noninfectious arteritis: systemic lupus erythematosus, polyarteritis nodosa, granulomatous angiitis, temporal arteritis, drug use and abuse including cocaine, heroin, amphetamine, phencyclidine, and lysergic acid diethylamide (LSD), irradiation arteritis, Wegener's granulomatosis, sarcoidosis, Behçet's disease
Hematologic diseases	Polycythemia, thrombocythemia, thrombotic thrombocytopenic purpura, sickle-cell disease, dysproteinemia, leukemia, disseminated intravascular coagulation, antiphospholipid antibody syndromes (lupus anticoagulant, anticardiolipin antibodies), protein C and protein S deficiency, resistance to activated protein C, antithrombin III deficiency

Table 8-2. Location and associated causes of hemorrhagic cerebrovascular disorders (intracranial hemorrhage)

Location of hemorrhage	Cause
Epidural hematoma	Head trauma; less commonly, anticoagulants, primary and metastatic neoplasm, bleeding diatheses
Subdural hematoma	Head trauma; less commonly, anticoagulants, primary and secondary neoplasm, arteriovenous malformation, bleeding diatheses
Subarachnoid hemorrhage	Intracranial aneurysm, arteriovenous malformation, head trauma, extension from intracerebral hemorrhage, bleeding diatheses, anticoagulant use, cerebral vasculitis, venous thrombosis, arterial dissection, primary and metastatic neoplasm, spinal lesions, drugs including alcohol abuse and cocaine use
Intracerebral (cerebral, intraparenchymal) hemorrhage	Hypertension, intracranial aneurysm, arteriovenous malformation, cerebral amyloid angiopathy, bleeding diatheses, anticoagulants, thrombolytic drugs, moyamoya disease, arterial dissection, infection, abscess, primary and metastatic brain neoplasm, venous thrombosis, drugs including cocaine, phenylpropanolamine, alcohol, and heroin use
Intraventricular hemorrhage	Hypertension, intracranial aneurysm, arteriovenous malformation, neoplasm of the choroid plexus, primary and metastatic brain neoplasms (see causes of intracerebral hemorrhage, above)

ness, seizures, or sensory or motor deficit in a single limb. Common clinical syndromes include pure motor hemiparesis with weakness in the face, arm, and leg and pure sensory stroke with numbness in the face, arm, and leg. Ataxic hemiparesis with dysmetria and weakness in the involved limbs characterizes another lacunar syndrome; dysarthria and nystagmus may also be noted. The dysarthria–clumsy hand syndrome leads to dysarthria, facial weakness, and slight weakness in the hand (see Chapter 16).

Hemorrhagic Cerebrovascular Disorders

Hemorrhagic cerebrovascular diseases can be categorized into five main categories according to location from outside to inside: epidural hematoma, subdural hematoma, subarachnoid hemorrhage, intracerebral (cerebral, intraparenchymal) hemorrhage, and intraventricular hemorrhage (Table 8-2). The clinical features of hemorrhagic cerebrovascular disease vary, depending on the site and size of the hemorrhage, but in many cases the location helps to define its cause (see Chapter 17).

Temporal Profile of Ischemic Cerebrovascular Diseases

The general description of focal cerebral ischemic events is based on the patient's temporal profile. The clinician should attempt to go beyond the profile, identify the underlying cause, and design a mechanism-based treatment approach. When the cause cannot be identified, treatment is less specific, again based on the temporal profile, results of available studies, probable cause given the patient's age and past history, and physical examination findings.

Transient Ischemic Attacks

Transient ischemic attacks (TIAs) are focal episodes of neurologic dysfunction caused by ischemia. They are typically rapid in onset, lasting 10 seconds to 15 minutes but occasionally as long as 24 hours. The longer the episode, the greater the likelihood of finding a cerebral infarction on computed tomography (CT) or magnetic resonance imaging (MRI). Overall, cerebral infarction in a distribution appropriate for the clinical symptoms is detected by radiologic imaging in about 10% to 15% of patients with TIA. TIAs can usually be localized to a portion of the brain supplied by a single vascular system. The symptoms usually reach maximal intensity within 2 minutes, often within a few seconds. Fleeting episodes that last only 1 or 2 seconds and symptoms such as unconsciousness without other symptoms of vertebrobasilar ischemia and a prolonged "marching" of symptoms are not likely to be TIAs. Positive symptoms such as tingling, repetitive rhythmic shaking of a limb, and scintillating scotomata are also uncommonly ischemic in nature. The frequency of episodes varies: some patients experience a single attack, but others experience multiple attacks at different intervals or at increasing frequency (crescendo TIAs).

Amaurosis fugax (transient monocular blindness) is included as part of the definition of carotid system TIA, but certain **isolated** symptoms, such as vertigo, light-headedness, syncope, dysarthria, dysphagia, diplopia, dizziness (or wooziness), bowel or bladder incontinence, loss of vision associated with alteration of level of consciousness, focal symptoms associated with migraine, amnesia, and confusion are not, by definition, considered TIA.

The duration, stereotyped nature, and frequency of repetitive spells may suggest a pathophysiologic mechanism. For example, repetitive (as many as 5–10/day), short-lived (<15 minutes), stereotyped spells suggest a hemodynamic mechanism with proximal arterial narrowing or occlusion associated with reduced cerebral perfusion (low flow) and inadequate collateral circulation or thrombosis at the low-flow arterial narrowing. Stereotyped focal spells may also result from seizures, migraine, positional vertigo, or other causes. Alternatively, a single spell that lasts from 2 to 24 hours is more characteristic of an embolic ischemic event, probably with some degree of infarction.

TIAs should be differentiated from other conditions that result in transient focal neurologic deficit. **Migraine** is often characterized by visual auras (particularly scintillating scotoma) that march or expand across the vision of both eyes during 10 to 30 minutes. Other focal neurologic symptoms associated with migraine include marching paresthesias that characteristically start in one hand, motor disturbances (hemiplegic migraine), unilateral visual disturbances (retinal migraine), ocular movement abnormalities (ophthalmoplegic migraine), and aphasia. These symptoms sometimes occur without associated headache (migraine equivalent or migraine cine cephalgia), but they are usually followed by a unilateral throbbing headache lasting hours to 1 or 2 days and are often associated with nausea or vomiting. Various combinations of posterior circulation symptoms evolving over minutes, such as dysarthria, vertigo, alteration in level of consciousness, bilateral visual obscuration, and motor weakness (often occurring in young women and typically followed by a severe, often throbbing occipital headache), are referred to as **basilar migraine.**

Focal seizures commonly produce episodes of repetitive jerking, tingling, visual phenomena, or speech arrest, any of which may be followed by a generalized seizure. Typical electroencephalographic findings provide additional evidence of seizure. **Postseizure states** may also mimic or follow TIA or stroke (a focal ischemic neurologic deficit may trigger a seizure and postictal state lasting as long as 24 hours).

Multiple sclerosis occurs mainly in young patients, usually characterized by recurrent fluctuating subacute onset (during hours or days) of symptoms with neurologic deficits lasting 1 day or longer. Less commonly, the condition may be associated with gradually progressive neurologic deficit; rarely, symptoms may involve sudden-onset, short-lived spells of neurologic dysfunction called paroxysmal symptoms of multiple sclerosis, including isolated recurrent dysarthria, ataxia with hemiparesis, hemisensory symptoms, and episodic tonic spasm of the limbs. The condition typically progresses to involve various parts of the white matter of the brain and spinal cord. The diagnosis is clinical in nature, but it may be aided by ancillary studies such as MRI.

Attacks that are clinically indistinguishable from TIA can result from **small cerebral infarction or intracerebral hemorrhage**. These attacks usually last hours rather than seconds or minutes. The diagnosis is established by CT or MRI. **Arteriovenous malformations, brain tumors** (for instance, meningiomas, gliomas, or metastases), or **subdural hematomas** may also be associated with TIA-like spells. Characteristic historical data and papilledema may or may not be present. The diagnosis is usually made with CT or MRI. Enlargement of a **saccular aneurysm** may present with transient symptoms and persistent, localized headache. Sometimes a clot that forms within the aneurysmal sac can embolize distally and cause TIAs; the diagnosis is based on arteriographic and CT or MRI findings.

Hypoglycemia with typical prodromal autonomic symptoms may mimic TIA. Prompt improvement after intravenous administration of 50% glucose helps establish the diagnosis. **Familial paroxysmal ataxia** may also be associated with transient focal neurologic deficit and is difficult to diagnose without the characteristic family history. Many patients with episodic vertigo alone have **benign positional vertigo** unrelated to cerebral or brain stem ischemia. These patients tend to hold their heads still or avoid certain head positions that exacerbate the vertigo, and the vertigo usually decreases with repeated actions that would typically precipitate the symptom (see Chapters 2 and 4). Episodic isolated diplopia seldom relates to cerebrovascular disease. A common ocular cause is **divergence insufficiency,** which tends to develop with increasing age (see Chapters 2 and 4).

Reversible Ischemic Neurologic Deficit

An ischemic stroke characterized by a focal neurologic deficit persisting for more than 24 hours but clearing within 3 weeks is sometimes referred to as a **reversible ischemic neurologic deficit (RIND).** Although the prognosis for subsequent stroke is slightly better than that of TIA, the management of TIA, RIND, and minor cerebral infarction is similar (see Appendix J-2).

Ischemic Stroke

When the hemodynamic disturbance resulting in stroke stabilizes, the stage of completed stroke occurs. Patients with completed ischemic stroke show no further deterioration or fluctuation of their focal neurologic deficit. Sometimes an apparently stable ischemic stroke may change abruptly (stuttering) or may progress within hours or during a few days and result in progressive ischemic stroke requiring appropriate treatment and having a different prognosis.

Progressive Ischemic Stroke

Progressive ischemic stroke refers to a neurologic deficit that progresses or fluctuates and occurs in about 20% of patients with infarction in the distribution of the carotid system and in about 40% with infarction in the vertebrobasilar distribution. The progression may last as long as 24 to 48 hours with infarction of the carotid system and as long as 96 hours with infarction of the vertebrobasilar system. It is critical that the physician attempt to identify the underlying mechanism responsible for the progression. In doing so, one must consider not only the possible ischemic mechanisms that may be responsible but also other disorders that may mimic this clinical picture.

In the area of cerebral infarction, vessels in the marginally ischemic zone are maximally vasodilated, and blood flow in this region depends mainly on the patient's systemic blood pressure. Some progression of the neurologic deficit as a result of widening of the marginally ischemic zone associated with a cerebral infarction may be attributed to a decrease in systemic blood pressure. In some cases, the infarction becomes hemorrhagic and the patient has a concomitant worsening deficit. Secondary hemorrhage into infarction is more frequent in large embolic infarction, especially when the infarction is treated with anticoagulants. Gradual neurologic deterioration a few hours to 2 weeks after an arterial occlusion is a common clinical feature; the diagnosis is established by CT or MRI.

Other patients have deterioration because of cerebral edema associated with the area of cerebral infarction. Edema, which may continue to increase 3 to 5 days after the event, should be suspected in a patient who has a large hemispheric infarction with alteration of consciousness and progressive deterioration. Patients with progressing infarction have propagation of an intra-arterial thrombus or subsequent additional embolization from a proximal source with associated failure of collateral circulation and a decrease in the blood supply to the ischemic area. In contrast to patients with cerebral edema, many of these patients have sudden, stepwise increases in neurologic deficits.

Some patients who have a progressive neurologic course that may initially appear to be related to cerebral infarction have other types of intracranial pathologic processes causing their symptoms. Such processes include intracerebral hemorrhage, subdural hematoma, neoplasms (particularly malignant gliomas and metastatic tumors), infectious or inflammatory processes (such as encephalitis, brain abscess, and demyelinating disease), and superimposed metabolic encephalopathies.

Suggested Reading for Part II

Bogousslavsky J, Regli F: Unilateral watershed cerebral infarcts. Neurology 36:373–377, 1986.

Bruno A: Ischemic stroke. Part 1: Early, accurate diagnosis. Geriatrics 48:26–28, 31–34, 1993.

Caplan L: Intracerebral hemorrhage revisited. Neurology 38:624–627, 1988.

Caplan LR, Pessin MS, Mohr JP: Vertebrobasilar occlusive disease. In: Barnett HJM, Mohr JP, Stein BM, et al, eds. Stroke: Pathophysiology, Diagnosis, and Management (2nd ed). New York: Churchill Livingstone, 1992, pp 443–515.

Celani MG, Righetti E, Migliacci R, et al: Comparability and validity of two clinical scores in the early differential diagnosis of acute stroke. BMJ 308:1674–1676, 1994.

Davidson E, Rotenbeg Z, Fuchs J, et al: Transient ischemic attack-related syncope. Clin Cardiol 14:141–144, 1991.

Falke P, Jerntorp P, Pessah-Rasmussen H: Differences in cardiac disease prevalence and in blood variables between major and minor stroke patients. Int Angiol 12:5–8, 1993.

Franke CL, van Swieten JC, van Gijn J: Residual lesions on computed tomography after intracerebral hemorrhage. Stroke 22:1530–1533, 1991.

Hart RG, Easton JD: Hemorrhagic infarcts. Stroke 17:586–589, 1986.

Kase CS: Diagnosis and management of intracerebral hemorrhage in elderly patients. Clin Geriatr Med 7:549–567, 1991.

Kelley RE, Berger JR: TIA and minor stroke: How to identify and treat patients at risk for recurrent cerebral ischemia. Postgrad Med 91:197–202, 211, 1992.

Koudstaal PJ, Algra A, Pop GA, et al: Risk of cardiac events in atypical transient ischaemic attack or minor stroke: The Dutch TIA Study Group. Lancet 340:630–633, 1992.

Koudstaal PJ, van Gijn J, Frenken CW, et al: TIA, RIND, minor stroke: A continuum, or different subgroups; Dutch TIA Study Group. J Neurol Neurosurg Psychiatry 55:95–97, 1992.

Lindsay KW, Bone I, Callander R: Neurology and Neurosurgery Illustrated (2nd ed). Edinburgh: Churchill Livingstone, 1991.

Mazagri R, Shuaib A, Denath F, et al: Very brief transient ischemic attack. South Med J 87:87–88, 1994.

National Institute of Neurological Disorders and Stroke: Classification of cerebrovascular diseases III. Stroke 21:637–676, 1990.

Norrving B, Cronqvist S: Clinical and radiologic features of lacunar versus nonlacunar minor stroke. Stroke 20:59–64, 1989.

van Swieten JC, Kappelle LJ, Algra A, et al: Hypodensity of the cerebral white matter in patients with transient ischemic attack or minor stroke: influence on the rate of subsequent stroke: Dutch TIA Trial Study Group. Ann Neurol 32:177–183, 1992.

Wain RA, Tuhrim S, D'Autrechy L, et al: The design and automated testing of an expert system for the differential diagnosis of acute stroke. Proc Annu Symp Comput Appl Med Care pp 94–98, 1991.

Whisnant JP, ed: Stroke: Populations, Cohorts, and Clinical Trials. Boston: Butterworth-Heinemann, 1993.

Wiebers DO, Whisnant JP, O'Fallon WM: Reversible ischemic neurologic deficit (RIND) in a community: Rochester, Minnesota, 1955–1974. Neurology 32:459–465, 1982.

Yasaka M, Yamaguchi T, Oita J, et al: Clinical features of recurrent embolization in acute cardioembolic stroke. Stroke 24:1681–1685, 1993.

Management Before Determination of the Mechanism of Cerebrovascular Disease

Telephone Interview and Triage

Although both the diagnostic evaluation and the initial care of many patients with acute cerebrovascular diseases are accomplished in the hospital, outpatient evaluation and treatment are provided for an increasing number of patients with cerebrovascular conditions. Outpatient management involves the efficient evaluation and treatment of underlying disease, the selection of appropriate therapy to lessen the risk of recurrence, and the treatment of physical or psychosocial complications of the disease. Many patients with transient ischemic attack (TIA), recent-onset mild-to-moderate symptoms from ischemic or hemorrhagic stroke, or even subarachnoid hemorrhage may initially present in an ambulatory setting. A patient with a probable acute cerebrovascular event needs prompt and efficient evaluation to decide whether immediate hospitalization is indicated and, if not, to plan appropriate outpatient evaluation and treatment.

Indications for Outpatient Management

In general, outpatient evaluation may be considered for the following patients with cerebrovascular diseases: (1) patients with fewer than 5 TIAs within 2 weeks of presentation, if the TIAs are unassociated with a probable cardioembolic source, if there is no evidence of a high-grade arterial stenosis as the probable cause, if there is no evidence of increasingly severe or frequent events, and if the deficit associated with the event(s) was mild; (2) those who have had TIA, reversible ischemic neurologic deficit, or cerebral infarctions more than 2 weeks before presentation; (3) those who have had recent ischemic cerebrovascular events that presented with transient monocular blindness alone; (4) those who have had a probable hemorrhagic stroke more than 30 days before presentation; (5) those who have chronic cerebrovascular disease, such as asymptomatic carotid or vertebral artery stenosis, asymptomatic and unruptured intracranial aneurysms or arteriovenous malformations, vascular dementia, and Binswanger's encephalopathy; and (6) those who refuse to be hospitalized. However, if symptoms of an acute cerebrovascular event recur during the period of diagnostic evaluation or treatment, immediate hospitalization is strongly recommended (the patient and family are requested to report any new symptoms immediately to the physician).

Telephone Evaluation and Triage

Although interviewing the patient by telephone is less optimal diagnostically than an in-person interview and examination, several circumstances call for at least some kind of preliminary judgment by the physician about the patient's condition. A growing number of physicians are being called on to make a triage decision about patients with possible cerebrovascular disorders on the basis of telephone interviews. An algorithm for the evaluation of a patient by telephone is depicted in Appendix J-1.

Patients should be instructed to call the physician if any of the following warning signs of acute cerebrovascular disease develop, especially if they occur as well-defined, acute-onset spells involving one or more of the following: (1) loss of strength (or development of clumsiness) in some part of the body, especially on one side, including the face, arm, or leg; (2) numbness (sensory loss) or other unusual sensations in some part of the body, especially if on one side; (3) unexplained visual disturbances; (4) inability to speak properly or to understand language; (5) unsteadiness or falling; (6) any other kind of transient spells (vertigo, dizziness, swallowing difficulties, or memory disturbances); (7) headache that is unusually severe, abrupt in onset, or of unusual character; and (8) convulsions or other unexplained alterations of consciousness.

If the physician is to make the right decision about sending an ambulance or instructing the patient to come to the office or hospital, the patient must be interviewed in a step-by-step manner to facilitate answering **two fundamental questions:** (1) Is the problem vascular? (2) If so, is the situation an emergency?

The answer to the first question is based primarily on the **temporal profile of the onset of the presenting symptoms and their character.** The physician should elicit a detailed description of the presenting complaint, including the course of the illness and how it developed. Time and mode of onset, character and severity of the symptoms, and whether any progression or improvement has occurred require clarification.

The rapid onset and evolution of focal neurologic symptoms are characteristic of most types of acute cerebrovascular disorders, although some disorders such as subarachnoid hemorrhage or mass effect from bilateral subdural hematoma may create generalized disturbances of neurologic function, regardless of the total duration or severity of the symptoms. Because of the acute onset, most patients with cerebrovascular events can recall accurately the actual time of onset of their symptoms and what activity they were engaged in at the time.

Some strokes (especially ischemic strokes) occur during sleep, and patients may recognize their new-onset focal neurologic dysfunction when they awaken. Unilateral monoparesis or hemiparesis with or without associated ipsilateral or contralateral numbness or sensory loss is characteristic of motor or sensory disorders caused by acute cerebrovascular disease.

However, one of the most dramatic acute cerebrovascular diseases, subarachnoid hemorrhage, may present with headache alone, without focal neurologic dysfunction or other associated symptoms. In this situation, it is critically important to obtain a **detailed history of the headache** to distinguish **subarachnoid hemorrhage** from other causes such as **migraine** (usually starts in childhood or early adulthood, with unilateral throbbing headache, often with nausea, vomiting, and photophobia), **temporal arteritis** (commonly occurs in elderly patients and is associated with an enlarged, painful, tender temporal artery and pain in the jaw during chewing), **cluster**

headache (usually unilateral, retro-orbital, searing pain, typically accompanied by unilateral lacrimation and nasal or conjunctival congestion), **muscle-contraction headache** (usually steady, deep, and generalized and associated with soreness of neck muscles), **brain tumor** (usually slowly progressive in frequency and severity and headache tends to occur when the person awakens in the morning), **meningitis or encephalitis** (usually generalized and associated with fever and meningismus), **subdural hematoma** (history of recent head trauma), and **ocular disease** (see Chapter 2).

Sudden severe headache commonly described by the patient as "like being hit over the head by a hammer" or "the worst headache of my life" with no apparent cause is strongly suggestive of **subarachnoid hemorrhage.** This type of headache is often accompanied by vomiting, stiff neck, or transient loss of consciousness. However, up to 30% of all subarachnoid hemorrhages may be atypical, and a small subarachnoid hemorrhage, especially in older persons, may not necessarily present with very severe headache or a catastrophic onset. In these cases, the element of abruptness in the new-onset headache suggests the diagnosis.

As outlined previously, it is important to distinguish **TIA,** defined as a temporary episode of focal ischemic neurologic deficit that completely resolves within 24 hours, from an episode of generalized cerebral ischemia **(syncope)** and from spells such as **seizures** and **migraine,** both of which may appear as episodes of transient focal neurologic dysfunction. The temporal profile of focal **seizures** generally involves progression and evolution within a few minutes (approximately 2–3 minutes), whereas the focal deficit that sometimes occurs with **migraine** usually builds or moves during 15 to 20 minutes before subsiding and often is associated with localized headache that normally occurs after the focal neurologic deficit. Another distinguishing characteristic of vascular spells is that they tend to produce negative phenomena (that is, weakness, difficulty in speaking or comprehending, or visual or sensory loss), but focal seizures tend to produce positive phenomena (tonic-clonic movements, tingling, visual hallucinations or scintillating scotomata); migraine may produce either (more commonly, positive phenomena).

Other symptoms of particular importance for differentiating cerebrovascular disorders from other types of illness are reviewed in Chapter 2.

Any pertinent **medical history** (general health before the onset of the current illness, operations, or injuries) and **family history** should be ascertained as needed. A recent history of head injury, even if minor, should raise the possibility of subdural or epidural hematoma. Patients with acute cerebrovascular disease may have a history of stroke or TIA, carotid artery stenosis, heart disease, hypertension, hematologic disorder, tobacco use, high cholesterol level, or use of illicit drugs and a family history of stroke.

Having determined that the problem is vascular, the physician must next decide whether to send an ambulance, have the patient report to the emergency room or hospital admission desk, or instruct the patient to come to the office for medical consultation and outpatient management. Patients with sudden weakness or clumsiness; numbness of the face, arm, and leg on one side of the body; sudden decrease or loss of vision (particularly in one eye) or double vision with other symptoms of potential posterior circulation ischemia (not diplopia alone); loss of speech or difficulty talking or understanding written or spoken language; sudden, severe headache with no apparent cause; sudden unexplained dizziness (not unsteadiness alone), or vertigo in combination with other brain stem symptoms; or sudden ataxia (especially associated with any of the symptoms noted above) within the 2 weeks before presentation probably have acute cerebrovascular disease and should be referred to the hospital immediately for initial evaluation and consideration of hospitalization (see Appendix J-1). If the deficit associated with the event is marked, associated with a decrease in the level of consciousness, seizure, or respiratory or circulatory insufficiency, an ambulance should be sent. Sending an ambulance is also advised for cases associated with worsening or fluctuating neurologic deficits, traumatic cerebrovascular disorders (for instance, subdural or epidural hematoma), and other suspected urgent noncerebrovascular neurologic disorders such as meningitis or encephalitis. In other cases, the patient may be instructed to come to the office.

Management of Acute
Stroke in Critically Ill Patients

While efforts are under way to determine the mechanism of acute cerebrovascular disease, the patient should be given supportive care to maintain general medical status. Particular attention should be directed to monitoring fluid intake and output and serum and urine electrolyte levels to ensure proper fluid balance. Constant observation in a neurologic intensive care unit (NICU) with monitoring of vital signs is advised for the first few days after large or progressive cerebral infarction and most intracerebral hemorrhages and subarachnoid hemorrhages (a NICU evaluation form is shown in Appendix D). In the absence of a NICU, admission to a medical intensive care unit is recommended.

The initial physical examination should include general and neurologic (including neurovascular) examinations (see Chapters 4–6). Cardiac monitoring and observations every 4 hours with recording of vital signs (level of consciousness, blood pressure, pulse, temperature, respiration), pupillary size and reaction, and limb movements are recommended during at least the first few days after onset of an uncomplicated, acute, persistent cerebrovascular event, but half-hourly clinical observations and monitoring of blood gases and intracranial pressure may be necessary for patients with severe stroke, especially those with impaired consciousness. Computed tomography should be performed as an emergency procedure for all critically ill patients with probable acute cerebrovascular disorders.

Immediate therapeutic measures for all comatose patients include establishing a good airway and insertion of a large-bore intravenous catheter to draw blood for studies and to maintain fluid and electrolyte balance. As noted in Chapter 6, for patients in whom the cause of coma is not readily known, naloxone, 0.4 mg intravenously, should be given with thiamine, 100 mg intravenously, followed by administration of 25 to 50 ml of 50% dextrose in water. Fluid administration should be kept to a minimum (usually 1000 ml normal saline/m^2 body surface area/day), unless the patient is hypotensive. If benzodiazepine overuse is suspected, flumazenil may be administered.

Airway Management

Maintenance of a patent airway is the first priority in the care of an unconscious patient or any alert patient with respiratory problems such as shallow and irregular respirations or labored breathing. The most common causes of airway obstruction are posterior displacement of oropharyngeal soft tissue structures, nasopharyngeal vomitus, and secretions. The airway should be suctioned as necessary, with the patient placed in a lateral position to prevent airway obstruction (an oropharyngeal or nasal airway may also be useful). These measures are helpful for preventing atelectasis and bronchopneumonia. Supplemental oxygen (2 to 4 liter/minute by nasal cannula) should be provided, especially in the presence of decreased blood oxygen levels (arterial O_2 tension < 90 mm Hg, O_2 saturation < 95%).

Endotracheal intubation or assisted respiration is rarely indicated for patients with stroke but should be considered in circumstances of obvious apnea, labored respiration, and likely aspiration. Endotracheal intubation and hyperventilation may also be considered for selected patients with increased intracranial pressure either alone or with other appropriate therapy for cerebral edema.

Management of Systemic Cardiovascular Disorders

Treatment of general circulatory problems includes control of arrhythmias, restoration of cardiac output, and treatment of acute shock or hypovolemia. Hypotension is rarely a problem in stroke or transient ischemic attack, except when there is coincident myocardial infarction, sepsis, or dehydration. To maintain normotension in these situations, plasma, low-molecular-weight dextran, or normal saline also may be administered. Volume expanders that contain an excessive amount of free water (such as D_5W) should be avoided. In patients with low blood pressure unresponsive to gentle volume expansion, sympathomimetic drugs (such as epinephrine) can be administered subcutaneously or intramuscularly to increase the systemic blood pressure and increase cerebral perfusion. In cases of myocardial infarction with vascular collapse, intravenously administered vasopressors are usually advised, with titration of the rate of infusion to maintain a stable, desired blood pressure. If clinical heart failure is present, immediate treatment with inotropic agents (such as dobutamine) is indicated.

In patients with type I or type II coma (see Chapter 6), arterial blood pressure usually is increased initially, but blood pressure is commonly decreased in patients with type III coma or in those who are in the terminal stages of type I or type II coma. Medical treatment of transient hypertension resulting from increased intracranial pressure associated with acute cerebrovascular disease (Cushing's reflex) is not usually required.

Persistent hypertension resulting from increased intracranial pressure requires lowering of the intracranial pressure rather than antihypertensive medication. However, in patients with acute ischemic stroke whose diastolic blood pressure is more than 140 mm Hg on two separate readings obtained 5 minutes or more apart, emergency antihypertensive therapy is usually started with a constant intravenous infusion of sodium nitroprusside (0.3–0.5 µg/kg/minute), which can then be titrated to the desired effect. The usual dose is 1 to 3 µg/kg/minute and should not exceed 10 µg/kg/minute. A gentle, carefully monitored reduction of blood pressure is also recommended for patients within 48 hours of onset of ischemic stroke and who have blood pressures of 230 mm Hg or more systolic or 121 to 140 mm Hg diastolic on two separate readings obtained 30 minutes or more apart or associated with documented intracerebral hemorrhage, acute myocardial infarction, left ventricular failure, renal failure due to accelerated hypertension, or dissection of the thoracic aorta. Reduction can be accomplished with intravenous agents such as labetalol, either in a constant infusion (2 mg/minute) or in an initial dosage of 10 to 20 mg intravenously during 1 to 2 minutes, repeated or doubled every 10 to 20 minutes until the desired blood pressure is achieved or until a cumulative dose of 300 mg is reached. If a satisfactory response is not obtained, sodium nitroprusside infusion should be considered.

Target blood pressures differ on the basis of the patient's history. In patients with no history of hypertension, the initial goal is usually from 160 to 170/95 to 100 mm Hg, whereas in those with a history of hypertension, an early goal of 170 to 180/100 to 110 mm Hg is more appropriate. Persistent (≥12 hours), milder levels (>180–230/105–120 mm Hg) of hypertension may be treated with intravenous labetalol (as outlined above) or oral agents, including labetalol and other beta-adrenergic blockers, angiotensin-converting enzyme inhibitors, or calcium channel blockers. Sublingual agents should be avoided, because the response is somewhat unpredictable and may lead to a precipitous decline in blood pressure.

Management of Increased Intracranial Pressure

Increased intracranial pressure often complicates moderate-sized to large intracerebral hemorrhages and large cerebral infarcts. Although associated edema tends to develop more rapidly with hemorrhage, edema related to infarction may also be fatal in the first 24 to 48 hours and often progresses during the first 3 to 7 days after infarction.

The generally recommended treatment for increased intracranial pressure caused by ischemic or hemorrhagic stroke includes osmotherapy, renal-loop diuretics, hyperventilation, glucocorticoids, hemicraniectomy and decompression, and ventricular drainage (Table 11-1). If repeated doses of hyperosmolar or other diuretic agents are provided, serum osmolality should be monitored as a guide to therapy (serum osmolality should be maintained in the 300 to 320 mOsm/liter range; acute elevation of the serum osmolality of more than 20 mOsm above the patient's usual level may result in an encephalopathy and should be avoided). However, the stable patient who remains awake and alert requires no antiedema therapy.

In patients with **cerebral infarction** and signs of increased intracranial pressure, such as a decreased level of consciousness, loss of spontaneous venous pulsations on ophthalmoscopic examination, or clinical features of herniation (pupillary enlargement ipsilateral to the infarcted hemisphere or pathologic corticospinal signs contralateral or ipsilateral to the hemispheric lesion), measures to control the edema should be initiated (see Table 11-1). Options include osmotic diuresis with hyperosmolar agents such as glycerol (administered orally, 10% solution in 0.4% normal saline at a dosage of 0.25–1 g/kg every 4–6 hours), 20% mannitol (administered intravenously at a dosage of 1 g/kg during a 30-minute period initially and then 0.25–0.5 g/kg every 2–6 hours, depending on the patient's intra-

Table 11-1. Options in management of cerebral edema and increased intracranial pressure

General measures
Elevate head of bed
Minimize stimulation

Fluids
Minimize free water (do not use D_5W)
Relative fluid restriction to 1000 ml/m² body surface area/day

Medical agent	Onset of action	Duration	Comments
Hyperventilation to P_{CO_2} 25–35 mm Hg	Immediate	24 hr	Monitor serum osmolarity (maintain 300–320 mOsm/liter), electrolytes, blood urea nitrogen
Hyperosmolar agents			
Mannitol, 20% solution, 1 g/kg IV during 5–30 min; repeat 0.25–0.5 g/kg every 2–6 hr*	30 min	Dose: hours Overall: 24–48 hr	Less potential for "rebound" increase in intracranial pressure at end of duration of action than with mannitol
Glycerol, 10% solution, 0.25–1 g/kg PO every 4–6 hr*	8–12 hr	Dose: hours Overall: 24–48 hr	
Steroids			
Dexamethasone, 10 mg IV, then 4 mg IV, every 6 hr	4–6 hr	Days	Works better for vasogenic edema (brain tumor) than for cytotoxic edema (ischemic stroke)

Surgery: See text
Barbiturate coma: In severe, life-threatening, increased intracranial pressure unresponsive to other treatment, barbiturate coma may be used. Intracranial pressure monitoring is typically used.

*Diuretics such as furosemide may be given with hyperosmolar agents, particularly if congestive heart failure is occurring as a side effect.

cranial pressure, cerebral perfusion pressure, serum osmolarity, and clinical findings), and free water restriction. Replacement fluids should be administered with attention to maintaining serum osmolality in the range of 300 to 320 mOsm/liter; hypotonic and glucose-containing solutions should be avoided. A combination of osmotic agents and renal-loop diuretics such as furosemide (20–80 mg every 4–12 hours intravenously) or ethacrynic acid can reduce intracranial pressure in some patients when osmotic diuretics alone are inadequate or produce dangerous side effects (especially in patients with congestive heart failure). In addition, hyperventilation may be considered for patients whose condition is deteriorating as a result of increased intracranial pressure, including those with herniation syndromes. If clinical or radiographic deterioration continues in patients with large hemispheric infarction, hemicraniectomy and decompression may be lifesaving and should be considered for selected patients.

In patients with **intracerebral hemorrhage** and an altered level of consciousness or evidence of herniation, intracranial pressure should be lowered emergently with intubation and mechanical hyperventilation, maintaining the Pco_2 at 25 to 30 mm Hg. Glycerol or mannitol (in the dosages discussed above) may also be used until emergency neurosurgical consultation is available. Dexamethasone, administered intravenously or intramuscularly in an initial bolus of 10 mg followed by 4 mg every 4 to 6 hours, has a more prolonged action but usually does not provide significant benefit during the initial 4 to 6 hours after administration. The benefit is greater in vasogenic edema, such as that associated with brain tumor, than with cytotoxic edema, which is the predominant edema subtype associated with cerebral infarction.

Cerebellar hemorrhage (or infarction) with any evidence of brain stem compression constitutes a neurosurgical emergency. Immediate neurosurgical consultation should be obtained and rapid consideration should be given to decompression, the alternative to which is often precipitous death.

In patients with **subarachnoid hemorrhage,** increased intracranial pressure is often caused by hydrocephalus and is typically treated by external ventricular drainage, with gradual pressure reduction. Other patients may have increased intracranial pressure without hydrocephalus as a result of diffuse cerebral edema. In this subgroup, pressure reduction may be achieved by administration of dexamethasone, glycerol, or mannitol (as discussed above) or by external ventricular drainage.

Nursing Care

Patients with impaired consciousness require special attention to nutritional status, bowel and bladder function, and care of the skin, eyes, and mouth.

In comatose patients or in patients with swallowing problems, nutrition may be provided initially by intravenous solutions, but feeding by a nasogastric tube should be considered when the patient is neurologically stable. A diet of 1300 to 1400 calories/day with vitamin supplements or liquid feeding systems (Ensure or Osmolite) by constant drip at a rate of 75 to 100 ml/hour (1–1.5 calories/ml) or bolus feedings may be used. Fluid replacement should be 2 liters/day; urine output should be monitored closely for balance with intake, and, in general, should be at least 500 to 1000 ml/day. If the patient is alert and able to swallow, oral feeding should be started with a liquid diet, followed by mechanical soft, bland, and regular diets. (Full liquid and soft diets may be easier to swallow without aspiration than clear liquids for patients with various degrees of dysphagia.) Percutaneous gastrostomy feeding should be considered after 1 to 2 weeks in patients with a poor prognosis for regaining an adequate and safe swallowing mechanism.

To soften stool and to prevent straining with bowel movements, stool softeners such as docusate sodium, 100 mg orally twice daily, or laxatives may be used, especially in patients with subarachnoid hemorrhage. An indwelling catheter should not be used in patients who are awake and able to cooperate with a voluntary voiding program. In comatose patients, the bladder should be emptied at regular intervals of every 4 to 6 hours by catheterization. If the patient is unconscious for more than 48 hours, an indwelling Foley catheter may be required to monitor the patient's urine output, but this method is associated with higher risk of urinary bacterial colonization and infection.

Comatose patients should be turned in bed every 1 to 2 hours on an air mattress with tightly drawn sheets and sponge padding of body prominences to prevent pressure neuropathy and decubitus ulcers. Deep vein thromboses may be prevented by using subcutaneously administered heparin (5000 U twice daily), antiembolism stockings, or intermittent pneumatic compression devices. The patient's skin should be kept dry and powdered, with daily inspections over pressure points for erythema or ulcers. Ophthalmic ointments, methylcellulose eyedrops, and eye patching help to prevent corneal ulceration and abrasion.

12

Transient Ischemic Attack and Minor Cerebral Infarction: General Evaluation and Treatment

A **transient ischemic attack** (TIA) is defined as an episode of loss of brain function caused by cerebral ischemia localized to a limited region of the brain, with symptoms lasting less than 24 hours. **Minor cerebral infarction** (MCI) may be defined as a persistent loss of brain function attributed to brain ischemia, again localized to a limited region of the brain. The residual deficit is nondisabling; affected persons are able to perform most of their usual activities and can ambulate without assistance. In a **reversible ischemic neurologic deficit** (RIND), the loss of function caused by focal brain ischemia resolves between 24 hours and 3 weeks. In general, for patients presenting with a TIA, RIND, or MCI, treatment may be initiated before determination of a definitive mechanism. The physician must choose from various therapeutic options while carefully considering the risk-benefit ratio as it applies to the specific circumstances involved. A systematic evaluation should then be undertaken to determine the specific mechanism for the cerebrovascular event(s) (see Appendix J-2).

Should a Patient Be Hospitalized?

Although in years past most patients with TIA or minor stroke were hospitalized, not all patients with TIA or minor stroke require inpatient evaluation. For patients with TIA, RIND, or MCI, hospitalization should be directed toward those at higher risk for early recurrent ischemic events and include those who may have favorable results with short-term anticoagulation with intravenously administered heparin. In general, the following patients usually are the best candidates for **hospitalization:** (1) those with more than four ischemic episodes within the 2 weeks preceding the initial presentation (particularly those without transient monocular blindness in isolation), and (2) those with a probable cardiac source of emboli (Tables 12-1 and 12-2), including atrial fibrillation, mechanical valve, dilated cardiomyopathy, known intracardiac thrombus, or recent myocardial infarction. In patients with fewer than five TIAs, the most recent of which occurred within 2 weeks before presentation, the issue of hospitalization is less clear. However, in general, if the deficit associated with the event was marked, if the events are increasing in frequency, severity, or duration, or if there are other factors that suggest a high risk for further events, including a carotid bruit ipsilateral to probable carotid symptoms, a patient is often hospitalized for assessment. For patients with TIA that occurred more than 2 weeks before the current assessment or with symptoms involving only transient monocular blindness, an expedited outpatient workup may be indicated. Specific clinical syndromes, including stroke in the young,

Table 12-1.   Proven cardiac risks for
transient ischemic attack or minor stroke

Atrial fibrillation
Mechanical valve
Dilated cardiomyopathy
Recent myocardial infarction
Intracardiac thrombus

Table 12-2.   Putative cardiac risks for
transient ischemic attack or minor stroke

Sick sinus syndrome
Patent foramen ovale
Atherosclerotic debris in thoracic aorta
Spontaneous echocardiographic contrast
Myocardial infarction 2–6 mo earlier
Hypokinetic or akinetic left ventricular segment
Calcification of mitral annulus

probable symptomatic carotid dissection, hypercoagulable state, inflammatory vasculopathies, stroke associated with illicit drug use, and cerebral venous thrombosis, usually lead to evaluation and treatment that is appropriate for the specific clinical entity.

In patients selected for hospitalization, consideration of short-term intravenous infusion of heparin is warranted. The rationale for use in this situation is based on theoretical and pharmacologic data, although there is evidence that patients with a cardiac source of emboli may benefit from heparin. The other clinical scenarios appropriate for hospitalization, including recurrent TIAs in the setting of a probable high-grade stenosis or crescendo TIAs, have not been subjected to a controlled trial of short-term heparin anticoagulation.

Heparin

Heparin, a heterogeneous mixture of sulfate and mucopolysaccharides, activates antithrombin III and inhibits regulation factors II, IX, X, XI, and XII. It also blocks the conversion of fibrinogen to fibrin, exerts both proplatelet and antiplatelet aggregation actions, and accelerates fibrinolysis and inactivates thrombin through heparin cofactor II. Intravenous infusion of heparin in appropriate patients with TIA or MCI may be initiated with a bolus of 5000 U followed by constant infusion of 800 to 1000 U/hour. The anticoagulant effect of heparin is immediate and can be quantified from measurements of activated partial thromboplastin time. The therapeutic range is typically 1.5 to 2 times the normal control value. The patient's activated partial thromboplastin time should be monitored every 6 hours until the therapeutic value has been documented and then daily during the time of infusion.

Hemorrhagic complications are the most frequent side effects of heparin therapy. These complications are related to the dose and duration of heparin therapy. They may be more common in patients with high systemic blood pressure, but this association has not been well documented. The frequency of intracerebral hemorrhage in patients who have had ischemic stroke is between 1% and 7%, but the risk is higher in patients with large ischemic stroke than in patients with TIA, RIND, or MCI.

Another complication associated with heparin involves heparin-induced **thrombocytopenia.** This complication is usually mild and transient (related to increased platelet aggregation), but it may be more serious in 1% to 2% of patients. The more serious form is related to an immunoglobulin G and immunoglobulin M (IgG- and IgM)-induced immune response that can be associated with "paradoxical" arterial occlusions, typically after 4 to 6 days of heparin treatment. For this reason, platelet counts should be determined every 2 days during heparin treatment. If heparin-induced thrombocytopenia develops and continued short-term parenteral anticoagulation is required, treatment sometimes includes low-molecular-weight heparins or heparinoids, which have less propensity for inducing thrombocytopenia than the usual unfractionated heparin. The **low-molecular-weight heparinoids** exert their anticoagulation effect in a more selective pattern, affecting almost exclusively the intrinsic clotting pathway and having little effect on platelets and thrombin.

Because of the potential risks with intravenous heparin therapy and because the reasons for use of heparin soon after TIA, RIND, or MCI are theoretical, with limited supporting scientific data, the use of heparin for patients with TIA, RIND, or MCI is typically restricted to those who meet the criteria for hospitalization as outlined above.

Initial Assessment

The initial evaluation in an inpatient setting is relatively similar to that in an expedited outpatient setting. Computed tomography (CT) of the head without contrast should be performed to quickly distinguish nonhemorrhagic from hemorrhagic cerebrovascular disease. CT of the head with contrast or magnetic resonance imaging (MRI) of the head may be required if the initial scan indicates a possible arteriovenous malformation, meningioma, or other mass lesion. Other baseline studies include complete blood cell count, activated partial thromboplastin time and prothrombin time, serum chemistry group tests, erythrocyte sedimentation rate, and lipid analyses, including high-density lipoprotein, low-density lipoprotein, and total cholesterol levels. Heparin may be indicated in patients selected for inpatient workup (as noted above), but if contraindications to its use exist, then urgent evaluation without heparin is indicated. In patients selected for expedited outpatient evaluation, unless there is a contraindication to use of antiplatelet agents, one aspirin/day may be initiated during the outpatient evaluation as the mechanism is defined.

Cardiac Evaluation

The patient's baseline medical history and neurologic history should have already been obtained and a neurologic examination performed (Chapters 1–6). A minimal cardiac evaluation includes elicitation of cardiac history (with specific attention to both ischemic symptoms and previous arrhythmias) and cardiac examination including careful auscultation for cardiac murmurs. Minimal laboratory investigations include electrocardiography, rhythm strip, and chest radiography. If one of the proven cardiac risks is identified (see Table 12-1), anticoagulation may be needed for long-term prophylaxis even if another potential mechanism for the TIA, RIND, or MCI is identified. The putative cardiac risks (see Table 12-2) also may require antiplatelet or anticoagulant therapy, but an alternative mechanism must be considered.

The remainder of the evaluation should be guided by the number and character of ischemic events. If a patient has stereotyped spells, which indicate recurrent events in the same vascular distribution, cardioembolic events are relatively less likely, although they are still part of the differential diagnosis. Alternatively, nonstereotyped spells implicating dissimilar symptoms during sequential spells and possible involvement of separate vascular territories lead to a different assessment.

Single Event or Multiple Spells in Same Vascular Distribution

In patients with multiple stereotyped spells or in those with only a single spell and no evidence of previous infarcts of large vessel distribution on CT or MRI, the evaluation should be tailored on the basis of the circulation implicated (Table 12-3).

ANTERIOR CIRCULATION

Clinical symptoms consistent with ischemia of the **carotid** distribution (see Table 12-3) should lead to evaluation of the extracranial carotid artery with carotid ultrasonography or ocular pneumoplethysmography; these tests can detect a high-grade stenosis in the carotid system with a high degree of sensitivity. Magnetic resonance angiography (MRA) is a subtype of MRI that can noninvasively visualize the extracranial and portions of the intracranial circulations. It has limited usefulness as a screening study because of its expense, difficulty in delineating between high-grade vessel stenosis and occlusion, tendency to overestimate the degree of carotid arterial stenosis, and limited usefulness for evaluating the intracranial circulation.

If the results of the noninvasive studies suggest the presence of a high-grade stenosis in a surgically accessible artery appropriate for the distribution of TIA, RIND, or MCI, cerebral arteriography should be considered if the patient is a surgical candidate. If arteriography verifies a high-grade stenosis, **carotid endarterectomy** should be strongly considered if there are no medical contraindications because its benefit has been clearly demonstrated in this

Table 12-3. Clinical symptoms associated with cerebral ischemia

Anterior circulation
    Motor dysfunction of contralateral extremities or face (or both)
        Clumsiness
        Weakness
        Paralysis
        Slurred speech
    Loss of vision in ipsilateral eye
    Homonymous hemianopia
    Aphasia if dominant hemisphere involved
    Sensory deficit of contralateral extremities or face (or both)
        Numbness or loss of sensation
        Paresthesias
Posterior circulation
    Motor dysfunction of any combination of extremities or face (or both)*
        Clumsiness
        Weakness
        Paralysis
    Loss of vision of one or both homonymous visual fields
    Sensory deficit of extremities or face (or both)*
        Numbness or loss of sensation
        Paresthesias
    The following typically occur but are nondiagnostic in isolation:
        Ataxic gait   Diplopia
        Ataxic extremities   Dysphagia
        Vertigo   Dysarthria

*Bilateral or alternating symptoms suggest involvement of the posterior circulation, and bilateral lower extremity symptoms may occur with unilateral carotid supply to both anterior cerebral arteries.

circumstance. If significant medical problems preclude carotid endarterectomy, **warfarin** anticoagulation should be considered. Patients with renal failure or significant allergy to contrast dye may be candidates for confirmation of the stenosis by MRA as a means to preclude the potential risk of cerebral arteriography, followed by endarterectomy. Even when cerebral arteriography is performed by experienced personnel, the associated risk of stroke is 0.5% to 1%.

For patients who are not surgical candidates, short-term (3–6 months) anticoagulation with warfarin followed by aspirin or ticlopidine is considered for those in whom a high-grade stenosis of the extracranial internal carotid artery is detected on noninvasive studies or for those in whom cerebral arteriography fails to reveal a high-grade stenosis at an extracranial site but instead indicates symptomatic stenosis of the distal internal carotid artery siphon or middle cerebral artery stem. Although these are indications that have not been evaluated with a randomized clinical trial, the type of clots that tend to form at sites of high-grade arterial stenosis may be affected favorably by warfarin anticoagulation. Furthermore, in randomized carotid endarterectomy trials, the high rate of stroke in patients assigned to medical therapy with aspirin suggests that antiplatelet treatment with **aspirin** is relatively ineffective in those with high-grade stenosis of the extracranial internal carotid artery. The medical management of cerebral ischemia is reviewed in Table 12-4.

The **coumarin anticoagulants** (warfarin and dicumarol) inhibit the clotting mechanism by interfering with synthesis of vitamin

Table 12-4.   Medical management of cerebral ischemia

Warfarin anticoagulation (INR 2.0–3.0)
   Short-term (3 mo), followed by antiplatelet agent
      Symptomatic low-grade stenosis in anterior or posterior circulation,
         symptoms while taking aspirin (use ticlopidine[a] if contraindication to
         warfarin)
      Symptomatic occlusion of carotid, vertebral, or basilar artery with
         associated thromboembolic symptoms (use warfarin for 4–6 wk)
   Consider longer-term (at least 3 mo) (INR 2.0–3.0)
      Symptomatic high-grade stenosis in intracranial carotid artery, verte-
         brobasilar system, or extracranial carotid artery, if not a surgical
         candidate[b]
      Cardiac source of emboli, level and duration of anticoagulation depend-
         ing on cause
Aspirin (80–1300 mg/day)
   Initial treatment in symptomatic low-grade stenosis in anterior or
      posterior circulation (ticlopidine[a] if intolerant of or allergic to aspirin)
   Initial treatment in symptomatic high-grade stenosis in intracranial
      carotid artery, vertebrobasilar system, or extracranial carotid artery, if
      not a candidate for operation or warfarin
Ticlopidine (250 mg twice a day)[a]
   Recurrent symptoms with aspirin, no mechanism detected that may be
      better treated with warfarin (such as high-grade arterial stenosis[b] or
      cardiac source of emboli)
   Recurrent symptoms with aspirin, contraindication to warfarin, in setting
      of high-grade arterial stenosis (nonsurgical candidate in anterior
      circulation ischemia)
   Initial treatment in selected patients with transient ischemic attack or
      minor stroke (nonsurgical candidate in anterior circulation ischemia)
   Allergic or sensitive to aspirin, requiring antiplatelet therapy

---

INR = International Normalized Ratio.
[a]Monitor complete blood cell counts every 2 wk for 3 mo.
[b]The use of warfarin as an initial agent in this setting is controversial. One may initiate therapy with aspirin or ticlopidine and reserve warfarin for recurrent symptoms while receiving an antiplatelet agent.

K-dependent factors II, VII, IX, and X. In addition, the coumarins also deplete protein C and protein S, two indigenous anticoagulant proteins. The half-life of the inhibited clotting factors ranges from approximately 6 to 60 hours, which produces a 1- to 3-day delay between peak plasma concentration and maximal effect.

Although in the past the usual therapeutic range of oral anticoagulation has been based on prothrombin time ratios, the intensity of coumarin anticoagulation is best measured by the **International Normalized Ratio (INR).** The INR is calculated by using the International Sensitivity Index (ISI) of the thromboplastin reagins, which are now supplied by most manufacturers, allowing calculation of an instrument-specific INR value for individual plasma samples. The formula for calculating the INR is

$$INR = (\text{prothrombin time ratio})^{ISI}$$

Both warfarin and dicumarol are usually given once daily. The starting dosage varies according to size, age, and hepatic status of the patient as well as the urgency of the situation. In an average-sized adult with normal liver function, a starting dosage of 10 mg/

Table 12-5. Intensity level of anticoagulation for major disease categories

Indication	PT ratio	INR
Atrial fibrillation	1.3–1.5	2–3
Ischemic heart disease	1.3–1.5	2–3
Craniocervical atherosclerotic disease	1.3–1.5	2–3
Myoprosthetic valve	1.3–1.5	2–3
Deep vein thrombosis	1.3–3.5	2–3
Valvular heart disease	1.3–1.5	2–3
Dilated cardiomyopathy	1.3–1.5	2–3
Recent myocardial infarction	1.3–1.5	2–3
Intracardiac thrombus	1.4–1.7	2.5–3.5
Mechanical heart valve	1.5–2.0	3.0–4.5
Recurrent cardiac embolus	1.5–2.0	3.0–4.5

INR = International Normalized Ratio; PT = prothrombin time; ratio of therapeutic PT to control PT.

day is often used for 2 days, followed by a 5-mg dosage, although the dosage after the first day should be tailored on the basis of prothrombin time or INR response, which is typically minimal, if any, after the first day of therapy. In outpatients, a dosage of 5 mg/day may be used from the onset, with daily monitoring of the INR and appropriate adjustment of the warfarin dose until the INR is stable in the therapeutic range.

The **usual therapeutic range** for oral anticoagulation is an INR between 2.0 and 3.0. Higher intensity anticoagulation (such as that for mechanical heart valves) usually involves keeping the INR between 3.0 and 4.5 (Table 12-5). This INR level is typically checked in the morning, and the warfarin or dicumarol is taken in the evening. Dose levels are estimated, based on the assumption of an approximate 2-day delay until maximal effect on the INR or prothrombin time from a given dosage and little or no effect within the first 24 hours.

When therapy is switched to oral anticoagulation in the setting of intravenous heparin use, the optimal timing for cessation of heparin is controversial. However, most experts advise that heparin should be used for at least 4 to 5 days after initiation of warfarin therapy or until the INR becomes therapeutic. The reason for the minimal delay of 4 to 5 days is that warfarin inhibits production of new clotting factors but does not eliminate clotting factors that are already present. The most important clotting factor for determining in vivo clotting is prothrombin, which has a half-life of approximately 2 days. It is necessary to go through at least 2 to 2.5 half-lives to reduce the existing level of prothrombin to an acceptable level of 25% to 35% or less.

Bleeding complications of the warfarin anticoagulants are related to the level of anticoagulation. Thus, it is important to check the prothrombin time or INR regularly (usually daily) until the level has stabilized. After stabilization, levels are checked every 2 to 3 days for a week, and eventually as infrequently as every 4 weeks if the patient has reached a maintenance dose and is otherwise stable. It is important to advise the patient not to take vitamin K, because it may greatly interfere with attempts at oral anticoagulation. Long-term anticoagulation has a complication rate from all bleeding episodes between 0.5% and 1% per 12 months. With careful monitoring in a controlled setting, such as in several recent atrial fibrillation trials, the bleeding complication rate is approximately 1.0% to 1.5% annually. In addition to a prothrombin time or INR higher than the therapeutic range, high systolic or diastolic blood pressure and age may be predictive features of an increased risk of hemorrhagic complications.

Antiplatelet therapy includes aspirin and ticlopidine. If abnormal findings on noninvasive arterial studies lead to cerebral angiography that fails to reveal a high-grade stenosis at either an extracranial site or an appropriate intracranial site, or if the initial noninvasive studies disclose no abnormalities, **aspirin** is often considered appropriate initial therapy in patients who have had a TIA or minor stroke. In patients who are to have carotid endarterectomy and are already taking aspirin, it is desirable for them to continue taking it up to and through the surgery unless contraindications exist.

Aspirin irreversibly limits platelet adhesion and aggregation, inhibiting production of cyclooxygenase and thromboxane A_2. Although aspirin has no effect on prothrombin time, partial thromboplastin time, or platelet count, it does prolong bleeding time with an effect that starts in 1 to 2 days and persists for 7 to 10 days.

The risk of nonfatal stroke is decreased by approximately 23% among patients with previous stroke or TIA who are treated with aspirin. The optimal dose of aspirin is controversial; the most common daily dosages range from 80 mg once daily to 650 mg twice daily. **Complications** including gastrointestinal irritation, ulceration, and bleeding are clearly reduced with lower doses, and some theoretical considerations involving differential aspirin effects on prostacyclin (related to prostacyclinol) indicate that lower doses of aspirin could be more efficacious than higher doses. Consequently, a starting dose of 325 mg daily is often recommended. Although no randomized trials have clearly documented any differences in efficacy between low-dose and high-dose aspirin for prevention of stroke, most of the treatment trials confirming a benefit from aspirin have used higher dosages, such as 650 mg twice daily, and some experts believe that these higher dosages should be used routinely unless individual contraindications exist.

Alternatively, therapy with **ticlopidine hydrochloride** could be considered, particularly for patients who are intolerant of or allergic to aspirin. Ticlopidine is an antiplatelet agent that prohibits platelet deposition by suppressing adenosine diphosphate-induced platelet aggregation and aggregation due to various other factors. Like aspirin, it prolongs bleeding time but does not affect platelet count, partial thromboplastin time, or prothrombin time. With the usual dosage of 250 mg twice per day, its effect begins within 1 to 2 days and persists for 7 to 10 days.

Ticlopidine is considerably more expensive than aspirin but also may be slightly more effective than aspirin in preventing future stroke among patients with TIA and ischemic stroke. **Side effects** from ticlopidine include severe neutropenia, which occurs in 0.5% to 1% of patients. This complication almost always occurs within the first 3 months of treatment and usually within the first 4 to 8 weeks. For this reason, patients given ticlopidine should have regular monitoring of complete blood cell counts every 2 weeks, especially during the first 3 months of therapy. Other side effects of ticlopidine include abdominal pain, diarrhea, and rash.

Overall, ticlopidine is usually considered for aspirin-intolerant or aspirin-allergic patients and for those who have recurrent spells during aspirin therapy but did not have an event that may be more appropriately treated with warfarin. Some authors have recommended the use of ticlopidine as a first-line antiplatelet agent, particularly for patients with initial ischemic stroke as opposed to TIA. Other antiplatelet agents including sulfinpyrazone and dipyridamole have not been shown to be effective in preventing stroke.

POSTERIOR CIRCULATION

Vertebrobasilar distribution ischemia often leads to symptoms that are related to brain stem, cerebellar, or occipital lobe dysfunction (see Table 12-3). Further evaluation of the posterior circulation may be performed noninvasively. Transcranial Doppler ultrasonography has a sensitivity of about 75% for detecting hemodynamically significant stenosis in the distal intracranial segments of the vertebral artery or the basilar artery. The sensitivity of MRA is less well-defined but may be similar to that of transcranial Doppler ultrasonography. Should findings with either of these two tests suggest the presence of a stenosis, therapeutic options include empiric warfarin anticoagulation (see pages 148–150) or consideration of arteriography in a selected group of patients. In patients with a **relative** contraindication to warfarin, cerebral arteriography may be performed to define the anatomy of the posterior circulation vasculature and to document the vertebrobasilar occlusive lesion potentially amenable to warfarin anticoagulation, although the risk of arteriographic complications is still 0.5% to 1%.

Again, the use of **warfarin anticoagulation** in this setting is somewhat controversial, although thrombin-dependent clots with fibrin as a primary component forming at low-flow arterial stenoses may be decreased with warfarin anticoagulation. Short-term warfarin anticoagulation is associated with relatively low risk. The optimal duration of warfarin anticoagulation in this setting is not clear. Patients with symptomatic high-grade stenosis in the basilar artery may require prolonged warfarin anticoagulation. In those with lesser grades of stenosis, 3 months of warfarin therapy followed by antiplatelet therapy is reasonable, and in an occlusion of the vertebral or basilar artery with thromboembolic symptoms, a short course of warfarin anticoagulation (4–6 weeks) may be followed by antiplatelet therapy with either aspirin or ticlopidine. If the vertebrobasilar noninvasive studies are normal or if arteriography fails to reveal high-grade stenosis, initial treatment with **antiplatelet therapy** may be indicated if a cardiac source of emboli was considered unlikely based on earlier evaluation.

Evaluation of a Probable
Embolic Event or Multiple Events
in Different Vascular Distributions

In patients without a proven cardiac risk documented on the initial evaluation, certain clinical findings may suggest an **embolic event,** although they do not exclude a different mechanism. These include multiple areas of vascular involvement, abnormal CT or MRI findings indicative of a large vessel infarction in a vascular distribution that would not explain the current symptoms, or an embolic syndrome, suggested by various findings including ischemia of the posterior cerebral artery distribution with homonymous hemianopia, ischemia of the lower middle cerebral artery division and receptive aphasia, top of the basilar syndrome, rapidly resolving severe deficit of abrupt onset, and spontaneous hemorrhagic transformation.

Should the multiple symptoms be explained by a large vessel distribution in the anterior circulation, screening of the anterior circulation with carotid ultrasonography or ocular pneumoplethysmography should be performed because of the proven success of carotid endarterectomy in such cases. High-grade stenosis on a noninvasive study in the internal carotid artery should prompt surgical consideration if a patient is a surgical candidate. Before surgical treatment, cerebral arteriography is normally performed. Because this is a subgroup of events that are not stereotyped or clearly associated with a proven cardiac risk (see Table 12-1), transesophageal echocardiography may need to be performed before carotid endarterectomy because the potential for a cardioembolic source remains in this subgroup of patients.

If the noninvasive arterial studies do not reveal a cause for the events, cardiac imaging with **transesophageal echocardiography** is usually performed, providing superior resolution of the left atrium, left atrial appendage, aortic arch, and other cardiac basal structures. Although results of transesophageal echocardiography prompt medical management changes in a relatively small number of patients overall, the proportion whose management is changed is higher among the subgroup of patients with no definite cause identified for their cerebrovascular symptoms by this point in the evaluation. **Holter monitoring** may also be useful in this setting. Patients with cerebral infarction of unknown cause may have underlying episodic arrhythmias known to be associated with an increased risk of systemic embolization, even in the presence of a normal electrocardiographic tracing.

If a **proven** cardiac risk factor (see Table 12-1) is detected with these studies, warfarin anticoagulation may be initiated depending on the specific finding (see Chapter 16). Detection of a **putative** cardiac risk factor (see Table 12-2) may also necessitate warfarin anticoagulation or antiplatelet therapy if no other mechanism is noted. If transesophageal echocardiography and Holter monitoring reveal normal findings and the other evaluation as outlined is normal, trial of an antiplatelet agent is indicated.

Recurrence with Aspirin Therapy

If spells recur with aspirin therapy, the distribution of the symptoms will be a guide to the most appropriate therapy. Symptoms recurring in the **anterior circulation** should promote carotid ultrasonography if the original study was not of sufficient quality or if it was performed more than 3 months earlier. If carotid ultrasonography is normal or has already been performed, ocular pneumoplethysmography may be done. If ocular pneumoplethysmography and carotid ultrasonography are normal, transcranial Doppler ultrasonography or MRA is the next appropriate step to evaluate the distal internal carotid artery and proximal middle cerebral artery. If one of these studies is abnormal, warfarin anticoagulation is usually indicated. If a patient is not a candidate for warfarin, the use of ticlopidine is reasonable. If the noninvasive studies, including ocular pneumoplethysmography, carotid ultrasonography, transcranial Doppler ultrasonography, MRA, transesophageal echocardiography, and possibly Holter monitoring, fail to reveal a cause for the event, additional evaluation, including special coagulation studies and arteriography, may be required. If results are negative, empiric treatment with either anticoagulation or ticlopidine is indicated. Increasing the aspirin dose may, theoretically, also be beneficial.

Recurrent symptoms in the distribution of the **posterior circulation** should prompt noninvasive imaging with either transcranial Doppler ultrasonography or MRA, if this was not performed earlier. If these studies fail to reveal a hemodynamically significant stenosis, cerebral arteriography should be considered because of the potential for a false-negative noninvasive study or a proximal vertebral stenosis. If the arteriogram reveals a high-grade stenosis, warfarin anticoagulation or ticlopidine is indicated if the patient is not a candidate for warfarin. Increasing the aspirin dose may, theoretically, also be beneficial in this context. If the arteriogram is negative, transesophageal echocardiography is indicated, and other evaluation to include Holter monitoring and special coagulation studies may follow if the cause is still unclear.

Recurrent clinical symptoms involving **multiple vascular territories** should prompt evaluation for a more proximal source of emboli. Evaluation might include transesophageal echocardiography and Holter monitoring. One may also consider alternative diagnoses, including cerebral vasculitis or a hypercoagulable state, which may cause symptoms in multiple distributions. Treatment issues for specific causes delineated by this additional evaluation are reviewed in Chapter 16.

Major Cerebral Infarction: General Evaluation and Treatment

General Management Considerations

Patients with acute stroke should be treated with the same sense of urgency as patients with an acute myocardial infarction. In the same sense that a heart attack indicates the need for emergency action because of a lack of blood supply to the heart muscle, an ischemic stroke (cerebral infarction) is a **brain attack** indicating an abrupt lack of blood supply to a region of the brain. Urgent medical or surgical intervention may be critical to long-term outcome. Most patients presenting with cerebral infarction should be hospitalized for **urgent evaluation and treatment**.

The initial evaluation of a patient presenting with **cerebral infarction** is similar to that outlined for transient ischemic attack and minor cerebral infarction (see Chapter 12). Computed tomography (CT) without contrast or magnetic resonance imaging (MRI) examination is indicated to quickly distinguish between nonhemorrhagic and hemorrhagic cerebrovascular disease. If CT without contrast is performed initially, CT with contrast or MRI may be required if the initial scan indicates a possible arteriovenous malformation, meningioma, or other mass lesion. Other baseline studies should include complete blood cell count, activated partial thromboplastin time, serum chemistry group, erythrocyte sedimentation rate, and lipid analyses, including high-density lipoprotein, low-density lipoprotein, and cholesterol levels. A chest radiograph, electrocardiogram, and rhythm strip should also be obtained.

Management of patients with acute cerebral infarction differs somewhat from that of patients with transient ischemic attack and minor stroke and includes (1) intensive general medical care, (2) treatment of the neurologic deficit, (3) prevention of subsequent neurologic event, and (4) prevention and treatment of secondary complications such as bronchial pneumonia, urinary tract infection, and deep vein thrombosis (see Appendix J-3). As with transient ischemic attack, minor cerebral infarction, and reversible ischemic neurologic deficit, cardiac evaluation should include cardiac history (with special attention to ischemic symptoms, arrhythmia, and murmurs) and cardiac examination.

Subsequent evaluation is typically based on the magnitude of the deficit, the patient's age and medical status, and candidacy for therapeutic intervention, including either operation or medical intervention. Early after the onset of a severe deficit, it is not possible to classify the deficit as a transient ischemic attack, reversible ischemic neurologic deficit, ischemic stroke, or progressive stroke because if and when the deficit will clear is uncertain.

Acute Therapeutic Considerations

The **initial therapeutic approach** to ischemic infarction is greatly dependent on the time from onset of symptoms to presentation for emergency medical care. If the history and examination verify that the probable cause of the symptoms is an ischemic stroke, and if the onset of symptoms was less than 3 to 6 hours before the evaluation, **emergent thrombolytic therapy** should be considered.

Thrombolytic agents such as tissue plasminogen activator (tPA), urokinase, and streptokinase given either intravenously or intraarterially dissolve thrombi and are designed to reopen arteries occluded by emboli or a primary thrombus and induce reperfusion of an ischemic area of the brain. Although such reperfusion may be associated with a return in neurologic function of the affected area, clinical improvement may not occur, and administration may be complicated by intracerebral hemorrhage.

The time of onset of the infarction must be sought from the patient or family; if a patient awakens from sleep with the deficit, thrombolytic therapy should not be considered unless the duration of the deficit is clearly less than 3 to 6 hours.

The result of the CT head scan is very important in selecting patients. The CT should not reveal any evidence of intracranial hemorrhage, mass effect, or midline shift. Clinical criteria that may exclude patients are (1) rapidly improving or mild deficits, (2) obtundation or coma, (3) presentation with seizure, (4) history of intracranial hemorrhage or bleeding diathesis, (5) blood pressure increase persistently more than 185/110 mm Hg, (6) gastrointestinal hemorrhage or urinary tract hemorrhage within 21 days, and (7) recent large ischemic stroke within 14 days or small ischemic stroke within 4 days. Laboratory abnormalities that may preclude treatment are (1) heparin use within 48 hours with increased activated partial thromboplastin time, (2) prothrombin time more than 15 seconds, and (3) serum glucose less than 50 or more than 400 mg/dl.

If the patient is a candidate for thrombolytic therapy, the patient and family should be counseled regarding the risks and benefits of such therapy. In a treatment trial of intravenous tPA published in 1995, the efficacy in improving neurologic status at 3 months was defined for tPA compared with placebo, with the agent administered within 3 hours of symptom onset. Although there was a greater proportion (12% greater) of people with minimal or no deficit in the tPA group at 3 months after the event, there was no increase in persons with severe deficits or disability. This finding is particularly important because there was an increased occurrence of symptomatic hemorrhage in the tPA group, and data from acute stroke trials of streptokinase reported before the intravenous tPA trial suggested that any improvement in outcome in patients receiving thrombolytic therapy may be offset by an increase in poor outcomes caused by hemorrhage.

An intracranial hemorrhage in the setting of thrombolytic therapy should be suspected if neurologic deterioration occurs or if there is new headache, acute hypertension, nausea, or vomiting. Use of tPA should be discontinued immediately if the infusion is ongoing, and a

CT scan should be obtained. In the meantime, prothrombin time, partial thromboplastin time, platelet count, and fibrinogen value should be determined emergently, and platelets (6 to 8 units) and fibrinogen in the form of cryoprecipitate containing factor VIII (6 to 8 units) should be prepared. If the CT scan confirms hemorrhage, neurosurgical consultation should be obtained. A hematologist may aid in outlining optimal replacement therapy with platelets and cryoprecipitate. Another CT scan can be obtained 6 hours later, or sooner if the deficit worsens.

The tPA should be administered intravenously in a dose of 0.9 mg/kg (maximum 90 mg), with 10% given as a bolus and the remainder over 60 minutes. Close monitoring in an intensive care unit should continue for 24 hours. Intravenous heparin should not be used for 24 hours, and blood pressure should be monitored closely, with the pressure kept at less than 180/105 mm Hg (see Chapter 11). Although administering tPA (or other thrombolytic agents) intra-arterially may ultimately be more helpful than giving these agents intravenously, the procedures require more time and expertise and are associated with greater risk.

In patients who are not candidates for thrombolytic therapy, or if 24 hours have passed since thrombolytic therapy, the initial therapeutic approach in ischemic infarction includes consideration of the use of heparin. In patients with mild-to-moderate cerebral infarction with the potential for marked worsening of the deficit in the distribution of the initial event, urgent initiation of **heparin** (intravenous) is considered. As described in Chapter 12, the rationale for heparin use in this situation is based on theoretical and pharmacologic data. The pharmacologic effect, complications, and dose initiation were described in Chapter 12. For patients with known or suspected ongoing sources for further embolization (for instance, cardiac embolic sources), the rationale for the use of heparin becomes stronger. In general, for patients with **small or moderate cerebral infarction** who are not candidates for a treatment protocol with one of the evolving therapeutic agents for acute stroke (discussed below), treatment with heparin or a heparinoid may be initiated. These two agents are particularly likely to be beneficial if the event was cardioembolic in nature.

Even though patients with embolic events are at greater risk of experiencing hemorrhagic transformation of an infarct, patients with small or moderate embolic infarcts may be safely anticoagulated if the activated partial thromboplastin time is monitored closely, as described in Chapter 12. For patients with **large cardioembolic infarcts** involving the entire middle cerebral artery or internal carotid artery distribution, heparin is usually withheld early and a CT scan is obtained several days after the onset of symptoms. If there is no evidence of hemorrhagic transformation, treatment usually involves intravenous heparin with no bolus and close monitoring of the activated partial thromboplastin time.

Use of heparin anticoagulation assumes that the patient has no contraindications such as bleeding peptic ulcer, uremia, hepatic failure, markedly increased blood pressure ($\geq$200/120 mm Hg), or strong suspicion or evidence of bacterial endocarditis or sepsis. Heparin is typically administered as an initial bolus of 5000 U, followed by a continuous drip of 1000 U/hour to maintain the activated partial thromboplastin time at 1.5 to 2 times normal (see Chapter 12 for more information on heparin anticoagulation). If heparin-related **hemorrhagic side effects** occur, protamine can be used to reverse the heparin anticoagulation at a dose of 5 ml of a 1% solution mixed with 20 ml of saline administered slowly intravenously, with no more than 50 mg given over a 10-minute period or 200 mg during 2 hours.

Low-molecular-weight heparin (LMWH) (see Chapter 12) may also be efficacious if initiated within 24 hours after stroke onset. In one study, at 6 months there was a 20% higher frequency of death or dependence outcomes in the placebo group compared with the group receiving high-dose LMWH.

In addition to the emergency initiation of heparin anticoagulation, other therapies currently under investigation may prove effective if given very early in the course of an ischemic event. Some of these agents are given before the mechanism for the infarction is clarified. Although ischemia may convert to irreversible cerebral infarction over a matter of minutes, marginal ischemic zones may possibly be affected by acute treatment during a period of hours or even days. This has led to the consideration of initiating these therapies as soon as possible after the onset of the event. At centers participating in treatment trials for acute stroke, a patient's candidacy for the trials should be considered as early as possible after the onset of symptoms.

Other emergency treatments of acute stroke include several categories of neuroprotective agents designed to limit or reverse parenchymal damage.

Calcium channel blocking agents (including nimodipine, nicardipine, nitrendipine, cinnarizine, and flunarizine) constitute one category of neuroprotective agents. These drugs prevent influx of calcium through voltage-operated channels with action at both cellular and vascular levels. Although treatment trials in ischemic stroke have not been conclusive, there is some suggestion that patients may benefit from these agents if treatment is started within several hours of the onset of ischemic stroke.

Another category of neuroprotective agents receiving considerable attention in recent years involves the **N-methyl-D-aspartate (NMDA) antagonists**. These drugs (dextromethorphan, dizocilpine, GS-19755, and others) block receptors of excitatory amino acids released during the ischemic cascade and provide another method of blocking influx effects of excessive amounts of calcium into the cell, which leads to cell death. Further studies are needed to assess the safety and tolerance of this class of drugs in the setting of acute ischemic stroke.

Another class of neuroprotective agents is the **free radical scavenger** agent group, which includes 21 amino steroids, allopurinol, and dimethyl thiouria. These drugs are designed to decrease cell damage by inhibiting the release of free radicals such as hydroxyl and superoxide. Because oxygen is required in the production of free radicals, the agents may be particularly useful in combination with agents used in reperfusion therapy, such as thrombolytic agents. However, definitive answers about effectiveness and toxicity await results of formal treatment trials.

Other agents, including **gangliosides, naloxone, clofibrate, hyperbaric oxygen, barbiturates, vasodilators** such as pentoxifylline, and various **hemodiluting agents** and **hypothermia,** have thus far not been shown to be of practical benefit in clinical situations involving humans. Other urgent medical therapies that have been evaluated with clinical trials include isovolemic hemodilution and the lowering of hematocrit to reduce the blood velocity. These measures have produced no convincing improvement in mortality or stroke severity. Hypervolemic hemodilution also has not been shown to be beneficial, and the mortality among patients receiving treatment is higher than that in controls, although some have questioned the design of the available studies. In patients with acute stroke, numerous randomized clinical trials have demonstrated no overall beneficial effect of hemodilution on survival or neurologic outcome.

The efficacy of **emergency surgical therapy** with carotid endarterectomy in patients with acute occlusion of the carotid artery or progressive cerebral infarction remains uncertain. Middle cerebral artery embolectomy also has been advocated by some, although the procedure has been performed in only a small subgroup of patients and has not been subjected to a clinical trial. The use of angioplasty in the setting of acute ischemic stroke is also unsupported at this time, although the procedure is undergoing further study.

Progressive Ischemic Stroke

Approximately 20% of patients with infarction in the distribution of the carotid system and about 30% to 40% of patients with infarction of the vertebrobasilar distribution have a progressive course (**progressive infarction**). Low blood pressure or perfusion pressure, recurrent emboli, propagation of intra-arterial thrombus, cerebral edema, and hemorrhagic infarction are the most common mechanisms of progression. Alternatively, other causes must also be considered, including tumor, subdural hematoma, demyelinating disease, toxic-metabolic encephalopathy, and infectious processes such as brain abscess or focal encephalitis. In patients with progression caused by evolving **cerebral edema**, treatment with mannitol, glycerol, hyperventilation, and dexamethasone (see Chapter 11) may be initiated, although these measures may be of limited value in this context.

If the intracranial process is still considered to be **ischemic,** resulting from either recurrent emboli or propagation of intra-arterial thrombus, and more than 3 to 6 hours have passed since the onset of symptoms, and the lesion is nonhemorrhagic on CT, intravenous heparin therapy (see Chapter 12 for initiation of therapy) should be considered if not already initiated, especially for events involving the vertebrobasilar circulation. If instituted, heparin treatment is usually continued for 3 to 5 days after the course has stabilized. If the worsening of the deficit occurs within 3 to 6 hours of onset of the original symptoms, intravenous tPA may be used, as outlined earlier.

For patients who continue to have progression of neurologic deficit despite anticoagulation therapy, cerebral arteriography should be considered to define the mechanism. A few patients in this group may be considered for emergency neurovascular surgical intervention, although no surgical trial has documented the efficacy of either carotid endarterectomy or cerebral arterial embolectomy. Urgent cerebral arteriography with intra-arterial thrombolytic treatment may also become a useful therapeutic option in this setting, although few data are available currently.

Particular attention should be paid to **hypotension** and any **metabolic abnormalities** that can accentuate the focal neurologic deficit. CT with contrast or MRI should be performed, if not done earlier, to identify **other types of intracranial pathologic processes** as a cause for the symptoms.

Treatment of Early Complications

Among the 20% of patients who die within 30 days of the first cerebral infarction, 50% die of potentially treatable medical causes. The frequency of **pneumonia, deep vein thrombosis, or pulmonary embolism** after a stroke has been estimated at 30%, 10%, and 5%, respectively. Approximately 30% of patients have deterioration during the first week after stroke; 70% of complications result from cerebral causes such as intracranial bleeding or rapidly progressive cerebral edema (see Chapter 11), and 30% result from systemic causes such as **cardiopulmonary failure** (including neurogenic pulmonary edema, myocardial damage, serious cardiac arrhythmias, and pulmonary embolism), **systemic infection, hyponatremia** (with inappropriate antidiuretic hormone syndrome or salt-wasting syndrome), side effects of **drugs** such as oversedation from tranquilizers, and other **metabolic causes** (including renal and hepatic failure). Early diagnosis and appropriate treatment of the specific cause of deterioration are essential. Urgent CT or MRI should be performed in patients with clinical deterioration to identify the aforementioned cerebral causes.

Nonneurologic Complications

Patients who are bedridden have an increased risk for development of **deep vein thrombosis and pulmonary embolism.** External pneumatic compression stockings, passive physical therapy, elevating the legs 6 to 10 degrees, and low-dose heparin therapy (5000 U subcutaneously every 12 hours) may help prevent deep vein thrombosis. Early heparin treatment in acute ischemic stroke has been associated with substantial reductions in deep vein thrombosis and with decreased mortality in several randomized trials. Evidence from randomized trials also suggests that antiplatelet therapy either alone or in addition to subcutaneously administered heparin should be considered for patients who are at substantial risk of venous thromboembolism. Because of the high risk of pulmonary embolism, which is fatal in 25% of cases, patients with acute deep vein thrombosis should be treated with heparin. The usual method of administration involves an intravenous bolus of 5000 to 10,000 U, followed by continuous intravenous infusion to maintain 1.5 to 2 times the monitored baseline activated partial thromboplastin time for 7 to 10 days, followed by warfarin therapy for at least 3 months. Endovascular placement of an inferior vena cava filter should be performed in patients with contraindications to anticoagulant therapy.

Because **pulmonary embolism** is responsible for approximately 10% of the deaths in cases of ischemic stroke, patients should be questioned daily about the occurrence of chest pain and dyspnea. For patients in whom pulmonary embolism is strongly suspected, initial intravenous therapy with heparin, given in a dose of approximately 5000 to 10,000 U, should be instituted immediately, even before diagnostic studies are completed if a patient is hemodynamically unstable. Arterial blood gas studies, chest radiography, electrocardiography, and ventilation-perfusion scanning (V/Q scan) also should be performed promptly to confirm the diagnosis. If the diagnosis is equivocal and the clinical suspicion is high, pulmonary angiography may be needed. In patients with nondiagnostic V/Q scans, impedance plethysmography or duplex ultrasonography should be performed. If the results are normal, further observation is indicated, but anticoagulation should be initiated if the study indicates thrombus. The intravenous bolus of heparin should be followed in 2 to 4 hours by continuous intravenous administration of heparin to maintain the activated partial thromboplastin time at 1.5 to 2 times baseline for 7 to 10 days, followed by warfarin therapy for at least 3 months, unless contraindications exist.

Pneumonia is also an important cause of death after ischemic stroke. Vigorous tracheobronchial toilet, deep-breathing exercises, and early mobilization are helpful preventive measures. To prevent aspiration pneumonia, swallowing should be tested before oral feeding is permitted. If there is any question about the safety of the patient's swallowing, a formal study with fluoroscopy may clarify the potential for aspiration and consistency of food necessary to prevent aspiration. Antibiotic therapy is used only for clinical infection and is not used prophylactically. In cases of infection, empiric antibiotic therapy should be instituted until the specific infectious agent and antibiotic sensitivities are established.

Urinary tract infection may be complicated by secondary septicemia in approximately 5% of patients. Indwelling catheters should be avoided; the alternative approach used is frequent, intermittent catheterization to minimize bladder distention. In patients with incontinence or urinary retention, anticholinergic drugs may help in the recovery of bladder function. In patients with hyperthermia, an antipyretic, such as acetaminophen, or cooling devices, such as cooling blankets or compresses, may be considered to maintain body temperature in the normal range.

Cardiovascular complications after stroke, such as cardiac arrhythmias, various types of myocardial damage (contraction bands, focal myocardial necrosis, subendocardial ischemia), and electrocardiographic abnormalities (ST- and T-segment changes, U-wave abnormalities, QT prolongation, sinus arrhythmias) should be treated whenever possible, with attention given to the underlying disease according to a cardiologist's suggestions. The treatment of cardiac ventricular arrhythmias after acute stroke often begins with beta-adrenergic blocking agents such as propranolol. Intravenous antiarrhythmic agents may be necessary in cases of malignant arrhythmias uncontrolled by oral agents.

Gastrointestinal alterations after an acute cerebrovascular event include nausea and vomiting, acute peptic ulceration, and fecal incontinence or impaction. Histamine blockers may be used for ulcer prophylaxis. Stool softeners, laxatives, and suppositories lessen the risk of impaction.

Decubitus ulcers are common and should be prevented with use of an air mattress on the bed, position adjustment every 1 to 2 hours, tight bed sheets, dry skin surfaces, and prevention of urinary and fecal incontinence.

For patients who are unable to fully close one or both eyes, artificial tears or blepharoplasty may be needed to maintain adequate corneal moisture and to prevent corneal clouding and ulceration.

Neurologic Complications

Seizures occur in approximately 10% of patients with cerebral infarction; 30% occur within the first 2 weeks and 75% within the first year after stroke onset. Intracerebral hemorrhages and embolic cortical infarcts are more frequently associated with seizures. Anticonvulsants are typically not given as prophylactic agents.

Initially, seizures resulting from an acute cerebrovascular event are treated with intravenously administered diazepam (5–10 mg, at a rate as high as 2 mg/minute, which may be repeated once in 5–15 minutes) followed by a loading dose of phenytoin given orally (15–20 mg/kg, given in a single dose, or split in three doses given every 8 hours) or intravenously administered phenytoin dissolved in normal saline (15–20 mg/kg at a rate as high as 50 mg/minute) or phenobarbital (20 mg/kg at a rate as high as 100 mg/minute). Instead of intravenous phenytoin, fosphenytoin may be used. Fosphenytoin, which is rapidly metabolized to phenytoin, is given intravenously (15–20 mg/kg phenytoin equivalents at a rate as high as 150 mg phenytoin equivalents/minute) or intramuscularly. Phenytoin, carbamazepine, or phenobarbital can subsequently be used for maintenance therapy.

Electrocardiographic and blood pressure monitoring should be used during and after acute intravenous administration of anticonvulsants because of concern about bradycardia and hypotension. If the duration of ventricular electrical activities (QT interval) widens, bradyarrhythmias occur, or hypotension appears, the infusion rate should be slowed. If seizures persist, addition of phenobarbital to phenytoin may be used initially, and if this approach is ineffective, general anesthesia with intravenously administered pentobarbital is recommended with electroencephalographic and blood pressure monitoring in a neurologic intensive care unit.

Subarachnoid Hemorrhage: General Evaluation and Treatment

Patient Evaluation

The diagnosis of subarachnoid hemorrhage (SAH) requires suspicion on the part of medical personnel in initial contact with the patient. Although the abrupt onset of a severe headache is a common presentation, less severe headache with or without an associated brief loss of consciousness, nausea, or vomiting may also signal SAH, and an initial, mild hemorrhage is sometimes missed. In any patient with new onset of an unusually severe or atypical headache, particularly if associated with a brief loss of consciousness, nausea, vomiting, stiff neck, or any focal neurologic findings, **computed tomography (CT) of the head** without contrast should be performed to determine whether intracranial hemorrhage is present (see algorithm for the management of SAH in Appendix J-4).

If obtained within 24 hours, the CT scan is abnormal in about 90% of cases of SAH and reveals the increased attenuation caused by hemorrhage in the subarachnoid space (Fig. 14-1). If the CT scan is negative, a **lumbar puncture** should be performed. If the CT scan shows evidence for SAH or intraparenchymal hemorrhage, a lumbar puncture will not contribute significant additional diagnostic information and can sometimes be dangerous, especially if parenchymal blood is present.

The typical patient with SAH has grossly bloody spinal fluid. However, **traumatic lumbar puncture** must be differentiated from true SAH. Three or four successive tubes of cerebrospinal fluid are collected, and, if the specimens show progressively less blood, a traumatic puncture is suggested. Clotting of the specimen virtually never occurs with true SAH. Xanthochromia is present in the supernatant within hours of SAH and remains in the spinal fluid for an average of 3 to 4 weeks. Erythrocytes often disappear within several days after SAH. The cerebrospinal fluid may not show xanthochromia if small numbers of erythrocytes are present from SAH (approximately ≤400), and xanthochromia has been reported in rare instances with traumatic lumbar puncture if the erythrocyte count is more than 200,000/µl. The D-dimer test may also be of value in distinguishing between traumatic lumbar puncture and true SAH, although this is still under evaluation.

In addition to a headache that varies from the classic severe, striking, generalized headache with meningismus to a much milder headache resolving within 24 to 48 hours, other aspects of the neurologic history and examination are important in clarifying the potential presence of SAH. Because aneurysms may cause a mass effect on adjacent structures, including the cranial nerves and brain stem, symptoms preceding SAH may include diplopia, facial weakness, extremity weakness, and unsteadiness. In addition, aneurysms can

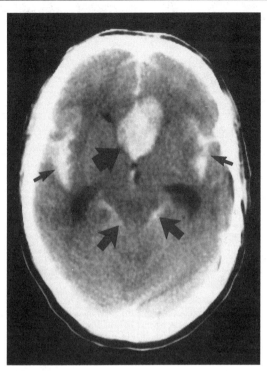

Fig. 14-1. CT scan of head without contrast: areas of increased attenuation consistent with subarachnoid hemorrhage in the sylvian fissures (small arrows), interhemispheric fissure (large arrow), and surrounding the brain stem (medium arrows). Hemorrhage was caused by an aneurysm of the anterior communicating artery.

occasionally present with transient symptoms caused by ischemia or seizures. Ischemic spells are typically thought to be caused by thrombus formation within or adjacent to the aneurysm and lead to distal embolization and ischemia. In addition to focal symptoms, more generalized symptoms, including transient loss of consciousness caused by a sudden increase in intracranial pressure, may also occur at the time of the hemorrhage.

A comprehensive neurologic examination should be performed in the patient with SAH, but profound muscle testing should be avoided because of the potential increased risk for rebleeding. On neurologic examination, the presence of any focal findings is important and may aid in localizing the aneurysm. Particular findings that may be useful include monocular visual deficits, which may indicate an ophthalmic artery aneurysm with optic nerve compression. Extraocular muscle abnormalities may indicate internal carotid artery, basilar artery, or ophthalmic aneurysms. A unilateral third cranial nerve palsy early in the course of the SAH strongly suggests an aneurysm of the posterior communicating artery. Sixth cranial nerve palsy may result from increased intracranial pressure or from a basilar artery aneurysm. Hemorrhage or mass effect from a middle cerebral artery

Table 14-1.   Laboratory investigations
for patients with subarachnoid hemorrhage

Complete blood cell count
Prothrombin time, activated partial thromboplastin time (APTT)
Erythrocyte sedimentation rate
Blood glucose
Serum electrolytes
Urinalysis
Chest radiography
Electrocardiography
Head CT or MRI; consider lumbar puncture (if hemorrhage is suspected and
    CT or MRI is negative)
Consider inpatient cardiac monitoring
Consider TCD (e.g., if vasospasm suspected)
Consider cerebral arteriography
Consider electroencephalography (if seizure is suspected)
Determination of arterial blood gas levels (if hypoxia is suspected)
Consider special coagulation studies (if cause is unclear despite
    arteriography)

CT = computed tomography; MRI = magnetic resonance imaging; TCD = transcranial Doppler ultrasonography.

aneurysm may cause aphasia and hemiparesis. Leg weakness and changes in behavior may be associated with rupture or mass effect from an anterior communicating artery or anterior cerebral artery aneurysm affecting the frontal lobe(s).

Initial CT scan may reveal the location of the hemorrhage as well as the possible source for the event, although standard CT imaging without contrast is unlikely to detect an uncalcified aneurysm, especially one less than 10 mm in size. An aneurysmal cause must be suspected in all cases of SAH or intracerebral hemorrhage that cannot be clearly explained by an alternative cause. Magnetic resonance imaging (MRI) and angiography (MRA) are more likely to show the underlying cause, including relatively small aneurysms, but MRI is less sensitive than CT for diagnosing acute SAH. After SAH is diagnosed and the patient is initially stabilized, urgent cerebral arteriography is typically indicated to attempt to define the cause for the SAH. Cerebral arteriography is the most sensitive study available; it reveals small saccular aneurysms and arteriovenous malformations as well as the associated morphology and anatomic characteristics. MRA is a noninvasive means of detecting small aneurysms with a relatively high sensitivity, especially if the lesion is more than 4 mm in maximal diameter, but this study alone is usually insufficient for surgical planning and is seldom used in the circumstance of acute SAH. Other studies (Table 14-1) are also typically undertaken to identify other potential underlying factors causing or exacerbating SAH, such as hypocoagulable states.

Treatment

Early treatment of patients with SAH is directed toward the prevention and management of major **neurologic complications,**

Table 14-2.   General management
measures for subarachnoid hemorrhage

1. Place patient on bed rest in quiet room
2. Provide ongoing monitoring of neurologic status (level of consciousness, focal deficit, Glasgow Coma Scale)
3. Consider cardiac monitoring
4. Elevate head of bed 30 degrees
5. Prevent straining (stool softeners and antitussive agents as needed)
6. Provide oral nutrition for alert patients with intact gag reflex
7. Provide enteral nutrition with nasogastric tube for patients with decreased level of consciousness or impaired gag reflex
8. Maintain normovolemia and normal sodium level by starting with administration of 2–3 liters/day of D_5W and 0.9 normal saline and adjusting accordingly (see Table 14-5)
9. Mildly sedate patient if agitated: phenobarbital (30–60 mg 2 times a day) or chloral hydrate (500 mg 3 times a day)
10. Control mild pain with acetaminophen or propoxyphene and severe pain with codeine (60 mg, IM or PO, every 3–4 hr); use morphine (1- to 2-mg increments IV) only as last resort
11. Reduce blood pressure conservatively and with careful monitoring if patient has extremely increased blood pressure or evidence of acute end-organ damage

including rebleeding, vasospasm and cerebral ischemia, hydrocephalus, and seizures. Early treatment of SAH also involves the management of various relatively common **systemic complications,** including electrolyte disturbances such as hyponatremia, cardiac arrhythmia and myocardial damage, and neurogenic pulmonary edema. The overall general treatment strategy is summarized in Table 14-2 and Appendix J-4. Specific management of aneurysms, arteriovenous malformations, and other underlying conditions such as hypocoagulable states is described in Chapter 17.

PREVENTION AND MANAGEMENT
OF NEUROLOGIC COMPLICATIONS

Rebleeding

The likelihood of **rebleeding** after SAH is greatest during the first few days after initial hemorrhage, particularly the first 24 hours. This time sequence and the associated mortality rate of approximately 50% make the prevention of rebleeding a major priority in the early treatment of patients with SAH.

Patients should be placed on **bed rest** in a **quiet room** and kept under **close observation** either in an intensive care unit or at least in a hospital room close to a nursing station. The head of the patient's bed should be elevated approximately 30 degrees to lower the patient's intracranial pressure. Straining should be prevented with stool softeners; coughing may be prevented with antitussive agents, such as codeine, as needed.

Serial assessments of level of consciousness by an experienced nursing staff are of great importance. The Glasgow Coma Scale (see Appendix B) may be used for this purpose.

Table 14-3. Indications for emergency surgical
intervention in patients with subarachnoid hemorrhage

1. Acute hydrocephalus causing substantial or progressive neurologic
   deficit
2. Large, surgically accessible intracerebral hematoma with significant mass
   effect
3. Rebleeding followed by partial or total recovery of neurologic function from
   a known aneurysm or arteriovenous malformation previously untreated or
   partially treated

If the patient is **agitated**, a sedative, phenobarbital (30–60 mg twice daily) or chloral hydrate (500 mg 3 times daily), is recommended. The patient should not be oversedated because the effect of medication may be indistinguishable from a depressed level of consciousness caused by rehemorrhage or other complications of SAH.

Analgesia should be provided for pain relief because extra pain often leads to agitation and an increased likelihood of additional hemorrhage. Mild pain can be managed with acetaminophen or propoxyphene. For severe pain, codeine (60 mg, intramuscularly or orally, every 3–4 hours) may be used as needed. Morphine should be used only as a last resort for otherwise uncontrollable pain (given in small increments of 1–2 mg intravenously) because it may depress respiration and level of consciousness.

The use of **antifibrinolytic agents** such as epsilon-aminocaproic acid (Amicar) (24–36 g/day in 1000 ml of 5% dextrose solution) or tranexamic acid (1 g intravenously or 1.5 g orally 4–6 times daily) may decrease mortality from rebleeding of aneurysms, but these agents are also associated with thrombotic side effects, including cerebral infarction, deep vein thrombosis, and pulmonary embolism. Consequently, administration of these antifibrinolytic agents does not appear to be warranted after a single SAH. However, the risk-benefit ratio is more likely to favor use of these agents if there is evidence of continued or recurrent hemorrhage after initial hemorrhage. Also, the use of antifibrinolytic agents in combination with a calcium channel blocking agent such as nimodipine may have the same benefit for preventing rebleeding while avoiding some of the untoward cerebral ischemic side effects.

Deterioration of neurologic status, including level of consciousness, in patients with SAH may signify an episode of rebleeding, especially early after the original SAH. However, several other possible causes of neurologic deterioration are (1) delayed ischemic neurologic deficits that may be related to vasospasm (most commonly 4–14 days after SAH), (2) acute hydrocephalus, (3) cerebral edema, (4) electrolyte imbalances, (5) neurogenic pulmonary edema, (6) seizures, and (7) severe cardiac dysrhythmia or ischemia. CT of the head should be performed in patients with deterioration of neurologic status as soon as possible to attempt to confirm the existence of rebleeding or acute hydrocephalus. In some cases, the appearance of acute hydrocephalus or intraparenchymal clot with mass effect may warrant emergency surgical intervention (Table 14-3). Repeated lumbar punctures are generally not of value in confirming the cause for neurologic deterioration and may be hazardous.

Many patients who rebleed experience a sudden respiratory arrest at the onset of the rebleeding episode. In general, vigorous attempts should be made to resuscitate these patients because recovery of complete neurologic function is quite possible in these circumstances, even after respiratory arrest.

After rebleeding, if the patient stabilizes and recovers, identification and clipping of an underlying aneurysm become even more urgent because further rebleeding episodes are common and associated with high mortality.

Vasospasm and Cerebral Ischemia

Another common and potentially serious complication of SAH hemorrhage is **cerebral vasospasm,** a narrowing of arteries in the intracranial segments of the carotid and vertebrobasilar circulations, typically most severe in areas of maximal hemorrhage. Vasospasm occurs in approximately 30% of patients with SAH, typically beginning about 3 to 5 days after the hemorrhage; maximal effect is at 5 to 14 days, and resolution occurs over 2 to 3 weeks.

Patients with suspected **cerebral ischemia** (a decrease in the level of consciousness, focal cerebral deficits, or both) should undergo CT, which may show evidence for cerebral infarction or evidence for other conditions that may mimic cerebral ischemia, including acute hydrocephalus, recurrent subarachnoid or intracerebral bleeding, or cerebral edema. Cerebral arteriography is the most sensitive means to evaluate vasospasm, although transcranial Doppler ultrasonographic examination often provides noninvasive detection of vasospasm and is a much more practical way to provide ongoing monitoring of the condition. The arteriographic or transcranial Doppler findings may not be associated with any clinical change because only about 50% of cases are associated with focal symptoms.

Several findings may be associated with an increased occurrence of vasospasm, such as an aneurysmal cause for the subarachnoid hemorrhage; a significant amount of subarachnoid blood, particularly at the base of the brain; and intraventricular hemorrhage. Measures that can help **prevent** cerebral ischemia include (1) maintenance of a normal fluid and sodium balance, (2) conservative use or avoidance of antihypertensive agents, and (3) the use of calcium channel blocking agents (Table 14-4).

Fluid management should seek to maintain normovolemia and a normal sodium level. Underhydration is associated with the development of vasospasm and cerebral ischemia, whereas overhydration may be associated with cerebral edema and increased intracranial pressure. In general, most patients should be started on approximately 2 to 3 liters/day of D_5W and 0.9 normal saline, with adjustments as needed, depending on body size, serial weights, intake and output measurements, central hemodynamic measurements, serum electrolyte levels, and general nutrition status. **Hyponatremia** is common in patients with SAH; its management is discussed later under Hyponatremia.

One must be cautious about the use of **antihypertensive agents** in patients with SAH because they may precipitate or accentuate cerebral ischemic complications. At least part of the hypertension observed is often the result of Cushing's reflex, in which intracranial

Table 14-4. Management of vasospasm and
cerebral ischemia associated with subarachnoid hemorrhage

1. Apply preventive measures, including adequate fluid and sodium intake,
   conservative use of antihypertensive agents and calcium channel blocking
   agents (nimodipine, 60 mg, PO, every 4 hr)
2. Provide volume expansion with 5% albumin (e.g., 250 ml 4–6 times daily),
   colloid, or packed erythrocytes
3. Maintain central venous pressure at 8–12 mm Hg and pulmonary wedge
   pressure at 16–20 mm Hg
4. Consider induction of hypertension with phenylephrine and/or dopamine
5. Consider balloon angioplasty, intra-arterial papaverine, or surgical
   drainage of clot and administration of tissue-plasminogen activator

hypertension leads to peripheral hypertension to maintain cerebral
perfusion. Alternatively, excessive hypertension may be associated
with an increased risk of rebleeding. Treatment of hypertension is
usually confined to careful, well-monitored, modest reductions in
blood pressure for patients with evidence of organ damage or very
high blood pressure (see Chapter 11). In general, a mean arterial
blood pressure

$$\left(\frac{2 \times \text{diastolic} + \text{systolic}}{3}\right)$$

of 130 mm Hg or more or systolic pressure of 180 mm Hg or more may
be treated with intermittent or continuous, intravenous administration of antihypertensive agents such as labetalol or sodium nitroprusside. The most appropriate goal blood pressures are controversial, although a mean arterial blood pressure of 120 mm Hg and a
systolic pressure of 160 mm Hg are reasonable.

Calcium channel blocking agents, such as nimodipine and
nicardipine, appear to have an inhibitory effect on smooth muscle
contraction as well as a separate neuroprotective effect. Nimodipine
reduces the frequency of cerebral infarction and poor outcomes in
aneurysmal SAH and should therefore be administered in a dosage
of 60 mg orally every 4 hours.

In patients with **confirmed symptomatic vasospasm,** despite
the described preventive measures, **blood volume expansion** is
indicated and may be accomplished by the administration of albumin solution (for instance, 5% albumin, 250 ml 4–6 times daily), colloid, or packed erythrocytes. Central venous pressures should be
maintained between 8 and 12 mm Hg, capillary wedge pressures
between 16 and 20 mm Hg, and the hematocrit value around 40%. If
treatment with calcium channel blocking agents has not already
been started, it should be instituted (nimodipine, 60 mg, orally every
6 hours or nicardipine, 0.01–0.15 mg/kg/hour, intravenously) and
continued for 10 to 21 days. If these measures are ineffective, pressor
agents such as dopamine (starting at 3–6 μg/kg/minute and titrating
based on blood pressure response) or phenylephrine are sometimes
given while maintaining the systolic blood pressure at or less than a
value of approximately 20 to 50 mm Hg above baseline.

Monitoring of cardiac output and serial transcranial Doppler ultrasonographic examinations are often helpful for following patients. If

clinically significant vasospasm persists despite the described measures, balloon angioplasty or intra-arterial injection of a vasodilator, such as papaverine, can be considered in centers with experience in these techniques, preferably in the setting of an ongoing randomized controlled trial because the efficacy and safety of these techniques have not been well established.

After clipping of the ruptured aneurysm, intrathecal injections of tissue-type plasminogen activator may hasten clot removal. The efficacy of this approach for preventing vasospasm and delayed ischemic deficit is being evaluated.

Acute Hydrocephalus

Subarachnoid blood may lead to ventricular enlargement and obstructive hydrocephalus. **Acute hydrocephalus** occurs in approximately 20% of patients with SAH, often presenting with either obtundation at the time of admission or increasing drowsiness within a few days of the SAH after an initial recovery. Paralysis of upward gaze and pupillary abnormalities may also be present. The diagnosis is confirmed by CT.

In patients who have small-to-moderate amounts of subarachnoid blood and who stabilize and remain alert, an attempt at **conservative management** is reasonable because approximately half these patients improve spontaneously without further intervention. In patients with neurologic impairment or deterioration resulting from the hydrocephalus, **neurosurgical intervention** should be urgently considered; this usually includes placement of an external ventricular drain. The amount of cerebrospinal fluid drainage should be carefully monitored because excessive decompression may be associated with rebleeding of an underlying aneurysm.

Seizures

Approximately 3% to 5% of patients with SAH have associated **seizures**. A single initial seizure at the time of hemorrhage does not predict the likelihood of future seizures, but patients with associated intracerebral hemorrhage are more likely to have early seizures. Patients with early seizures are usually treated with intravenously administered diazepam (5–10 mg at a rate as high as 2 mg/minute, which may be repeated once in 5–15 minutes), followed by an intravenous or oral loading dose of phenytoin in normal saline (15–20 mg/kg at a rate as high as 50 mg/minute), fosphenytoin (see p. 162), or phenobarbital (20 mg/kg at a rate as high as 100 mg). Electrocardiographic and blood pressure monitoring should be used during and after acute administration. Phenytoin, fosphenytoin, or phenobarbital may be used for maintenance therapy.

PREVENTION AND MANAGEMENT OF NONNEUROLOGIC COMPLICATIONS

Various systemic complications arise in patients with SAH, the identification and treatment of which may substantially alter long- and short-term outcomes.

Hyponatremia

By far the most common electrolyte disturbance associated with SAH is **hyponatremia,** which is present to some extent in up to 30%

Table 14-5. Management of hyponatremia

1. Avoid overhydration with hypotonic fluids
2. Look for evidence of salt-wasting syndrome or syndrome of inappropriate antidiuretic hormone (SIADH)
3. If salt-wasting syndrome is associated with hypovolemia, give isotonic saline, Ringer's lactate, or colloid to correct hyponatremia
4. If SIADH is present, manage with fluid restriction (<1 liter/day) and furosemide (40 mg/day) or demeclocycline (300–600 mg, PO, twice a day)
5. Consider adding fludrocortisone acetate (1 mg twice a day)
6. In rare instances of symptomatic, severe hyponatremia (<120 mEq/liter), consider infusion of 3% saline at rate of 25–50 ml/hr
7. Avoid excessively rapid correction or overcorrection of sodium levels (≤20 mEq/liter during 24 hr or 1.5–2 mEq/liter/hr)

to 35% of cases and to a severe extent in approximately 5% of cases. Clinical manifestations including minor alterations in level of consciousness, seizures, asterixis, and coma usually do not develop until the sodium value is 120 mmol/liter or less. Hyponatremia usually develops between 2 and 10 days after SAH.

Treatment of the hyponatremia is based on identification of the underlying mechanism of the disorder, which may vary from patient to patient. Most cases of mild hyponatremia associated with SAH are the result of overhydration with hypotonic fluids and may be corrected by switching to smaller amounts of isotonic fluids without major manipulations in therapy (Table 14-5).

In many patients with substantial hyponatremia after SAH, the underlying cause is a **salt-wasting syndrome.** These patients tend to have a negative fluid balance, low central venous and pulmonary wedge pressures, decreasing weight, negative sodium balance, and excessive natriuresis. In these patients, hyponatremia is best corrected with isotonic saline, Ringer's lactate, or colloid while keeping the central venous pressure between 8 and 12 mm Hg. It may also be helpful to use fludrocortisone acetate (1 mg twice a day) to help reduce or eliminate a negative sodium balance.

Patients with hyponatremia caused by the **syndrome of inappropriate antidiuretic hormone (SIADH)** have a stable or positive fluid balance with normal-to-high central venous and pulmonary wedge pressures and stable to increasing body weight. These patients also have increased urine sodium and osmolality levels. For patients with SIADH, treatment usually involves fluid restriction (<1 liter/day) and a loop diuretic such as furosemide (40 mg/day) or a drug that inhibits the ability of ADH to increase water reabsorption, such as demeclocycline (300–600 mg twice daily).

Regardless of the cause of the hyponatremia, it is generally advised that the abnormality be corrected slowly, not exceeding 20 mEq/liter within 24 hours or 1.5 to 2 mEq/liter/hour. In rare cases of severe, symptomatic hyponatremia and a sodium level less than 120 mEq/liter, it is necessary to administer a 3% saline solution (25–50 ml/hour) with or without a loop diuretic to increase the plasma sodium concentration by approximately 10%.

Cardiac Dysfunction

SAH is also associated with various **cardiac arrhythmias** and other electrocardiographic changes resulting from **myocardial ischemia, infarction,** or other mechanical damage. Patients with known or suspected cardiac arrhythmias, other ongoing cardiac dysfunction, a history of cardiac disease, or intracranial hemorrhages causing significant or progressive neurologic deficits should be considered for continuous cardiac monitoring.

The treatment of cardiac ventricular arrhythmia often involves beta-adrenergic blocking agents such as propranolol. Intravenously administered antiarrhythmic agents may be required in cases of malignant arrhythmias or those uncontrolled by oral agents. However, one must be careful because of the propensity of these agents to decrease blood pressure. Life-threatening arrhythmias, such as ventricular fibrillation, are rare and usually of short duration. Patients with arrhythmias require ongoing cardiac monitoring and should be questioned daily about the occurrence of chest pain and dyspnea.

Other Nonneurologic Complications

Another less common complication of SAH is **neurogenic pulmonary edema,** which may present with sudden or subacute onset of dyspnea, cyanosis, and pink, frothy sputum. Treatment usually involves positive end-expiratory pressure ventilation and diuretics.

The most common **acid-base disorders** associated with SAH are **metabolic alkalosis and respiratory alkalosis,** the former caused by excessive vomiting, diuretics, and bicarbonate administration and the latter caused by hyperventilation. Potassium depletion is common in patients with metabolic acidosis and requires replacement with potassium chloride.

Adequate **nutrition** is important and is often accomplished by means of a nasogastric tube for patients who cannot be fed orally because of a decreased level of consciousness or impaired gag reflex. The caloric intake should be maintained at approximately 2000 to 3000 calories/day, or more in the setting of fever. Enteric feeding can be accomplished with various commercially available preparations (Ensure, Ensure Plus), which are usually given at half strength or full strength and better tolerated with a continuous-infusion feeding pump, if available. To avoid **aspiration,** patients are usually fed with head elevated 30 degrees; hourly checks should be made for gastric residue. For intubated patients, the endotracheal cuff should be inflated during feeding. Oral medications may be crushed and given through the enteral tube.

Prophylaxis for **deep vein thrombosis and pulmonary embolism** can be accomplished by intermittent pneumatic compression devices applied to the legs, compression stockings, or mild range-of-motion foot exercises for patients who are awake and alert.

15

Intracerebral Hemorrhage: General Evaluation and Treatment

As noted in Chapter 1, patients with **intracerebral (intraparenchymal) hemorrhage** typically present with relatively abrupt onset of focal neurologic symptoms and signs that may be associated with early decreased level of alertness, headache, nausea, and vomiting. In patients with this abrupt onset of symptoms, clinically suspected intracranial hemorrhage should prompt urgent computed tomography (CT) or magnetic resonance imaging (MRI) to determine the location and size of the hemorrhage (Fig. 15-1) and possibly to reveal other intracranial disease processes (see algorithm for management of intracerebral hemorrhage in Appendix J-5). The location of the hemorrhage may guide further evaluation necessary to define the mechanism. In addition to the five main locations for **intracranial hemorrhage** outlined in Chapter 8, the specific location of an intracerebral (intraparenchymal) hemorrhage may further define the likely mechanism of the hemorrhage.

Lobar intracerebral hemorrhages are characterized by bleeding into the cortex or subcortical white matter. Common features at the onset include vomiting and localized headache (frontal hemorrhage usually afflicts the forehead area; temporal hemorrhage, the area around or anterior to the ipsilateral ear; parietal hemorrhage, the temple area; and occipital hemorrhage, the area around or over the ipsilateral eye).

In lobar intracerebral hemorrhages, unlike deep supratentorial hemorrhages, the neurologic deficits are often more restricted and variable (frontal hematoma usually produces contralateral arm weakness; left temporal hematoma, aphasia, and delirium; parietal hematoma, contralateral hemisensory loss; and occipital hematoma, contralateral homonymous hemianopia). Disturbances of the level of consciousness occur later in the clinical course, and a history of hypertension is less frequent. The neurologic deficit appears rapidly, within one to several minutes, but not instantaneously as it usually does with an embolus. Stiff neck or seizures at the onset are uncommon, and more than half the patients are drowsy. However, a large lobar hemorrhage may affect two or more lobes and may produce stupor or coma associated with severe neurologic deficit.

Most patients with **lobar hematoma** require further evaluation with arteriography because of the potential for underlying intracranial aneurysm or arteriovenous malformation (AVM). If aneurysm or AVM is highly suspected, arteriography is necessary; if aneurysm is not detected, MRI with gadolinium may further clarify a cause for the hemorrhage. Underlying neoplasm, arteriographically occult vascular malformation, bleeding diathesis, anticoagulant use, and amyloid angiopathy are other primary considerations for hemorrhage at that site. Magnetic resonance angiography (MRA) and MRI may aid in revealing an underlying cause, including aneurysm, AVM or other vascular malformation, neoplasm, or multiple infarcts con-

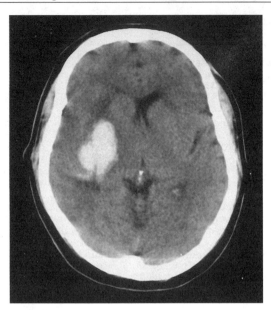

Fig. 15-1.   CT scan of head without contrast: right basal ganglia hemorrhage.

sistent with an inflammatory vascular disorder. Although surgical therapy is reasonable in certain cases of lobar hemorrhage, medical treatment alone results in a good recovery in most patients.

Supratentorial deep hemorrhages into the basal ganglia and internal capsule are usually characterized by sudden onset of headache followed by acute or subacute (as long as 48 hours) loss of consciousness associated with contralateral hemiparesis, hemisensory loss, homonymous hemianopia, and, if the dominant hemisphere is involved, aphasia. Vomiting is common. In comatose patients, signs of uncal herniation (ipsilateral third cranial nerve palsy) or upper brain stem compression may appear (deep, irregular, or intermittent respiration, ipsilaterally dilated and fixed pupil, and decerebrate posturing).

The presence of upward gaze palsy with unreactive miotic pupils, sometimes associated with convergence paralysis, is characteristic of **thalamic hemorrhage** and helps to differentiate it from putaminal hemorrhage. Besides characteristic oculomotor abnormalities, thalamic hemorrhage often produces contralateral eye deviation, aphasia (dominant hemisphere involvement), neglect (nondominant hemisphere involvement), unilateral hemiplegia or hemiparesis, and unusual sensory syndromes (distressing dysesthesias and spontaneous pain occurring with a latency of days to weeks from onset).

In **putaminal hemorrhage**, the eyes are conjugately deviated to the side of the lesion, the pupillary size and reactivity are normal unless uncal herniation has occurred, and focal neurologic signs (dense, flaccid hemiplegia or hemiparesis, hemisensory loss, homonymous hemianopia, global aphasia [dominant hemisphere involvement], or hemi-inattention [nondominant hemisphere involvement]) and level of consciousness tend to gradually worsen within minutes to hours.

Caudate hemorrhages are characterized by headache, nausea, vomiting, and various types of behavioral abnormalities (such as disorientation or confusion), occasionally accompanied by a prominent short-term memory loss, transient gaze paresis, and contralateral hemiparesis without language disorders.

Basal ganglia hemorrhage is typically caused by chronic hypertension with associated lipohyalinosis and Charcot-Bouchard aneurysms in the small, perforating vasculature. In the presence of chronic hypertension, MRI with gadolinium may be performed to be certain that there is no underlying neoplasm, vascular malformation, or alternative cause. If there is no history of hypertension, it is more likely that an underlying neoplasm, vascular malformation, or other cause is present, and further evaluation with MRI is indicated. Hematomas in the putamen with signs of deterioration or progressive neurologic deficit are usually amenable to surgical therapy; those in the thalamus and caudate are rarely operable. If the deficit is stable, hemorrhage into these subcortical locations is typically treated medically.

Primary brain stem hemorrhage usually occurs in the **pons** and results in early coma, quadriplegia, prominent decerebrate rigidity, pinpoint (1 mm) pupils that react to light, and the locked-in-syndrome with some persistent ability to move the eyelids and eyes up and down. The eyes are often in midposition and have an impaired or absent response to caloric tests. Hyperpnea, hyperhidrosis, and hyperthermia are common. Primary **midbrain and medullary hemorrhages** are rare. When midbrain hemorrhage occurs, it often results in homolateral oculomotor paralysis with crossed hemiplegia (Weber's syndrome). If the hemorrhage enlarges, quadriplegia and coma often occur. Medullary hemorrhage usually produces early coma and rapid death.

Cerebellar hemorrhage usually develops in one of the cerebellar hemispheres (origination in the region of the dentate nucleus is common) within a period of several hours; loss of consciousness at the onset is uncommon. Repeated vomiting, nausea, severe occipital headache, and vertigo with inability to walk or stand (dysequilibrium, limb ataxia) are common early features. Often, the following signs or symptoms occur: mild peripheral facial palsy, dizziness, nystagmus, miosis, decreased corneal reflex, paresis of conjugate lateral gaze of the eyes to the side of the hemorrhage, forced deviation of the eyes to the side opposite the lesion, or an ipsilateral abducens palsy, which indicates both cerebellar and pontine dysfunction (hemiplegia usually does not occur).

Pontine and cerebellar hemorrhage are also commonly a result of chronic hypertension. If the patient does not have a history of hypertension, MRI of the head with gadolinium should be performed. If a vascular malformation or other vascular lesion is suggested on the scan, arteriography may need to be performed to clarify an underlying AVM. Hematomas in the brain stem are usually inoperable, but evacuation is occasionally attempted when there is evidence for neurologic deterioration in an otherwise healthy patient with a good life expectancy.

Because moderate-to-large cerebellar hematomas (2–3 cm or more in diameter) often lead to a life-threatening, downhill course with unpredictable deterioration caused by brain stem compression, it is important to monitor patients closely and to remove the hematoma before compression causes alteration in the level of consciousness and an unstable clinical situation. Often, immediate surgical intervention is indicated. However, alert patients with smaller lesions who have no signs of brain stem compression may be treated medically under close observation in the neurologic intensive care unit. The same treatment approach applies to a patient with a stable neurologic course and unimpaired consciousness who is seen later than 1 week after the cerebellar hemorrhage. However, once a patient shows signs of brain stem compression or deterioration, such as a diminution in the level of consciousness, immediate evacuation of the clot is indicated as a potentially lifesaving treatment, even if the patient is in a deep coma.

Patients with **subarachnoid and intracerebral hemorrhage** are likely to have an underlying structural abnormality, such as a saccular aneurysm, and should have cerebral arteriography. Lumbar puncture should not be performed in patients suspected of having intracerebral hemorrhage because CT or MRI yields much more information; lumbar puncture, in the presence of a central nervous system mass lesion, may lead to herniation.

Other laboratory tests are usually performed (as listed for subarachnoid hemorrhage in Table 14-1) to further assess for underlying causes of the hemorrhage and associated complications. In severely impaired patients, the laboratory evaluation is usually not extensive because 80% to 90% of such patients have a progressive and ultimately fatal clinical course. Specific treatment options relating to identified underlying causes are discussed in Chapter 17.

Surgical Interventions

After initial medical and neurologic stabilization of the patient (see Chapter 11), the first general treatment consideration involves whether to undertake surgical intervention. A decision regarding immediate surgical intervention should be made on the basis of the size and location of the hemorrhage and the condition of the patient (see Appendix J-5).

In general, when clinical and computed tomography criteria are considered in combination, **three categories** of patients emerge:

1. those who have a profound neurologic deficit with associated brain stem involvement and a large hemorrhage noted on CT
2. those who have a focal neurologic deficit with little or no evidence of brain stem compression or increased intracranial pressure and a small, well-localized hemorrhage on CT
3. those who have a focal deficit referable to their hemorrhage with minimal-to-mild signs of brain stem dysfunction but a moderate-to-large lesion on CT

Patients in the **first category** have a nearly uniform fatal course and, with the exception of patients with cerebellar hematomas, are generally not considered to be surgical candidates. The few patients who survive the initial days of their illness and who show stabilization and improvement with supportive medical treatment may be considered for surgical evacuation of the hemorrhage.

Patients in the **second category** are treated medically with appropriate attention to ventilation, fluid intake, electrolyte balance, and blood pressure, as delineated below. Most patients in this category stabilize, and their neurologic deficit improves without surgical intervention.

Patients in the **third category** frequently have progressive deterioration and worsening during their clinical course and therefore should be considered for surgical therapy.

The location of the lesion is also an important determinant in the decision regarding surgical evacuation of the hematoma. Patients in the third group, and even in the first group, with **cerebellar hemorrhage**s and evidence of brain stem compression or deterioration usually have an operation as soon as the anatomic diagnosis is established. Patients in the third group with **laterally situated lobar hemispheric lesions** are also good surgical candidates and are also usually operated on as soon as the diagnosis is established. Patients with **supratentorial deep hemorrhage** (often with intraventricular extension) are less frequently considered to be operative candidates. Some patients with supratentorial deep hemorrhage in the third group undergo surgical evacuation, and although occasional dramatic results are noted, most do not survive or are left with severe, persistent deficits. Patients with **primary brain stem hemorrhage** usually have a devastating course and are seldom operative candidates.

Medical Treatment

INTRACRANIAL PRESSURE AND CEREBRAL EDEMA

The medical management of patients with intracerebral hemorrhage (Table 15-1) often includes measures to decrease **cerebral edema** and **intracranial pressure,** as described in Chapter 11. In addition to osmotherapy with mannitol or glycerol and corticosteroids in the form of dexamethasone, many patients are hyperventilated in an attempt to decrease intracranial pressure.

BLOOD PRESSURE

It is important to stabilize and control blood pressure in patients with intracerebral hemorrhage. As seen with subarachnoid hemorrhage, blood pressure is often increased, at least partly in response to increased intracranial pressure. Unlike subarachnoid hemorrhage, isolated intracerebral hemorrhage does not have the same propensity to induce cerebral vasospasm; consequently, the lowering of blood pressure can be somewhat more aggressive without undue concern about precipitating vasospasm. However, substantial overcorrection could result in decreased cerebral perfusion.

**Table 15-1.   General principles of caring
for patients with intracerebral hemorrhage**

1. Place patient on bed rest in quiet room
2. Provide ongoing monitoring of neurologic status (level of consciousness, focal deficit, Glasgow Coma Scale)
3. Consider cardiac monitoring
4. Elevate head of bed 30 degrees
5. Prevent straining (stool softeners and antitussive agents as needed)
6. Provide oral nutrition for alert patients with intact gag reflex
7. Provide enteral nutrition with nasogastric tube for patients with decreased level of consciousness or impaired gag reflex
8. Maintain normovolemia and normal sodium level by starting with administration of 2–3 liters/day of D_5W and 0.9 normal saline and adjusting accordingly (see Table 14-5 and pages 168–169)
9. Mildly sedate patient if agitated: phenobarbital (30–60 mg 2 times a day) or chloral hydrate (500 mg 3 times a day)
10. Control mild pain with acetaminophen or propoxyphene and severe pain with codeine (60 mg, IM or PO, every 3–4 hr); use morphine (1- to 2-mg increments, IV) only as last resort
11. Reduce blood pressure conservatively and with careful monitoring if patient has extremely increased blood pressure or evidence of acute end-organ damage
12. Treat increased intracranial pressure as needed (see Table 11-1 and pages 139–141)

Target blood pressure in this situation is usually about 150/90 mm Hg. Pressures much higher than this can be controlled with a sodium nitroprusside drip titrated to the desired level or labetolol given intravenously (see Chapter 11). The intravenous infusion subsequently can be tapered in conjunction with intravenous or oral medication, including centrally acting adrenergic agents such as methyldopa, beta-adrenergic antagonists such as propranolol, labetalol, or metoprolol, calcium channel blockers such as nifedipine, or angiotensin-converting enzyme inhibitors.

In some patients, hypotension is a problem, and this can be controlled by a constant infusion of dopamine (starting at 3–6 µg/kg/minute and titrating based on blood pressure response) or phenylephrine to reach target levels of 120 to 140/80 to 90 mm Hg.

ANTICONVULSANTS

Patients with evidence of seizure activity are treated with anticonvulsants. Patients with ongoing seizures are usually treated with intravenously administered diazepam (5–10 mg, at a rate as high as 2 mg/minute, which may be repeated once in 5–15 minutes) or lorazepam followed by a loading dose of phenytoin given orally (15–20 mg/kg, given in a single dose, or split in three doses given every 8 hours) or intravenously administered phenytoin dissolved in normal saline (15–20 mg/kg, at a rate as high as 50 mg/minute), fosphenytoin (see p. 162), or phenobarbital (20 mg/kg at a rate as high as 100 mg/minute). Maintenance therapy with phenytoin or fosphenytoin can be given either orally through a nasogastric tube or intravenously. Most patients with lobar hematomas are treated prophylactically with phenytoin or phenobarbital.

OTHER GENERAL CARE

Patients with intracerebral hemorrhage require **close observation,** particularly those who have signs of intracranial pressure, high blood pressure, or brain stem compression soon after the onset of hemorrhage. This is best accomplished in an **intensive care unit** with a nursing staff experienced in performing serial neurologic assessments, including assessment of level of consciousness and focal deficits, and a standardized coma scale such as the Glasgow Coma Scale (see Appendix B).

The patient should be kept on **bed rest** until neurologically and medically stable and alert for 24 to 48 hours.

Most patients require an **indwelling urinary catheter** or intermittent catheterization every 4 to 6 hours, and all patients require careful assessment of **fluid balance** and **daily weights.**

The clinician should be alert to the possibility of serious **cardiac arrhythmias,** such as ventricular tachycardia and severe bradycardia. Patients with preexisting cardiac disease and those with hemorrhages causing significant or progressive clinical deficits should be monitored with a continuous cardiac monitoring system.

Nutrition should be provided orally if the patient is alert and has a normal gag reflex. Otherwise, feeding should be accomplished by means of a nasogastric tube. Caloric intake should be approximately 2000 to 3000 calories/day, or more if the patient is febrile. Feeding is usually begun with a full liquid diet or with a liquid feeding system (Ensure, Ensure Plus), as described in Chapter 11.

Prevention of deep vein thrombosis and pulmonary emboli is assisted by the use of lower-extremity intermittent pneumatic compression devices, compression stockings, and range-of-motion exercises.

Pain control is accomplished with acetaminophen or propoxyphene. Salicylates and nonsteroidal anti-inflammatory drugs should be avoided, as for other types of intracranial hemorrhage, because of their inhibitory effect on coagulation. More severe pain can be controlled with codeine, 60 mg orally or intravenously every 4 to 6 hours. **Agitation** is controlled with phenobarbital, 30 to 60 mg twice a day, or chloral hydrate, 500 mg three times a day, but the clinician must be careful not to oversedate the patient. **Nausea and vomiting** are controlled with prochlorperazine, 10 mg intramuscularly or orally every 4 to 6 hours as needed.

Skin care is also important in the general care of patients with intracerebral hemorrhage, particularly those who are not alert. Patients should be turned at least once each hour, and their skin should be kept dry and powdered and be regularly inspected for erythema.

Suggested Reading for Part III

Adams HP Jr, Brott TG, Crowell RM, et al: Guidelines for the management of patients with acute ischemic stroke: A statement for healthcare professionals from a special writing group of the Stroke Council, American Heart Association. Stroke 25:1901–1914, 1994.

The American Nimodipine Study Group: Clinical trial of nimodipine in acute ischemic stroke. Stroke 23:3–8, 1992.

Anderson DC, Bottini AG, Jagiella WM, et al: The pilot study of hyperbaric oxygen in the treatment of human stroke. Stroke 22:1137–1142, 1991.

Arron MJ, McDermott MM, Dolan N, et al: Management of medical complications associated with stroke. Heart Dis Stroke 3:103–109, 1994.

Asplund K: Hemodilution in acute stroke. Cerebrovasc Dis 1(Suppl 1): 129–138, 1991.

Axelsson K, Asplund K, Norberg A, et al: Nutritional status in patients with acute stroke. Acta Med Scand 224:217–224, 1988.

Bayer AJ, Pathy MS, Newcombe R: Double-blind randomised trial of intravenous glycerol in acute stroke. Lancet 1:405–408, 1987.

Borges LF: Management of nontraumatic brain hemorrhage. In Ropper AH, ed. Neurological and Neurosurgical Intensive Care (3rd ed). New York; Raven, 1993, pp 279–289.

Bounds JV, Wiebers DO, Whisnant JP, et al: Mechanisms and timing of deaths from cerebral infarction. Stroke 12:474–477, 1981.

Brott T: Prevention and management of medical complications of the hospitalized elderly stroke patient. Clin Geriatr Med 7:475–482, 1991.

Brott T: Urgent evaluation and management of stroke. In: Adams HP, ed. Handbook of Cerebrovascular Diseases. New York: Marcel Dekker, 1993, pp 385–400.

Brott T, Reed RL: Intensive care for acute stroke in the community hospital setting: The first 24 hours. Stroke 20:694–697, 1989.

Caplan LR: Anticoagulation for cerebral ischemia. Clin Neuropharmacol 9:399–414, 1986.

Clagget GP, Salzman EW, Wheeler HB, et al: Prevention of venous thromboembolism. Chest 102 (Suppl):391S–407S, 1992.

Coletta EM, Murphy JB: The complications of immobility in the elderly stroke patient. J Am Board Fam Pract 5:389–397, 1992.

Delashaw JB, Broaddus WC, Kassell NF, et al: Treatment of right hemispheric cerebral infarction by hemicraniectomy. Stroke 21:874–881, 1990.

Dromerick A, Reding M: Medical and neurological complications during inpatient stroke rehabilitation. Stroke 25:358–361, 1994.

Dyken ML: Overview of trends in management and prognosis of stroke. Ann Epidemiol 3:535–540, 1993.

Emergency Cardiac Care Committee and Subcommittees, American Heart Association: Guidelines for cardiopulmonary resuscitation and emergency cardiac care. Part IV. Special resuscitation situations. JAMA 268:2242–2250, 1992.

Fieschi C, Argentino C, Lenzi GL, et al: Clinical and instrumental evaluation of patients with ischemic stroke within the first six hours. J Neurol Sci 91:311–321, 1989.

Gelmers HJ, Gorter K, de Weerdt CJ, et al: A controlled trial of nimodipine in acute ischemic stroke. N Engl J Med 318:203–207, 1988.

Gelmers HJ, Hennerici M: Effect of nimodipine on acute ischemic stroke:

pooled results from five randomized trials. Stroke 12(Suppl 21):IV81–IV84, 1990.

Gladman JR, Lomas S, Lincoln NB: Provision of physiotherapy and occupational therapy in outpatient departments and day hospitals for stroke patients in Nottingham. Int Disabil Stud 13:38–41, 1991.

Haley EC Jr, Brott TG, Sheppard GL, et al: Pilot randomized trial of tissue plasminogen activator in acute ischemic stroke. The TPA Bridging Study Group. Stroke 24:1000–1004, 1993.

Horner J, Brazer SR, Massey EW: Aspiration in bilateral stroke patients: A validation study. Neurology 43:430–433, 1993.

Kay R, Wong KS, Yu YL, et al: Low-molecular-weight heparin for the treatment of acute ischemic stroke. N Engl J Med 333:1588–1593, 1995.

Kelley RE: Cerebrovascular disorders. In: Weiner WJ, ed. Emergent and Urgent Neurology. Philadelphia: Lippincott, 1992, pp 79–107.

Kilpatrick CJ, Davis SM, Tress BM, et al: Epileptic seizures in acute stroke. Arch Neurol 47:157–160, 1990.

Leahy NM: Complications in the acute stages of stroke: Nursing's pivotal role. Nurs Clin North Am 26:971–983, 1991.

Levine SR: Acute cerebral ischemia in a critical care unit: A review of diagnosis and management. Arch Intern Med 149:90–98, 1989.

Lewis SL, Topel JL: Coma. In: Weiner WJ, ed. Emergent and Urgent Neurology. Philadelphia: Lippincott, 1992, pp 1–25.

Lisk DR, Grotta JC, Lamki LM, et al: Should hypertension be treated after acute stroke? A randomized controlled trial using single photon emission computed tomography. Arch Neurol 50:855–862, 1993.

Marler JR, Brott T, Broderick J, et al: Tissue plasminogen activator for acute ischemic stroke. N Engl J Med 333:1581–1587, 1995.

Olinger CP, Adams HP Jr, Brott TG, et al: High-dose intravenous naloxone for the treatment of acute ischemic stroke. Stroke 21:721–725, 1990.

Patel RV, Kertland HR, Jahns BE, et al: Labetalol: Response and safety in critically ill hemorrhagic stroke patients. Ann Pharmacother 27:180–181, 1993.

Prins MH, Gelsema R, Sing AK, et al: Prophylaxis of deep venous thrombosis with a low-molecular-weight heparin (Kabi 2165/Fragmin) in stroke patients. Haemostasis 19:245–250, 1989.

Rieke K, Krieger D, Adams HP, et al: Therapeutic strategies in a space-occupying cerebellar infarction based on clinical, neuroradiological and neurophysiological data. Cerebrovasc Dis 3:45–55, 1993.

Rosenbaum D, Zabramski J, Frey J, et al: Early treatment of ischemic stroke with a calcium antagonist. Stroke 22:437–441, 1991.

Siesjo BK: Calcium and ischemic brain damage. Eur Neurol 1(Suppl 25):45–56, 1986.

Stern BJ: Outpatient care of the stroke patient. Semin Neurol 7:352–360, 1987.

Stone SP, Whincup P: Standards for the hospital management of stroke patients. J R Coll Physicians Lond 28:52–58, 1994.

Trust Study Group: Randomised, double-blind, placebo-controlled trial of nimodipine in acute stroke. Lancet 336:1205–1209, 1990.

Villanueva P: Intensive care unit monitoring. In: Andrews BT, ed. Neurosurgical Intensive Care. New York: McGraw-Hill, 1993, pp 43–55.

Wade DT: Stroke: Rehabilitation and long-term care. Lancet 339:791–793, 1992.

Wagner JH: Neurologic Disorders of Ambulatory Patients. Philadelphia: Lea & Febiger, 1989.

Wechsler LR, Koroshetz W: Therapy for acute ischemic stroke. In: Ropper AH, ed. Neurological and Neurosurgical Intensive Care (3rd ed). New York: Raven, 1993, pp 265–278.

Wiebers DO: Intracranial aneurysm. Curr Ther Neurol Dis 3:192–194, 1990.

IV

Medical and Surgical Management Based on Specific Mechanisms of Cerebrovascular Disease

Whenever possible, management of a patient is based on precise definition of the underlying pathophysiologic mechanism for the cerebrovascular condition. After general medical and neurologic examinations, certain diagnostic studies are usually performed to help identify the underlying pathophysiologic mechanism for the cerebrovascular symptoms. If the responsible pathophysiologic mechanism can be identified, appropriate treatment is established. One way of categorizing the various **ischemic pathophysiologic mechanisms** is by four major groupings, progressing from proximal to distal in the vascular system, as follows: (1) cardiac disease, (2) large vessel disease, (3) small vessel disease, and (4) hematologic disease. **Hemorrhagic mechanisms** can be categorized best according to location of the hemorrhage.

Four Major Categories of Ischemic Cerebrovascular Disease: Identification and Treatment

Cardiac Disease

Cerebrovascular conditions resulting from cardiac disorders include cerebral infarction, transient ischemic attack (TIA), syncope, and global anoxia. Heart disease may produce cerebral ischemic symptoms by means of several mechanisms. It is useful to group these into

1. disturbances associated with **pump failure** resulting in generalized cerebral ischemia (syncope) or infarction (anoxic encephalopathy)
2. conditions that more frequently predispose to **thromboembolism** associated with focal cerebral ischemic events

Disturbances associated with pump failure consist primarily of cardiac arrhythmias, including cardiac arrest and congestive heart failure. **Embolic cerebral infarction or TIA** from a cardiac source (Fig. 16-1) may result from any of three basic mechanisms:

1. Generation of embolic fragments from heart valves
2. Production of intracardiac thrombi from local stagnation and endocardial alterations
3. Shunting of systemic venous thrombi into the arterial circulation

Patients with ischemic cerebrovascular disease or retinal ischemic events should be examined for evidence of cardiac rhythm disorders (such as atrial fibrillation and sick sinus syndrome), valvular lesions (such as mitral stenosis, mitral valve prolapse, mitral annular calcification, and subacute bacterial endocarditis), and lesions of the myocardium (such as recent infarction, old infarction with segmental akinesia or aneurysmal dilatation, and cardiomyopathy) (see Table 8-1).

The most common cardiac disorders implicated in cerebrovascular ischemia can be divided into **proven and putative cardiac risks** based on the available epidemiologic and clinical evidence substantiating the role of these disorders in cerebrovascular disease (Table 16-1).

Cardioembolic infarction is the cause of about 20% to 25% of all ischemic strokes. The onset of focal neurologic deficit is typically very sudden and most often maximal at onset, but sometimes the neurologic deficit may be incomplete or may worsen significantly after onset. Focal or generalized seizures tend to occur early after embolic cerebral infarction with cortical involvement but may also commence many months after the acute ischemic episode. Some cases of "idiopathic" epilepsy in the elderly may result from this kind of clinically silent cortical cerebral infarction.

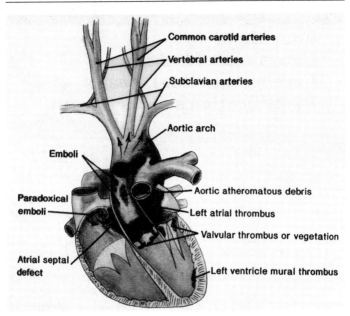

Fig. 16-1. Emboli originating from the heart.

Table 16-1.   Cardiac risks for cerebrovascular ischemia

Proven cardiac risks
    Atrial fibrillation
    Mechanical valve
    Dilated cardiomyopathy
    Recent myocardial infarction
    Intracardiac thrombus
    Intracardiac mass
Putative cardiac risks
    Sick sinus syndrome
    Patent foramen ovale
    Atherosclerotic debris in the thoracic aorta
    Spontaneous echocardiographic contrast
    Myocardial infarction 2–6 mo earlier
    Hypokinetic or akinetic left ventricular segment
    Calcification of mitral annulus

The basis for clinical diagnosis is the demonstration of a cardiac source of embolus or right-to-left shunt with a venous source of emboli and no evidence for other causes of ischemic stroke. Evidence of emboli in other locations such as the retina, kidney, or spleen and multiple cerebral infarctions in different vascular distributions make the diagnosis even more certain. In addition, certain clinical syndromes and radiographic findings may suggest embolism as the underlying mechanism, although they are not specific for an embolic cause.

Most cardioembolic infarcts involve the cortex and are commonly in the distribution of the cortical branches of the middle cerebral artery. They produce symptoms such as unilateral lower facial weakness associated with severe dysphasia; contralateral brachial or hand monoplegia or paresis with or without cortical sensory loss; and relatively isolated Broca's aphasia or motor speech apraxia or Wernicke's aphasia. A sudden, isolated homonymous hemianopia apparent to the patient may occur with a posterior cerebral territory embolus; sudden unilateral foot weakness or incoordination may be caused by an anterior cerebral territory embolus. Cardioembolic ischemic strokes affecting the brain stem are relatively uncommon.

Septic cerebral embolism with bacterial endocarditis often produces a focal neurologic deficit associated with nonfocal symptoms such as confusion, agitation, or delirium caused by tiny septic infarcts with microscopic abscesses. However, depression of consciousness caused by a large arterial embolus may also occur. Computed tomography (CT) or magnetic resonance imaging (MRI) often reveals some degree of hemorrhagic transformation, and multiple brain or systemic infarcts are typically present.

The **differential diagnosis** of embolic ischemic events includes other subtypes of cerebral infarction as well as primary intracerebral hemorrhage, complicated migraine, primary seizure disorders, and functional disorders. Noncardiac causes of cerebral embolism include atherosclerosis of the aorta and craniocervical arteries and, in the presence of right-to-left cardiac shunting, pulmonary or peripheral venous thrombosis, or tumor, fat (after major fractures), or air (after neck or chest injury or operation) emboli.

VALVE-RELATED CEREBRAL EMBOLI

Valve-related cerebral emboli may result from various conditions, including rheumatic heart disease, other aortic and mitral valvular diseases, prosthetic valves, cardiac procedures, and infective and noninfective endocarditis. Cerebral embolization in **rheumatic heart disease** may occur during the acute illness, when inflammatory vegetations on the heart valves may detach and embolize, or, more commonly, during the chronic phase of the disease, when valvular deformity, atrial enlargement, and abnormal cardiac rhythm have developed. The greatest risk of cerebral infarction from chronic rheumatic heart disease occurs within 1 year after the onset of atrial fibrillation. In clinical series, the brain is the site of emboli in roughly 30% of patients, but in autopsy series, nearly 50% of patients show cerebral infarction presumably related to emboli. Mitral stenosis has been present in most of these patients.

Anticoagulation treatment with intravenously administered heparin followed by warfarin anticoagulation or valve repair is recommended for all embolic cerebral events associated with rheumatic heart disease, particularly in patients with an audible murmur or those in whom surgical therapy is to be delayed or cannot be done.

Spontaneous calcium embolization occasionally occurs with **calcific aortic stenosis,** but more commonly such embolization produces symptomatic retinal rather than cerebral ischemia. Cerebral ischemic events unrelated to other recognized risk factors have been noted in patients with **mitral valve prolapse.** The causative role of mitral valve prolapse in stroke has not been defined, and the overall importance is uncertain. Embolic material may arise from the surface of the prolapsed, degenerated mitral valve. In patients with embolic cerebral events associated with mitral valve prolapse, antiplatelet therapy or anticoagulation with warfarin should be considered. **Mitral annulus calcification** is another possible risk factor for cardioembolic events, and this is still under study.

Prosthetic and porcine heart valves are associated with an increased occurrence of cerebral and systemic emboli. The risk is higher with prosthetic valves, and chronic anticoagulation is used in this setting. Even with therapeutic warfarin (International Normalized Ratio, 3.0–4.5), the rate of stroke is 2%–4%/year, and the risk is higher with prosthetic mitral valves than with prosthetic valves. In addition to warfarin, some investigators advocate concurrent use of dipyridamole and cite recent evidence indicating a potential reduction in the risk of stroke.

Cardiac catheterization and arteriography, performed in nearly all patients before cardiac surgery, are associated with a low risk of cerebrovascular complications (approximately 0.2%). Such complications may occur from direct displacement of clot or atheromatous material or from trauma to the arterial intima, which causes subsequent embolization.

Cardiac operation of all types is associated with an increased risk of cerebral ischemia. This may be caused by manipulation leading to clot formation and embolization, nonfocal encephalopathic syndromes caused by either hypotension or anoxia, or multifocal ischemic syndromes caused by embolization of air, fibrin, calcium, or fat globules. Focal ischemic deficits are observed more frequently after valve operations than they are after coronary bypass procedures. Late embolization is a complication of valve replacement and is more common with mitral valve replacement than it is with aortic valve prostheses.

Cerebral embolization occurs in about 20% of patients with **infective endocarditis** and may be the presenting symptom of the disorder. The probability of embolization is highest in patients with mitral valve involvement. Four distinct clinical and pathologic syndromes are observed: (1) focal cerebral infarction (the most common) resulting from embolic occlusion of large arteries, (2) multiple small areas of cerebral infarction producing a diffuse encephalopathy with or without alteration in consciousness, (3) meningitis from small infected emboli lodging in meningeal arteries, and (4) mycotic aneurysm formation resulting from septic embolization with subsequent aneurysmal rupture and intracranial hemorrhage.

Management of patients with **infective endocarditis** includes appropriate antimicrobial therapy, usually guided by culture results. Anticoagulants are not used, at least during the period of active infection, because of the increased risk of hemorrhagic infarction. If mycotic aneurysm is detected on cerebral arteriography, repeat arteriography is necessary after antimicrobial therapy, and surgical intervention may be necessary if an aneurysm persists.

Nonbacterial thrombotic endocarditis, also called marantic endocarditis, usually occurs in cachectic, debilitated elderly patients with some underlying systemic disease, most commonly carcinoma. Pathologically, nonbacterial thrombotic endocarditis vegetations consist of amorphous, acellular material composed of a mixture of fibrin and platelets. Less than half the patients with this condition have heart murmurs. As with infective endocarditis, many patients show signs of diffuse cerebral dysfunction, either alone or in association with recognizable focal deficits.

Although the value of antithrombotic therapy is still undetermined in patients with **marantic (nonbacterial thrombotic) endocarditis**, the use of anticoagulants followed by antiplatelet therapy is usually advised for patients with focal cerebral ischemic events. Disseminated intravascular coagulation, often associated with nonbacterial endocarditis, may independently produce multiple small areas of cerebral infarction.

Noninfectious valvular deposits called **Libman-Sacks endocarditis** may occur in patients with systemic lupus erythematosus. Patients with cerebral or systemic emboli in this context are typically treated with at least short-term warfarin anticoagulation. Therapy is often switched to an antiplatelet agent, especially if serial echocardiographic studies demonstrate lesion resolution.

INTRACARDIAC THROMBI

Atrial fibrillation is the cardiac arrhythmia most frequently associated with embolic brain infarction. In this condition, the atria do not contract effectively, and the resultant stagnation of blood predisposes to intraluminal thrombi. The risk of cerebral embolization increases with longer duration of the dysrhythmia, an enlarged left atrium, previous systemic thromboembolism, history of hypertension or congestive heart failure, and associated valvular heart disease, especially mitral stenosis.

If atrial fibrillation is a **new finding** at the time of presentation with an ischemic event, conversion to normal sinus rhythm with either electrical or chemical cardioversion may be indicated. Conversion of atrial fibrillation to a normal rhythm is associated with a risk of embolization, which often occurs within 48 hours. Anticoagulant therapy should precede conversion, especially in high-risk patients (those with recent or recurrent embolization, cardiac enlargement, heart failure, or associated mitral valve disease).

In patients with **chronic atrial fibrillation,** medical therapy is indicated to prevent systemic embolic events. Long-term oral anticoagulation is recommended (International Normalized Ratio, 2.0–3.0; a lower range of 1.8–2.5 may also be efficacious), except in patients younger than 60 years with no associated cardiovascular disease, including hypertension, recent congestive heart failure, left atrial enlargement, left ventricular dysfunction, or previous thromboembolic events. The recommendation for anticoagulation becomes even stronger for patients who have had focal cerebrovascular ischemic events within the previous 2 years. Aspirin may be a useful prophylactic agent in patients with a contraindication to warfarin or in elderly patients.

Sick sinus syndrome is a common dysrhythmia among the elderly, occurring in 2% to 3% of people older than 75 years. The risk of cerebral ischemia in persons with sick sinus syndrome is controversial. Although some investigators believe this is a relatively benign condition, others have documented an increased risk of cerebral embolism, particularly among those with a bradycardia-tachycardia syndrome.

The most appropriate therapy for primary prevention of stroke in sick sinus syndrome is unknown. Some have advocated dual-chamber pacing, whereas others believe that long-term anticoagulation is necessary. Further study is necessary to better define the risk of stroke and clarify the most efficacious prophylactic treatment approach. In patients with cerebral ischemic events related to sick sinus syndrome, a pacemaker should be implanted.

Patients who experience transient loss of consciousness and syncopal events associated with **other serious rhythm disorders,** such as complete heart block or serious paroxysmal ventricular rhythm disturbances, usually do not require antithrombotic therapy because of the relatively low risk of thromboembolism.

Brain infarction occurs in approximately 2% of patients with **myocardial infarction**. Although systemic hypotension may be responsible for some ischemic brain deficits, clinical and autopsy studies have shown that most focal brain lesions are caused by the formation of mural thrombus and subsequent embolization. Autopsy studies reveal that left ventricular thrombus may occur in up to 44% of patients after myocardial infarction, especially in those with large areas of infarcted tissue and congestive heart failure. If cerebral embolization occurs, it is usually within the first 2 weeks after acute myocardial infarction and may be the presenting symptom. In addition, because a ventricular aneurysm develops as an additional source of thrombus formation in 5% to 20% of patients with myocardial infarction, cerebral events that occur later should be carefully evaluated for a possible cardiac source. In this situation, long-term anticoagulant therapy should be instituted unless contraindications exist. Recent published data indicate that after myocardial infarction, patients receiving warfarin had reduction in recurrent myocardial infarction and cerebrovascular events compared with those treated with placebo. After a patient has had myocardial infarction, anticoagulation should begin with intravenously administered heparin followed by oral anticoagulant therapy (warfarin) alone, and use of heparin may be discontinued when the International Normalized Ratio is therapeutic (2.0–3.0) (see Chapter 12). Although the most efficacious duration of therapy is not known, warfarin therapy is usually continued for several months and then replaced with an antiplatelet agent such as aspirin.

Congestive heart failure is characterized by cardiac enlargement, poor myocardial contractility, and decreased cardiac output that predisposes to blood stagnation and intracardiac thrombi. Any pathologic condition that interferes with cardiac filling or emptying may be associated with congestive heart failure. Although occasionally congestive heart failure is the only identifiable cause of intracardiac or pulmonary venous thrombus formation, other identifiable cardiac disorders, such as myocardial infarction, generalized cardiomyopathy, valvular disease, or arrhythmia, may also contribute to thrombus at these sites.

In patients with focal cerebral ischemic events associated with **cardiomyopathy** in whom the ejection fraction is less than 30% or if definite mural thrombi are seen on echocardiography, anticoagulants are used. Among these patients, as well as in patients with various **congenital heart diseases,** decisions regarding long-term anticoagulant therapy should be considered on an individual basis.

SYSTEMIC VENOUS THROMBI

The foramen ovale is anatomically patent in 15% of persons and retains the functional capacity of patency in an additional 15%. In these situations, venous emboli can enter the cerebral circulation (paradoxical embolism), especially after pulmonary embolization with an associated increase in pulmonary and right atrial pressures. The clinical syndrome is uncommon, but the diagnosis should be suspected in patients with thrombophlebitis or pulmonary embolism in whom acute focal cerebral deficit subsequently develops. Other cardiac deficits producing right-to-left shunts also may cause paradoxical emboli. About 5% of children with cyanotic congenital heart disease have cerebral infarction. In most cases these infarcts are embolic, occurring in the first 2 years of life. Associated hematologic deficits may also predispose these children to cerebral ischemia.

Patients with embolic cerebral infarction or transient ischemic attack resulting from **systemic venous thrombi,** including patients with **interatrial or interventricular septal defects,** should receive warfarin for at least 3 months, even if the primary cardiac disorder is surgically corrected. If the defect is not surgically corrected, chronic therapy with warfarin should be considered. Recurrent embolic cerebrovascular events after cessation of anticoagulation or hemodynamic evidence of pulmonary hypertension indicate the need for longer-term warfarin therapy. If **pulmonary vein thrombosis** is suspected as the cause of a cerebrovascular ischemic event, heparin therapy should be given, followed by warfarin for 3 months.

Approximately 25% of patients with stroke who have a cardioembolic source have another potential cause for the ischemic event. If one of the proven cardiac risks (see Table 16-1) is identified in a patient with an ischemic cerebrovascular event, long-term anticoagulation with warfarin may be needed for prophylaxis even if another potential mechanism for the current ischemic event is identified. In patients with cardioembolic stroke, heparin is typically given in the acute stage, followed by warfarin therapy in nonhypertensive patients with small or moderate strokes. In patients with a small cerebral infarct, use of heparin is usually not delayed, but use of heparin should be delayed in those with a moderate stroke until CT performed 24 to 48 hours after the event reveals no significant hemorrhagic transformation. Anticoagulant therapy may be postponed (a few days to 2 weeks) or not used if the stroke is large or if a patient is severely hypertensive.

Large Vessel Disease

ATHEROSCLEROSIS

The most commonly identified disease process producing retinal or cerebral ischemia is atherosclerosis. Atherosclerosis may produce cerebral symptoms through a hemodynamic or thromboembolic mechanism or both (Fig. 16-2). The lumen of an involved artery may become progressively narrowed and eventually occluded by athero-

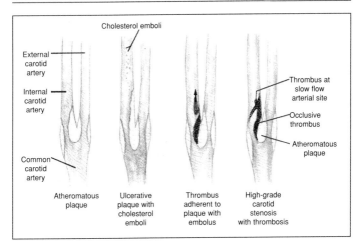

External carotid artery

Internal carotid artery

Common carotid artery

Cholesterol emboli

Thrombus at slow flow arterial site

Occlusive thrombus

Atheromatous plaque

| Atheromatous plaque | Ulcerative plaque with cholesterol emboli | Thrombus adherent to plaque with embolus | High-grade carotid stenosis with thrombosis |

Fig. 16-2. Thrombus formation in atherosclerosis.

sclerotic deposits. Blood flow across the stenotic area becomes impaired when more than 75% of the luminal area becomes compromised. This process usually progresses slowly during years or decades, often allowing time to establish collateral blood flow distal to the lesion. Consequently, not uncommonly, asymptomatic patients have occlusion of one or more major cranial cervical arteries. When collateral circulation distal to the lesion is insufficient, **hemodynamic** compromise occurs and produces symptoms of cerebral ischemia. The terminal branches (watershed areas) of the anterior, middle, and posterior cerebral arteries are most frequently involved.

Thromboembolism is another mechanism whereby atherosclerosis may produce cerebral ischemic symptoms. Atherosclerotic deposits in the process of evolution tend to ulcerate and form necrotic areas capable of attracting blood products, and clot formation results. This atherothrombotic material may either stenose or occlude the vessel lumen, or it may break off to embolize distally in the arterial tree. When either mechanism is combined with systemic factors such as hypotension, hypoxia, anemia, abnormal blood viscosity, and hypoglycemia, focal or multifocal cerebral ischemia may result.

Pathologic changes of atherosclerosis are characterized by focal proliferation of smooth muscle cells within the intima of medium-sized to large arteries and associated deposits of lipids (including cholesterol), blood products, calcium, and fibrous tissue. Although atherosclerosis is usually found diffusely in multiple areas of the body, the primary sources for cerebrovascular symptoms are atherosclerotic deposits, usually localized at cervical artery bifurcations. The most commonly affected areas (Fig. 16-3) in the neck are (1) the proximal portions of the internal carotid arteries and (2) the proximal portions of the vertebral arteries. Intracranially, the circle of Willis and the basilar artery are the areas of maximal involvement. With the increasing use of transesophageal echocardiography, aortic arch atherosclerosis has become recognized as a frequent finding in

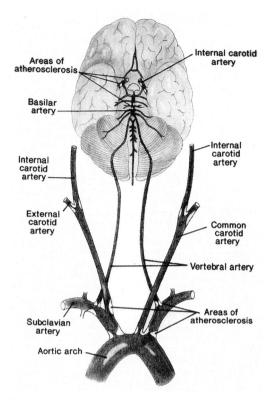

Fig. 16-3. Typical sites for atherosclerosis in the craniocervical arteries.

association with cerebral ischemia. The clinical significance of this finding is still under study.

Epidemiologic studies have identified several factors that seem to contribute to the formation of atherosclerosis. Among these risk factors, cigarette smoking and hypertension are the most clearly implicated. Diabetes mellitus and elevated serum total cholesterol, low-density lipoprotein cholesterol, and triglyceride levels have also been implicated. Atherosclerosis and its complications are especially likely to develop in patients with combinations of these risk factors (see Chapters 23 and 25–27).

Cerebral infarction caused by atherosclerosis is the cause of 15% to 30% of all ischemic strokes, resulting from primary arterial occlusion by atherosclerotic plaque enlargement, thrombus formation at a site of stenosis, or embolism of thrombus or plaque fragments. Artery-to-artery emboli may cause infarcts indistinguishable from cardiac embolic infarcts.

Extracranial vertebral artery occlusive disease resulting from atherosclerosis or other etiologies uncommonly causes brain stem or posterior circulation strokes because of compensatory flow from the contralateral vertebral artery or rostral cervical arteries and retrograde flow down the basilar artery from the carotid-posterior communicating artery system. More often atherosclerosis causes a syndrome of vertebrobasilar insufficiency or may result in TIAs, including symptoms such as dizziness, presyncopal sensation, blurred vision, diplopia, vertigo, dysarthria, extremity weakness, incoordination, sensory loss, facial weakness or loss of sensation, and imbalance.

A history of TIAs and cervical bruit is more frequent in patients with atherothrombotic infarction than it is in those with other types of stroke. In addition to atherosclerosis, causes of craniocervical occlusive disease with associated thrombosis include arteritis; hematologic disorders; carotid, vertebrobasilar, or cerebral arterial dissection; and systemic or central nervous system (CNS) infections (see Table 8-1). Many patients with thrombotic infarction have sudden or stepwise (stuttering) onset of their neurologic deficits. The clinical diagnosis is established by evidence of arterial stenosis or occlusion at one or more sites (see Chapters 12 and 13).

Laboratory evaluation of patients with possible atherosclerotic carotid artery occlusive disease must include tests that define the presence, location, and severity of the lesion. The evaluation approach for patients with TIA and ischemic stroke is outlined in Chapters 12 and 13. Initial noninvasive screening for the presence of "pressure-significant" or "hemodynamically significant" stenoses in the carotid system is usually done with oculopneumoplethysmography or carotid ultrasonographic/duplex studies. The ultrasonographic/duplex studies are more widely used and available, but oculopneumoplethysmography may be more cost effective and reproducible. Other studies that further define the location and severity of carotid lesions include magnetic resonance angiography (MRA) and cerebral arteriography. Intracranial arterial lesions may be identified by transcranial Doppler ultrasonography, MRA, and cerebral arteriography. Ophthalmic and intracranial carotid artery hemodynamics may be evaluated with oculopneumoplethysmography and transcranial Doppler ultrasonography.

If an appropriate, surgically correctable atherosclerotic lesion is defined, **carotid endarterectomy** is considered (Fig. 16-4). Carotid endarterectomy is performed with the goal of preventing cerebral ischemia in the territory of the artery subjected to the procedure and should generally be considered only by surgeons whose combined stroke morbidity and mortality from arteriography and the surgical procedure is less than 3% for asymptomatic patients and less than 6% for symptomatic patients. Medical management becomes more of a consideration in the presence of one or more of the following conditions: (1) evidence of severe or progressive renal, hepatic, pulmonary, or cardiac failure; (2) uncontrolled diabetes mellitus or unregulated hypertension; (3) cancer that confers a low 5-year survival rate; (4) the coexistence of other (such as cardiac) sources for cerebral emboli; (5) symptoms that are of unknown origin, contralateral to the stenotic artery, or in the vertebrobasilar territory; or (6) the presence of a tandem lesion distally in the same arterial distribution of equal or greater severity compared with the carotid bifurcation area lesion. Carotid endarterectomy is generally not considered in the circumstance of known carotid occlusion, except in rare instances of acute occlusion when endarterectomy can be performed immediately (for

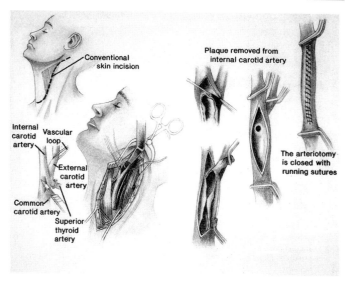

Fig. 16-4. Basic techniques of carotid endarterectomy.

instance, an occlusion occurring during arteriography in a hospital setting).

The overall effect of carotid endarterectomy on the immediate and subsequent risk of stroke is influenced by patient selection and the availability of a surgeon able to perform the procedure with low morbidity and mortality. Patients who have undergone successful carotid endarterectomy for TIA or minor stroke continue to be at risk for subsequent ipsilateral hemispheric stroke with a cumulative risk of about 9.5% over the first 4 years after the operation.

Symptomatic carotid artery stenosis that reduces the diameter of the artery **70% or more** and is associated with single or multiple TIAs, minor cerebral infarction (within a 6-month interval), or crescendo TIAs (with or without antiplatelet therapy) is a **proven indication** for carotid endarterectomy (Table 16-2). Antiplatelet therapy should not be discontinued preoperatively if it is already being given. Patients with cerebral infarction and moderate to severe deficit were not eligible for the major trials evaluating carotid endarterectomy in symptomatic patients. In general, a surgeon will wait 2 to 6 weeks after the patient has had a significant cerebral infarction to decrease the risk of hemorrhagic transformation. In this subgroup, the procedure is typically reserved for patients who have a reasonable functional recovery.

For **symptomatic patients** with TIAs or minor cerebral infarction associated with a moderate carotid artery stenosis of **30% to 69%,** carotid endarterectomy should be considered **acceptable but not yet of proven value** for the prevention of stroke (see Table 16-2). (Two large international treatment trials are currently investigating this issue.) Whether carotid endarterectomy is indicated in the setting of progressing stroke related to carotid stenosis is contro-

Table 16-2. **Indications for carotid endarterectomy**

Symptomatic
Proven
Symptomatic carotid stenosis, ≥70%
Unproven but acceptable
Acute carotid occlusion, symptomatic
Stroke in evolution
Simultaneous coronary artery bypass grafting
Acute carotid dissection, with recurrent symptoms of cerebral ischemia
while patient is treated with anticoagulation
Symptomatic carotid stenosis, 30% to 69%
Uncertain
Symptomatic carotid stenosis, ≤30% on aspirin
Unacceptable
Symptomatic carotid stenosis, ≤30% not on aspirin
Long-standing carotid occlusion
Asymptomatic
Proven
Selected patients with carotid stenosis, ≥60%*
Unproven but acceptable
Selected patients with carotid stenosis ≥60%, who are mild to moderate
surgical risks, are women, or have multiple or diffuse atherosclerotic
lesions
Unacceptable
Asymptomatic carotid stenosis, ≤60%
Long-standing carotid occlusion
Carotid dissection (asymptomatic or asymptomatic after initiation of
medical treatment)
Patients with carotid stenosis, ≥60%, who are moderately high or high
surgical risks

---

*Patients who appear to benefit the most: (1) men appear to benefit more than women; (2) patients with no major organ failure, including cardiac, pulmonary, or renal disease; (3) patients with no other relative or absolute contraindications to operation or arteriography; (4) patients with relatively isolated, high-grade, easily accessible lesions in area of the carotid bifurcation.

versial and has not been adequately studied. At this time, many investigators consider the procedure to be **acceptable but not of proven value** for patients with **progressive ischemic stroke** related to carotid stenosis of 70% or more, with or without ulceration.

Patients who do not undergo carotid endarterectomy are treated medically (anticoagulants or antiplatelet agents). Ischemic cerebrovascular events associated with a stenosis in the extracranial carotid artery in a patient who is not a surgical candidate are generally managed with heparin therapy followed by warfarin for 3 months. After warfarin therapy, daily aspirin (81–1300 mg) is often recommended for an indefinite period (see Table 12-4). Those with symptomatic stenosis in the distal internal carotid artery, middle cerebral artery, vertebral artery, or basilar artery are also typically treated with warfarin for at least 3 months, followed by antiplatelet therapy. In those with a contraindication to warfarin, aspirin or ticlopidine is indicated. Transluminal balloon angioplasty of the vertebral and basilar arteries may be considered in selected patients who have symptomatic stenotic lesions of both vertebral arteries, severe narrowing of the basilar artery, severe narrowing of the distal internal carotid artery or middle cerebral artery, or long segments of stenosis with irregularity and evidence of thromboemboli, who are not candidates for a bypass procedure, and who fail medical therapy consisting of anticoagulation and antiplatelet medication.

Ipsilateral carotid endarterectomy in **combination with coronary artery bypass grafting** is also generally considered to be **acceptable but not yet proven** in a symptomatic patient experiencing TIAs or minor cerebral infarction in the presence of unilateral or bilateral stenosis of 70% or more and who is in need of coronary artery bypass grafting. Another surgical procedure, **extracranial-to-intracranial bypass,** has been found to be generally ineffective for preventing ischemic stroke among patients with focal cerebral ischemic symptoms and various underlying craniocervical occlusive lesions. However, rare patients may be candidates for such a procedure, such as patients with incapacitating recurrent, reproducible, hemodynamic (postural) cerebral ischemic events or progressive visual loss from venous stasis retinopathy in the setting of inoperable internal carotid system occlusive disease. (Chapter 24 and Table 16-2 address asymptomatic carotid stenosis.)

FIBROMUSCULAR DYSPLASIA

Fibromuscular dysplasia is a noninflammatory disease usually affecting one or both internal carotid arteries above the carotid bifurcation. Cerebral arteriography (often performed for unrelated symptoms) usually shows a characteristic beaded-lumen appearance, with multiple stenoses, elongation and kinking, and, occasionally, aneurysm formation. The hyperplastic changes of the arterial intima and media may stenose or occlude the arterial lumen and predispose to thromboembolism. The involved segments of the carotid artery may dissect and lead to vessel stenosis or aneurysmal dilatation with blood stagnation and thrombus formation.

In patients with cerebrovascular symptoms associated with fibromuscular dysplasia, aggressive intervention options such as endarterectomy or endovascular arterial dilation are rarely necessary. On the basis of available information, managing these patients conservatively (antiplatelet therapy) is usually preferable because of the relatively benign natural history of the condition. Medical treatment with warfarin for 3 to 6 months may be considered in patients with hemodynamically significant carotid artery stenosis associated with ipsilateral TIA, reversible ischemic neurologic deficit, minor cerebral infarction, or recurrent focal ischemic events. If fibromuscular dysplasia is complicated by dissecting aneurysm associated with recurrent ischemic cerebrovascular symptoms, anticoagulant or antiplatelet therapy followed by operation should be considered.

CAROTID ARTERY DISSECTION

Carotid artery dissection may be related to trauma, fibromuscular dysplasia, or collagen disorders, or it may occur spontaneously. This disorder is noted primarily in young women. The clinical syndrome includes ocular pain, ipsilateral Horner's syndrome, and hemicranial discomfort with or without focal ischemic cerebrovascular deficits. Cerebral arteriography or MRA demonstrates an elongated narrowing, often with a conical tapering and sometimes with an accompanying "distal pouch." Some authors believe that fibromuscular dysplasia and spontaneous carotid artery dissection are part of the clinical spectrum of one disease process. However, the cause for each of these conditions remains unknown.

Anticoagulation therapy with heparin followed by approximately 3 months of warfarin therapy is generally recommended for **extracranial internal carotid artery dissection** associated with focal cerebral ischemic events. However, the use of heparin is controversial if the disorder involves hemorrhage into the arterial wall. In this setting, or if warfarin therapy is contraindicated because of other medical problems, antiplatelet therapy is considered. Surgical treatment is typically not used for carotid dissection because partial or complete resolution of the dissection and thrombosis with recanalization during a period of several months generally occurs.

Management of **intracranial carotid artery dissection** is still controversial. Antiplatelet therapy is often recommended (especially in situations without focal cerebral ischemic symptoms or when such symptoms have not occurred within the past week). Although there is some risk of arterial rupture, early therapy with heparin and warfarin is typically given if cerebral ischemic symptoms have occurred within the past week, particularly if they are recurrent. If embolic symptoms recur during heparin therapy, surgical options should be considered. Hemodynamic events often resolve with recanalization of the thrombosed vessel; thus, a delay in surgical intervention is prudent. Patients with brain stem ischemia caused by vertebral or basilar artery dissection should be treated medically with early heparin anticoagulation if they have no evidence of intracranial bleeding. Warfarin is typically then used for about 3 to 6 months, followed by antiplatelet therapy.

RADIATION

Sometimes, intensive **brain or neck radiation** (for example, for brain tumors, lymphoma, and carcinoma of the larynx) may result in arterial, capillary, or venous vasculopathy and lead to ischemic or hemorrhagic stroke or TIA. In these patients, the time from radiation to cerebrovascular complications is usually 6 months to 2 years. Radiation may also promote premature and rapidly worsening atherosclerosis, which may lead to large vessel occlusive disease.

HOMOCYSTINURIA

Homocystinuria is also associated with thromboembolic infarcts and should be considered in the differential diagnosis of stroke in the young. Although the usual mechanism is premature atherosclerotic narrowing of large vessels, occlusion without preceding stenosis may also occur. The administration of a low-methionine diet and large doses of pyridoxine, vitamin B_{12}, and folate may be helpful.

Small Vessel Disease

HYPERTENSION

Hypertension (systolic blood pressure of 160 mm Hg or more or diastolic blood pressure of 95 mm Hg or more) may affect brain performance indirectly by contributing to the development of impaired cardiac function or directly by producing physiologic and pathologic changes in the cerebral circulation. Although atherosclerosis is regularly encountered in normotensive patients, it occurs with increased frequency and severity in patients with hypertension. Thus, atherosclerotic cerebrovascular disease causes many of the stroke syndromes that develop in patients with hypertension. However, the more specific cerebrovascular abnormality in patients with sustained hypertension consists of fibrinoid necrosis, lipohyalinosis, and miliary microaneurysms, resulting in a nonatherosclerotic segmental degeneration in the walls of penetrating arteries. These lesions, found almost exclusively in the brains of patients with hypertension, are located primarily in the basal ganglia, thalamus, pons, cerebellum, and subcortex—the same regions in which both lacunar infarction and intracerebral hemorrhage predominate.

Lacunar infarctions cause 10% to 15% of all ischemic strokes and tend to be associated with certain clinical syndromes. Lacunar infarctions are small (less than 1.5 cm in greatest diameter) and result from involvement of deep, small, penetrating branches of the major intracranial arteries without involvement of the cortex. Because these arterial branches have poor collateral connections, obstruction of blood flow caused by fibrin deposition, lipohyalinosis, microatheroma, or thrombus leads to infarction in the limited distribution of one of these arteries. Other possible causes of these clinical syndromes are a small hemorrhage or a very small embolic infarct.

Lacunar infarcts are the single most frequent cerebrovascular lesion found in elderly patients with hypertension and may or may not be symptomatic, depending on their location. Lacunes typically do not cause deficits such as aphasia, homonymous hemianopia, coma, seizures, isolated memory impairment, monoplegia, or loss of consciousness. They may occur during sleep, and progression in a stepwise fashion during 1 to 4 days is not uncommon. The **five most common recognizable syndromes** described are

1. **Pure motor hemiparesis** with weakness involving face, arm, and leg on one side of the body caused by a lesion in the contralateral internal capsule or base of the pons
2. **Pure sensory stroke** with numbness of the face, arm, and leg on one side of the body caused by a lesion in or near the contralateral thalamus
3. **Dysarthria clumsy hand syndrome,** with severe dysarthria, mild hand weakness and clumsiness, facial weakness, and dysphagia caused by a lesion in the base of the pons
4. **Ataxic hemiparesis,** with pure motor hemiparesis and ataxia in the affected limbs, caused by a lesion in the base of the upper pons
5. Dementia, pseudobulbar palsy, and bilateral motor system deficit caused by multiple bilateral lesions involving the basal ganglia, subcortex, and brain stem (referred to as **lacunar state,** or état lacunaire)

Although all these syndromes usually indicate lacunar disease, other ischemic mechanisms may be involved.

Lacunar infarction is suspected when the clinical symptoms correspond to one of the five syndromes. CT is positive in only about 50% of cases; MRI is often more useful for characterizing the topography of the lesion. When performed, electroencephalography is typically normal, and cerebral arteriography shows no visible arterial occlusion. Sometimes these infarctions are asymptomatic, revealed incidentally by brain imaging or autopsy.

Lacunar infarction occurring in the distribution of the anterior circulation should be evaluated with carotid duplex or oculopneumoplethysmography. Lacunar infarctions in the posterior circulation may be evaluated with MRA or transcranial Doppler ultrasonography of the vertebrobasilar system. The evaluation of lacunar events is somewhat controversial. Many studies support the concept that up to 90% of lacunar infarcts occur in the setting of chronic hypertension and its associated pathologic changes of the arterial system, but others have reported a lower prevalence of hypertension in such patients, which makes a comprehensive evaluation for a thrombotic or embolic cause more likely to define an alternative cause. If doubt exists about the kind of vascular lesion responsible, echocardiography and cerebral arteriography may be necessary to help eliminate other causes of infarction.

Lacunar infarction generally has a good prognosis, and rehabilitation efforts are usually successful. Treatment should be directed at gradual reduction of blood pressure. Antiplatelet therapy with aspirin or ticlopidine is of unclear benefit in this setting, but warfarin anticoagulation is relatively contraindicated.

Cerebrovascular diseases also may be associated with acute elevation of blood pressure, referred to as **hypertensive crises.** Clinical syndromes include hypertensive encephalopathy (see Chapter 19), hypertensive hemorrhagic stroke (see Chapter 17), and severe hypertension associated with pregnancy (see Chapter 22).

ARTERITIS

Intracranial arteritis may or may not be associated with an identifiable infectious cause. **Infectious** conditions include those in which the arteritis seems to be due to meningeal involvement (bacterial, fungal, tuberculous, and syphilitic meningitis) and those in which the arteritis occurs independent of meningitis (aspergillosis, mucormycosis, herpes zoster, malaria, trichinosis, rickettsial diseases, and schistosomiasis). The **noninfectiou**s processes often involve the brain parenchyma in addition to cerebral arteries of a given caliber.

Infectious Arteritis

Several different CNS infective processes result in a reactive change in the cerebral blood vessels, known as **obliterative endarteritis.** The condition is characterized by an inflammatory cellular infiltrate and thickening of the arterial intima, which may stenose or occlude the lumen or serve as a nidus for thromboembolism. Bacterial, fungal, and tuberculous meningitides that bathe the smaller leptomeningeal arteries in purulent or granulomatous exudate may lead to obliterative endarteritis in the vessels. The process may remain focal but usually becomes more generalized and causes numerous, small, superficial areas of cerebral infarction. With rare exception, the patient appears very ill and has clear-cut signs of meningeal irritation before any ischemic symptoms develop.

Once a common cause of ischemic stroke in young adults, **tertiary syphilis** is now rare. All forms of tertiary syphilis may be associated with vascular involvement, but clinical cerebrovascular symptoms are most prominent with meningovascular syphilis, which usually develops 5 to 10 years after the initial infection. The endarteritis is usually confined to the intracranial arteries, but the aorta and major cervical arteries also may be affected. Multifocal cerebral ischemic symptoms in the territories of the middle and posterior cerebral arteries are the most common.

Other rare infectious causes of cerebral endarteritis include **malaria** and **rickettsial diseases,** in which cerebral ischemic symptoms are often preceded by convulsions, psychosis, or depressed levels of consciousness. These infections include **aspergillosis,** which usually occurs in association with systemic disease, especially involving the respiratory system; **mucormycosis**, occurring in patients with diabetes mellitus who have periorbital and cavernous sinus infections; **herpes zoster,** which leads to involvement of the distal internal carotid artery and proximal cerebral arteries, with delayed contralateral hemiplegia being the most common syndrome; **trichinosis**, which is associated with an inflammatory myopathy and, less frequently, with meningoencephalitis; and **schistosomiasis mansoni,** with lymphadenopathy, hepatosplenomegaly, eosinophilia, gastrointestinal hemorrhages and obstructions, and transverse myelitis.

Appropriate antimicrobial therapy should be provided for the treatment of cerebral vasculitis caused by **bacterial meningitis**. In patients with pneumococcal or meningococcal meningitis, penicillin G (20–24 million U, intravenously, daily in four to six divided doses) or chloramphenicol (4–6 g/day) for adults and penicillin G in a dosage of 300,000 U/kg of body weight for children are recommended. Cefotaxime or moxalactam (2 g every 4 hours), or gentamicin (5 mg/kg/day) in divided doses at 6-hour intervals, is effective for the treatment of patients with gram-negative enteric bacillus. For adults with *Staphylococcus aureus*, nafcillin or oxacillin (12–18 g/day) or methicillin (18–20 g/day) in divided doses, intravenously, alone or in combination with rifampin (600 mg daily), is usually prescribed.

Amphotericin B (0.5–0.6 mg/kg/day) alone or in combination with flucytosine (150 mg/kg/day) in divided doses every 6 hours is effective in the treatment of patients with cryptococcal **fungal meningitis** complicated by cerebral vasculitis. Intravenously administered amphotericin B usually is prescribed for the treatment of patients with candidiasis, aspergillosis (often combined with 5-fluorocytosine and amidazole drugs and surgical removal of the infected material), and coccidioidomycosis (often combined with intraventricular administration).

A combination of isoniazid (5 mg/kg once daily in adults; 10 mg/kg in children), rifampin (600 mg daily for adults; 15 mg/kg for children), and a third drug (ethambutol, 15 mg/kg once daily; ethionamide, 750–1000 mg, 3 times daily after meals for adults; or pyrazinamide, in a single dose of 30–50 mg/kg daily) is used for the treatment of cerebral vasculitis associated with **tuberculous meningitis**.

Penicillin G (aqueous penicillin G, 18–24 million U, intravenously in six divided doses every 4 hours for 14 days, followed by benzathine penicillin G, 2.4 million U, intramuscularly weekly for three doses) is the drug of choice for **meningovascular syphilis**. In patients who are allergic to penicillin, erythromycin or tetracycline (500 mg orally every 6 hours for 20–30 days) is usually prescribed. Treatment of patients with cerebral vasculitis caused by **leptospirosis** usually consists of the administration of tetracyclines, such as doxycycline (100 mg orally) given twice daily for 7 days.

For the treatment of patients with cerebral vasculitis caused by **Lyme disease**, penicillin G (20 million U intravenously in six divided doses daily for 10–14 days) or ceftriaxone (2 g/day intravenously) is usually effective. Patients who are allergic to these drugs may be treated with tetracycline, 500 mg orally, four times a day for 30 days.

Noninfectious Arteritis

The noninfectious inflammatory angiopathies include those that primarily affect the arterioles and capillaries (systemic lupus erythematosus), those that primarily affect small or medium-sized arteries (polyarteritis nodosa, isolated CNS angiitis), and those that primarily affect medium-sized to large arteries (temporal arteritis, Takayasu's disease). Takayasu's disease is discussed here in the context of inflammatory angiopathies, but the primary site of involvement is near the origin of the major vessels of the aortic arch.

Systemic lupus erythematosus is a diffuse, connective tissue disorder in which 50% to 75% of patients have CNS involvement sometime during the course of the disease. However, only about 2% of patients with systemic lupus erythematosus have neurologic manifestations when first examined. Most of these patients already have prominent clinical systemic involvement (skin, bone marrow, heart, liver, kidneys, lungs, muscle, peripheral nerves). CNS findings are usually those of a diffuse encephalopathy with delirium, seizures, acute psychosis, and increased intracranial pressure. Focal or multifocal cerebral and brain stem infarcts occur, but they rarely produce recognizable arterial syndromes. The cause of the CNS findings in systemic lupus erythematosus may be multifactorial. Multifocal infarction with inflammatory vasculitis is uncommonly noted on histologic examination; small-vessel vasculopathy without inflammation is typically seen. When systemic lupus erythematosus is associated with hypertension, intracerebral hemorrhage or small-vessel hypertensive occlusive changes may result. Treatment with high-dose corticosteroids is recommended for cerebrovascular disease caused by systemic lupus erythematosus (in pregnant patients, this treatment is advised throughout pregnancy and during the first 2 months postpartum to limit puerperal exacerbations).

From 10% to 20% of patients with **polyarteritis nodosa** have CNS involvement, almost invariably after systemic manifestation of the disease. The pathologic findings vary from multifocal infarction or (especially when associated with hypertension) intracerebral hemorrhage to isolated large cerebral infarction resulting from occlusion of a major cerebral artery. The clinical features, therefore, may be those of diffuse disease of the CNS, such as headache, dementia, psychosis, generalized seizures, or focal or multifocal disease with facial paralysis, deafness, ocular nerve palsies, cerebellar abnormalities, or focal seizures. Corticosteroids such as prednisone (1 mg/kg/day in three to four divided doses) with or without immunosuppressive agents, such as cyclophosphamide (2–4 mg/kg/day in a single morning dose followed by a generous amount of water to avoid hemorrhagic cystitis), appear to improve the survival of patients with polyarteritis nodosa.

A rare vasculitis, **isolated CNS angiitis (granulomatous angiitis)**, unlike systemic lupus erythematosus and periarteritis nodosa, is usually confined to the CNS. Symptoms result from widespread occlusion of small parenchymal and leptomeningeal arteries and veins. The condition is often heralded by a flu-like illness, with headache and generalized weakness, followed by confusion, seizures, or multifocal neurologic deficits. MRI or CT may demonstrate single or multiple cerebral infarctions, meningeal enhancement, or subcortical enhancement with administration of contrast agent, or, less commonly, show subarachnoid or intracerebral hemorrhage. Cerebrospinal fluid examination may reveal increased protein and lymphocytic pleocytosis. Findings on cerebral arteriography are usually abnormal and demonstrate alternating dilation and constriction (beading) of medium-sized and small intracranial arteries.

Meningeal and cortical biopsy are necessary in patients with equivocal or atypical arteriographic findings or in those not responding to treatment. There is no standard treatment of cerebrovascular disease associated with isolated CNS angiitis, although treatment with prednisone (60–100 mg/day orally) alone or in combination with cyclophosphamide in a single morning dose of 1 to 2 mg/kg orally (adjusted to avoid severe leukopenia) is the most common initial treatment approach. Patients who do not tolerate cyclophosphamide may be given azathioprine (2 mg/kg/day).

A generalized granulomatous vascular disease, **temporal arteritis** (cranial arteritis, giant cell arteritis) usually involves the superficial temporal and extracranial scalp arteries and ophthalmic arteries in patients older than 55 years. The inflammatory reaction within the superficial temporal arteries often makes these arteries tender to palpation and gives them a swollen, erythematous, beaded appearance. An unremitting unilateral or bilateral temporal headache is common, but any distribution of head and face pain may occur. Painful chewing may be caused by jaw muscle ischemia with claudication or by contact between moving skin and temporalis muscles. Occlusion of the ophthalmic artery or its branches, which occurs in 20% to 25% of patients, results in ipsilateral eye pain and visual impairment progressing to complete blindness. In 10% to 20% of patients, both eyes are affected. Cerebral infarction is a rare complication but may occur in both carotid and vertebrobasilar artery distributions.

Most patients also have features of a more generalized vasculitis, including fever, malaise, weight loss, and polymyalgia rheumatica. Laboratory findings show elevated erythrocyte sedimentation rate, slightly increased leukocyte count, and mild anemia. Temporal artery biopsy is indicated to make a definitive diagnosis. Clinical findings most strongly correlated with a positive biopsy include jaw claudication and abnormality of the superficial temporal arteries, including erythema, tenderness, or beading.

If temporal arteritis is suspected, corticosteroid treatment (60–100 mg prednisone daily) is initiated, even before the biopsy can be arranged. This dose is typically maintained for 1 month, with a slow reduction in dose, depending on the patient's clinical response and decrease in erythrocyte sedimentation rate. Daily corticosteroid therapy may be required for 2 years or longer, depending on response to the treatment.

A chronic inflammatory arteriopathy of unknown origin, **Takayasu's arteritis** (pulseless disease) most commonly affects young women. Involvement of the aortic arch and its branches results in narrowing of major-vessel ostia and cerebral ischemic symptoms, including ischemic Takayasu's retinopathy. Clinically, there may be reduction or absence of subclavian, carotid, brachial, and radial pulses, with bruits over affected or collateral vessels and neurologic symptoms of cerebrovascular insufficiency such as blurred vision (especially with activity), dizziness, decreased visual acuity, memory loss, and hemiparetic and hemisensory syndromes. Systemic complications include secondary hypertension caused by renal artery involvement; systemic symptoms such as malaise, arthralgias, fever, anorexia, weight loss, and night sweats; aortic regurgitation; aortic aneurysm; and laboratory abnormalities (such as elevated erythrocyte sedimentation rate, anemia, leukocytosis, and elevated C-reactive protein level). Arteriography of the aortic arch demonstrates diffuse narrowing and occlusion of multiple large arteries as they originate from the aortic arch, with or without fusiform aortic dilatation and calcification.

In the early stages of the disease, corticosteroid therapy with prednisone is recommended. Initial doses as large as 100 mg daily are continued until inflammatory factors are controlled, usually 2 to 4 weeks, with subsequent reduction of the dose. For chronic symptomatic lesions such as renovascular hypertension, cerebrovascular or limb ischemia, dilatation of the ascending aorta with aortic insufficiency, or thoracic or abdominal aortic aneurysms, a reconstructive procedure on severely involved vessels may be necessary to restore flow and prevent further ischemia and infarction.

Behçet's disease is an uncommon, recurrent, inflammatory disorder affecting the CNS, occasionally complicated by ischemic stroke. Episodes characteristically resolve completely during several weeks and tend to involve the brain stem. Men are affected more often than women. Typical clinical features usually include recurrent aphthous or herpetiform oral ulceration, recurrent genital ulceration, anterior or posterior uveitis, retinal vasculitis, erythema nodosum, papulopustular lesions, recurrent (aseptic) meningoencephalitis, cranial nerve (particularly abducens) palsies, and cerebellar ataxia. Because the cause of the disease is assumed to be autoimmune, treatment with corticosteroids or other immunosuppressive agents has been recommended.

Other systemic vasculitic syndromes have been rarely associated with cerebral ischemia or infarction. These include **Wegener's granulomatosis** with primary involvement of the lungs, kidneys, and upper respiratory tract. **Rheumatoid arthritis** is more commonly associated with neuropathy, but cerebral infarction has been described. **Sjögren's syndrome** may cause dementia, cranial neuropathies, especially of the trigeminal nerves, and, less commonly, cerebral ischemia. **Sarcoidosis** of the nervous system may cause a cerebral vasculitis with cerebral infarction. Aseptic meningitis, cranial nerve palsies (especially cranial nerve VII), and hypothalamic dysfunction are also typically present.

Hematologic Disease

Abnormalities in blood cell constituents and plasma proteins may result in a hypercoagulable or hypocoagulable state, with corresponding abnormalities in blood viscosity and stasis, which predispose the patient to cerebral ischemia or cerebral hemorrhage.

POLYCYTHEMIA

Patients with primary or secondary polycythemia may have neurologic symptoms on the basis of increased red blood cell mass with hyperviscosity and increased vascular resistance. Cerebral arterial or venous thrombosis involving both small and large vessels may occur with focal areas of infarction or hemorrhagic infarction. From 10% to 20% of patients have clear-cut focal cerebral ischemic events (usually TIAs) that correlate with the values of the hematocrit and regress partially or totally after adequate therapy. In contrast, the reduction in red blood cell mass and oxygen-carrying capacity that occurs with various anemic states is rarely associated with focal cerebral ischemia.

Management of patients with polycythemia is complex and typically includes reduction of blood volume with phlebotomy (especially with hematocrit value ≥55%), with a goal hematocrit value of 40% to 45%. Thrombocytosis should be controlled with myelosuppression (alkylating agents, hydroxyurea, or radioactive phosphorus). Young patients may be treated with phlebotomy alone to avoid the long-term risk of myelosuppressive agents.

THROMBOCYTHEMIA

Thrombocythemia also has been associated with focal ischemic neurologic lesions. This disorder may be primary or secondary to other forms of myeloproliferative disease, such as polycythemia vera. Megakaryocyte hyperplasia and increased platelet production result in elevation of the platelet count. Even in the absence of preexistent atherosclerosis, spontaneous platelet aggregation occurs with thromboembolic ischemic manifestations. In symptomatic patients, maintained suppression of platelet counts to lower than $500 \times 10^9/$ liter may prevent recurrence of serious events. Treatment of acute cerebrovascular events in patients with thrombocythemia (essential thrombocytosis) should begin with emergency plateletpheresis. Lowering the platelet count also may be achieved by therapy with hydroxyurea, alkylating agents, or ^{32}P radiotherapy followed by administration of antiplatelet agents such as aspirin or dipyridamole to reduce the risk of recurrent thromboses.

THROMBOCYTOPENIC PURPURA

An uncommon disorder, thrombotic thrombocytopenic purpura is likely a multicentric vasculitis. The hematologic and cerebrovascular manifestations are the result of secondary mechanical damage to erythrocytes. The damage causes hemolytic anemia, fever, and increased utilization of platelets to form diffuse microthrombi. Occlusion of terminal arterioles in the brain produces multiple small infarcts and a fluctuating encephalopathy, focal neurologic signs and symptoms, and coma; the neurologic findings are often reversible. The clinical picture may also include intracerebral (often multiple) hemorrhage.

Laboratory evaluation includes looking for evidence of Coombs-negative hemolytic anemia, fragmented erythrocytes, decreased platelet count, and erythroid hyperplasia with increased megakaryocytes in the bone marrow. Proteinuria, hematuria, and abnormal results of liver function studies also are found.

No consistently effective treatment of thrombotic thrombocytopenic purpura is available, although plasmapheresis (1.5 plasma volume removal in 4 days), infusions of fresh frozen plasma, and high-dose corticosteroids (prednisone, 1–2 mg/kg/day) may be helpful. Splenectomy or use of vincristine sulfate (Oncovin, Vincasar PFS) may lessen the plasma dependency, which can become protracted in some patients. Platelet inhibitors (such as aspirin, dipyridamole) are of unclear benefit and are generally not used if a patient is severely thrombocytopenic.

SICKLE-CELL DISEASE

Occurring in about 1 in 600 black Americans at birth, sickle-cell disease is inherited as an autosomal dominant trait. When red blood cells containing hemoglobin SS are exposed to low oxygen tension, their structure is altered in a way that increases blood viscosity and leads to multiple small vessel occlusions. When large arteries are involved through vessel wall ischemia from occlusion of nutrient arteries, large focal cerebral infarctions may occur. Other cerebrovascular lesions associated with sickle-cell disease include multiple small cortical and subcortical hemorrhages or hemorrhagic infarcts, cortical vein and venous sinus thrombosis, massive intracerebral hemorrhage, and, rarely, subarachnoid hemorrhage. Sickle cell crises are often precipitated by stress, physical exertion, hypoxia, or acute infection and are rarely manifested as a thrombotic crisis associated with fever and abdominal, bone, or chest pain. Children younger than 15 years are at greater risk for cerebrovascular complications. Patients with cerebrovascular disorders associated with sickle-cell disease are usually treated with repeated red cell transfusions.

DYSPROTEINEMIA

The various dysproteinemias, including macroglobulinemia, cryoglobulinemia, and multiple myeloma, also may be associated with thrombotic cerebrovascular complications. The usual picture is that of a diffuse encephalopathic disorder caused by the disseminated vascular lesions that form at the capillary, arteriolar, and venous levels and produce multifocal microinfarction and hemorrhage. Large areas of focal infarction are less common and may be the result of dural sinus thrombosis. Plasma exchange (large-volume plasmapheresis) seems to be efficacious in the acute treatment of at least some dysproteinemia-related hyperviscosity syndromes, although persistent control may require more prolonged treatment with chemotherapeutic agents.

ANTIPHOSPHOLIPID ANTIBODY SYNDROMES

Antiphospholipid antibodies, including lupus anticoagulant and anticardiolipin antibodies, have been associated with an increased occurrence of cerebral infarction. A previous history of frequent miscarriages, previous ischemic stroke, or other recurrent arterial or venous thromboses may be detected. Arterial infarct patterns vary widely, including both cortical and subcortical locations. Venous sinus thrombosis may also occur. The diagnosis is made on the basis of the combination of clinical and laboratory findings. In addition to direct measurement of circulating lupus anticoagulant and anticardiolipin antibody levels, a prolonged activated partial thromboplastin time or false-positive Venereal Disease Research Laboratory (VDRL) test may also indicate the presence of a circulating antiphospholipid antibody. Other laboratory findings that may be associated with these syndromes are hemolytic anemia, decreased serum complement (C4), thrombocytopenia, and positive antinuclear antibody level.

Treatment is controversial, and the benefits of various therapies remain unproven. For patients with focal cerebral ischemic symptoms, warfarin is commonly used, although aspirin and ticlopidine are other options. Others have advocated high doses (60–100 mg/day) of prednisone, which can sometimes suppress antiphospholipid antibody levels, particularly those related to lupus anticoagulant. Prednisone (or other immunosuppressant) therapy has sometimes been added to anticoagulant or antiplatelet therapy in patients with continuing cerebral ischemic events. Rarely, plasmapheresis has been used in patients with acute encephalopathy or disseminated intravascular coagulation.

Sneddon's syndrome, characterized by recurrent strokes and livedo reticularis in younger patients, may be associated with antiphospholipid antibodies.

Deficiencies of protein C, protein S, and antithrombin III or resistance to activated protein C may also occur on either a hereditary or an acquired basis. Although venous occlusive disease of the extremities typically occurs, patients may also present with arterial occlusions, including cerebral vessels, causing infarction.

LEUKEMIA

Leukemia and its attendant leukocytosis and hyperviscosity may be accompanied by cerebral arterial or venous thrombosis. However, cerebral symptoms developing during the course of the disease are more commonly the result of intracranial hemorrhage or infection. Treatment of myelogenous or lymphocytic leukemia involves different regimens for distinct phases and is directed toward complete eradication of the leukemic cells or control of cell counts by means of cytotoxic drugs and bone marrow transplantation from a human leukocyte antigen (HLA)-compatible donor.

DISSEMINATED INTRAVASCULAR COAGULATION

Disseminated intravascular coagulation may be associated with virtually any pathologic process that produces tissue damage (such as massive tissue trauma, obstetrical complications, cardiothoracic operation, burns, severe infections, heat stroke, incompatible blood transfusions, disseminated malignancy, shock from many causes, massive brain damage including stroke) and results in the release of tissue thromboplastins into the circulation with subsequent activation of the coagulation process, thrombin formation, subsequent platelet and clotting factor consumption, and the formation of fibrin thrombi and emboli throughout the microvasculature. The early thrombotic phase of disseminated intravascular coagulation leads to widespread small infarctions in many organs (including the brain) followed by a phase of secondary fibrinolysis that results in petechial hemorrhages around small penetrating vessels. The mortality rate in patients with disseminated intravascular coagulation varies, depending on the underlying disorder.

The clinical presentation of disseminated intravascular coagulation is dependent on the stage and severity of the syndrome. The neurologic complications include (1) a syndrome of acute encephalopathy characterized by fluctuating focal neurologic symptoms usually associated with altered levels of consciousness, (2) venous sinus thrombosis, (3) intracerebral hemorrhage (usually subcortical petechial hemorrhages), and (4) cerebral arterial occlusions (small- to medium-sized arteries are frequently involved). Extensive skin and mucous membrane bleeding are common. The diagnosis is confirmed by blood test results revealing thrombocytopenia; presence of schistocytes or fragmented red blood cells; prolonged prothrombin, partial thromboplastin, and thrombin times; reduced plasma fibrinogen level; and elevated fibrin degradation products.

Treatment of disseminated intravascular coagulation should include control of the underlying disease and maintenance of adequate oxygenation and blood pressure. If significant hemorrhagic or ischemic complications are present, treatment should be initiated. In patients with thrombosis, heparin therapy (intravenous bolus followed by continuous intravenous infusion and a target activated partial thromboplastin time of 2 times control) is usually added, and hemorrhage is aggressively treated with platelets and fresh frozen plasma. (Disseminated intravascular coagulation associated with fulminant liver failure is generally considered a contraindication for heparin therapy.) The target platelet count during therapy is generally around 50×10^9/L. Increasing fibrinogen and platelet levels indicate that the process is coming under control and often correlate with a reduction in hemorrhagic complications. In patients with ongoing hemorrhage and lack of platelet or fibrinogen response to the transfusions, addition of antithrombotic treatment with heparin should be considered to impede fibrin formation.

Five Major Categories of Hemorrhagic Disease: Treatment of Specific Underlying Mechanisms

Hemorrhagic cerebrovascular disorders cause approximately 20% of all strokes. These conditions can be divided into five subgroups based on the location of the primary hemorrhage, including (from superficial to deep) epidural, subdural, subarachnoid, intracerebral, and intraventricular hemorrhage (see Fig. 1-1 and Table 8-2).

The clinical features of hemorrhagic cerebrovascular disease vary, depending on the site and size of the hemorrhage, and occasionally may not be clinically distinguishable from other types of stroke. Computed tomography (CT) or magnetic resonance imaging (MRI) allows precise differentiation and localization of brain hemorrhage and also helps to determine the extent of damage. When performed, cerebral arteriography may show an avascular mass in the region of hemorrhage.

Deterioration of a patient with hemorrhagic stroke is usually attributed to rebleeding (most commonly with saccular aneurysms and arteriovenous malformations), progressive cerebral edema, or other systemic causes such as heart, renal, or hepatic failure; serious cardiac arrhythmias; recurrent cardiac emboli; acute myocardial infarction; pneumonia; pulmonary embolism; septicemia; drug effects; or electrolyte disturbances such as hyponatremia (associated with salt-wasting syndrome or inappropriate antidiuretic hormone syndrome).

Epidural Hematoma

Epidural hematoma is a collection of blood between the skull and dura and commonly results from a parietal or temporal skull fracture with laceration of the middle meningeal artery and, occasionally, from a dural sinus tear. Because the dura becomes adherent to the skull with age, epidural hematoma rarely occurs in the elderly. A lucid interval, of several minutes to a few hours, followed by increasing severity of headache associated with nausea, vomiting, progressive impairment of consciousness, and contralateral hemiparesis is the classic clinical course. Pupillary dilatation on the side of the hematoma is often an indication of transtentorial herniation. In this situation, the head injury and hemorrhage are ipsilateral to the dilated pupil in 90% of patients, and the pulse is often less than 60 beats/minute, with a concomitant increase in systolic blood pressure.

Radiography of the skull may reveal a fracture line that crosses the groove associated with the middle meningeal artery. CT or MRI reveals a lenticular-shaped (biconvex) (Fig. 17-1) or, rarely, a crescent-shaped clot with a smooth inner margin, and cerebral arteriog-

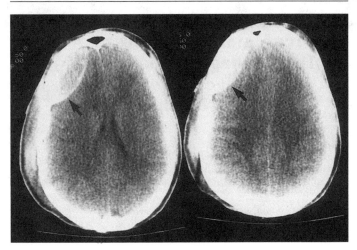

Fig. 17-1. CT scan of the head without contrast: lenticular-shaped clot consistent with an epidural hematoma (arrows).

raphy shows inward displacement of the surface arteries. Lumbar puncture may precipitate transtentorial herniation and is contraindicated in this setting. Early diagnosis and immediate neurosurgical consultation may be lifesaving. Treatment typically involves placement of several burr holes, evacuation of the hematoma, and identification and ligation of the bleeding vessel.

Subdural Hematoma

Subdural hematoma occurs 10 times more often than epidural hematoma. Subdural hematoma results from head trauma with a tear in a vein as it crosses the subdural space. Because the blood is collected between the dura and the underlying brain, nonfocal neurologic symptoms such as headache, nausea, vomiting, and altered consciousness are often more prominent than focal or lateralizing signs. Symptoms may fluctuate and, when focal, may (rarely) resemble transient ischemic attacks. A lucid interval between the trauma and comatose state is usually absent or brief. CT or MRI (Fig. 17-2) demonstrates a crescent-shaped (or, less commonly, lenticular-shaped) high-intensity mass consistent with hemorrhage, typically located over one or both (10% of cases) hemispheres. At 1 to 3 weeks after the appearance of subdural blood, the lesion changes from hyperdense to isodense on CT and thereafter becomes hypodense. Cerebral arteriography shows displacement of the brain away from the inner table of the skull.

Depending on the interval between the head injury and the onset of symptoms, subdural hematomas may be acute (within 24 hours), subacute (1–14 days), or chronic (>14 days). **Acute or subacute subdural hematoma** may be unilateral or bilateral and frequently result from a severe, high-speed head injury. A combination of sub-

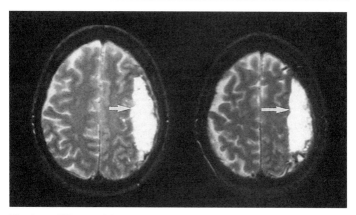

Fig. 17-2. MRI scan of the head: high-intensity mass consistent with a subdural hematoma (arrows).

dural hematoma, cerebral contusion, and laceration is common. Surgical treatment with placement of burr holes and evacuation of the subdural hematoma is usually indicated to prevent the development of deep coma.

In contrast to acute or subacute subdural hematoma, **chronic subdural hematoma** usually results from a less severe head injury, which may have been trivial or even forgotten. A gradual drift into drowsiness, inattentiveness, incoherence of thinking, confusion, stupor, and coma may be associated with increasing headache and, rarely, a seizure. Mental deterioration may be prominent, resembling dementia, brain tumor, drug intoxication, or depressive illness. Focal signs may include ipsilateral dilated pupil and hemiparesis, which may be contralateral, ipsilateral, or both. In infants and children, vomiting and seizures are prominent manifestations of chronic subdural hematoma. In these age groups, retinal hemorrhage in association with subdural hematoma may be manifestations of the so-called shaken-infant syndrome.

Patients with small chronic subdural hematomas without severe or progressive deficit in whom follow-up with serial neurologic examination and CT is possible can be managed conservatively. In cases of chronic subdural hematoma with severe or progressive deficit, surgical treatment is recommended.

Subarachnoid Hemorrhage

Subarachnoid hemorrhage causes 5% to 10% of all strokes, affecting females more often than males (1.5–2:1). The disorder usually presents with the very sudden onset of a new, severe headache, which is commonly associated with vomiting and follows a rapid alteration of the level of consciousness, including unconsciousness with recovery in a few minutes. Subarachnoid hemorrhage may be caused by a ruptured intracranial saccular aneurysm (about 60% of all cases), arte-

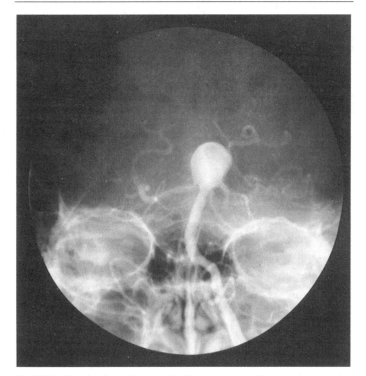

Fig. 17-3.   Cerebral arteriogram: basilar caput saccular aneurysm.

riovenous malformation (about 5% of all cases), or other conditions, including mycotic, atherosclerotic, traumatic, dissecting, or neoplastic aneurysms or vasculitis (about 5% of all cases). Subarachnoid hemorrhage is of unknown cause in approximately 30% of all cases (see Table 8-2).

INTRACRANIAL ANEURYSM

The most common cause of subarachnoid hemorrhage is a ruptured **intracranial aneurysm** (Fig. 17-3). Saccular or berry aneurysms represent 80% to 90% of all intracranial aneurysms and normally appear as small, rounded, berry-like arterial outpouchings, but other shapes (sessile, pedunculated, multilobed) are also seen. The size of saccular aneurysms ranges from 2 mm to several centimeters in diameter, and most lesions are between 2 and 10 mm in greatest diameter.

Intracranial aneurysms usually go undetected until rupture results in a clinical picture of subarachnoid hemorrhage, intracerebral hemorrhage, or both. The clinical features associated with subarachnoid hemorrhage and intracerebral hemorrhage are described in detail in Chapters 14 and 15. In some instances, however, the aneurysm is diagnosed before rupture on the basis of clinical signs and symptoms unrelated to intracranial hemorrhage, including cranial nerve compression, compression of other central nervous system structures, seizures, focal headaches, and cerebral ischemic events resulting from embolism of thrombus within large aneurysms. Alternatively, the diagnosis may be fortuitous after CT, MRI, or cerebral arteriographic studies done for an unrelated disorder.

On the basis of existing evidence, it appears that most aneurysms probably form over a relatively short time (hours, days, or weeks), and attain a size allowed by the limits of elasticity in the elastic components of the walls of the aneurysm. At that point, either the aneurysm ruptures or, if the limits of elasticity are not exceeded and the aneurysm maintains itself intact, the walls undergo a process of compensatory hardening, similar to the process in other vascular walls that are subjected to arterial blood pressures, in which excessive amounts of collagen are formed. The tensile strength of collagen is several hundred times that of elastic fibers. With this added tensile strength, which continues to accumulate over time, the likelihood of rupture decreases unless the aneurysm is large at the time it initially stabilizes. Aneurysms 1 cm or more in size at the time of initial stabilization are much more likely to undergo subsequent growth and rupture, because the stress on the wall increases with the square of the diameter of the aneurysm. Therefore, it follows that the critical size for aneurysm rupture is lower if rupture occurs at the time of or soon after formation, as appears to be the case for most aneurysms that rupture. The mean size of aneurysms discovered after rupture is approximately 7.5 mm; the mean size of aneurysms discovered before rupture, which then go on to rupture, is approximately 20 mm.

Unruptured intracranial aneurysms less than 1 cm in diameter in patients with no history of subarachnoid hemorrhage from a different source have a very low likelihood of subsequent rupture. Unruptured intracranial aneurysms in patients with a history of subarachnoid hemorrhage from a separate aneurysm may be more likely to rupture than aneurysms in patients with no previous subarachnoid hemorrhage, but this point requires further clarification. Ruptured aneurysms are more likely to be associated with small aneurysmal structures attached to the main aneurysm, called "daughter sacs."

Intracranial aneurysms are typically located at large artery bifurcations involving the circle of Willis and its major branches (Fig. 17-4): internal carotid-posterior communicating artery junction, approximately 30%; anterior communicating artery, 30%; proximal middle cerebral artery, 20% to 25%; and posterior circulation, 10% to 15%.

Intracranial aneurysms are rare in childhood, and the incidence of aneurysmal subarachnoid hemorrhage is higher in women than in men (ratio, approximately 3:2). Approximately 10% to 15% of patients with saccular aneurysms have a family history of subarachnoid hemorrhage or intracranial aneurysm, and 10% to 20% of patients have multiple aneurysms.

The pathogenesis of intracranial saccular aneurysms is controversial and may be multifactorial. There is convincing evidence that these are not congenital lesions but, rather, that they develop with increasing age. This possibility does not, however, preclude a genetic predisposition for these lesions to develop. Various environmental factors (cigarette smoking, use of oral contraceptives, acute hypertension, use of stimulant drugs, physical stress, and alcohol con-

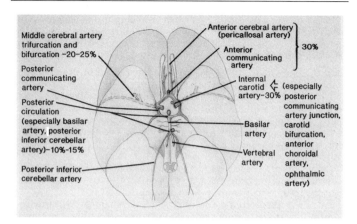

Fig. 17-4. Most common sites of saccular aneurysms.

sumption) may also have some role in the pathogenesis of intracranial aneurysms. Medical conditions that have been associated with intracranial aneurysm include autosomal dominant polycystic kidney disease, intracranial arteriovenous malformation, coarctation of the aorta, Marfan's syndrome, Ehlers-Danlos syndrome, fibromuscular dysplasia, pseudoxanthoma elasticum, moyamoya disease, neurofibromatosis, and pituitary tumors.

Several large autopsy studies have shown a wide range in overall frequency (0.2%–9.9%) of intracranial aneurysms in the general population; the mean frequency is about 5%. The incidence of aneurysmal subarachnoid hemorrhage increases progressively with age, and the average annual incidence is approximately 10/100,000 population/year. These data suggest that most intracranial aneurysms never rupture.

About 5% of all cerebral aneurysms are **mycotic cerebral aneurysms.** They commonly result from infected arterial emboli, primarily as a complication of acute or subacute bacterial endocarditis, and lead to septic degeneration of the elastic lamina and the muscular coats of the arterial wall. The most common sites of mycotic aneurysm formation are the distal middle cerebral artery branches, as seen in 2% of all cases of bacterial endocarditis. The lesions often resolve with antibiotic treatment, although some symptomatic lesions require surgical clipping.

Dissecting and traumatic intracranial aneurysms are rare. The clinical presentation of **dissecting intracranial aneurysms** in a relatively young patient may consist of a focal and severe headache followed by progressive stroke, brain swelling, and death. Typically, **traumatic intracranial aneurysms** develop after neck or head trauma (penetrating trauma, bony fractures), and occur most commonly in the internal carotid, middle cerebral, and anterior cerebral arteries.

Neoplastic cerebral aneurysms may be caused by arterial emboli from a cardiac (atrial) myxoma. Cerebral arteriography shows irregular filling defects in major and minor cerebral arterial branches, fusiform and saccular aneurysms, and occlusion of vessels. Systemic emboli often occur.

Arteriosclerotic intracerebral aneurysms may develop in patients with widespread atherosclerosis and hypertension and affect primarily the basilar, internal carotid, middle cerebral, and anterior cerebral arteries. These lesions are usually **fusiform.** Radiographic abnormalities include tortuosity, widening, and elongation of the affected arteries. In contrast to saccular or mycotic aneurysms, these aneurysms only rarely present with subarachnoid hemorrhage, but they may cause cerebral ischemia or mass effect. They are typically treated conservatively, although antiplatelet agents or even anticoagulants may be needed if thromboembolic events from the fusiform aneurysm occur.

Early **investigation and treatment** of intracranial aneurysms are important, particularly when the aneurysm has produced intracranial hemorrhage (see Appendix J-4). Even in pregnant patients, radiologic and therapeutic or surgical procedures should not be delayed or avoided, although special shielding during radiography is required (see Chapter 22). The clinical decisions involved in managing these patients vary with the type of aneurysm, but in patients who present with subarachnoid hemorrhage, CT should be performed as soon as possible. CT may confirm the presence of subarachnoid blood, detect associated intracerebral and intraventricular hemorrhage, and, in some instances, demonstrate the aneurysm. If CT is nondiagnostic, lumbar puncture may confirm the diagnosis of subarachnoid hemorrhage (see Chapter 14). MRI and magnetic resonance angiography (MRA) may also reveal the aneurysm, particularly if it is more than 4 mm in maximal diameter.

Arteriography of all intracranial vessels should be performed to identify the bleeding source as early as possible. In patients with subarachnoid hemorrhage of unknown cause and initially negative arteriography, repeat arteriography to search for an occult intracranial aneurysm should be considered if the first arteriogram shows significant vasospasm or fails to demonstrate the entire vascular tree, or if CT demonstrates a large amount of subarachnoid blood, especially when the blood is located diffusely or anteriorly. Arteriography may be delayed in patients who show extensive alteration in consciousness with or without focal neurologic deficits (Hunt and Hess clinical grade 4 or 5 [Appendix C-4]) because their prognosis is very poor (80%–90% mortality rate in the first 30 days) and the early operative mortality rate is high (15%–30%). In these patients, supportive treatment is generally indicated. If the patients improve with supportive treatment, more aggressive diagnostic and therapeutic procedures are generally pursued. Alternatively, patients with little or no neurologic deficit (Hunt and Hess clinical grade 1, 2, or 3) have a more favorable prognosis (10%–30% mortality rate during 30 days), but many of the deaths in this group result from rebleeding in the first 2 weeks after initial subarachnoid hemorrhage.

The potential advantages of early operation (including direct surgical clipping of the neck of the aneurysm [Fig. 17-5] and, if this is not feasible, other techniques such as endovascular placement of metallic coils into the aneurysm, endovascular balloon occlusion of the aneurysm or parent artery, proximal arterial ligation, aneurysmal

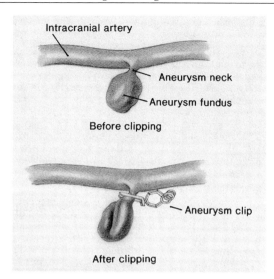

Fig. 17-5. Basic technique of clipping of saccular aneurysm.

trapping, or, rarely, wrapping or coating of aneurysms) must be weighed against the increased operative mortality rate during the first week after subarachnoid hemorrhage. Internal carotid artery ligation alone or in combination with extracranial-intracranial arterial bypass has become less popular because of high complication rates, but it is still occasionally used as treatment for large internal carotid system aneurysms.

Early aneurysm operation (within the first 3 days after hemorrhage) is especially indicated for patients who are alert, have little or no neurologic deficit (a Hunt and Hess clinical grade of 1, 2, or 3), have no CT evidence of brain swelling, have an aneurysm that can be approached without excessive retraction, and are considered to be medically stable. After operation, the patient is usually followed in the neurointensive care unit until neurologically stable, with transcranial Doppler ultrasonography every 1 to 2 days. The patient should be kept well hydrated, be maintained on oxygen, and have central venous access for monitoring of central venous pressure. (Pages 168–169 and Table 14-4 discuss prevention and treatment of vasospasm.)

Although direct surgical clipping has long been and remains the preferred form of early treatment for ruptured aneurysms, the efficacy of early endovascular treatment with coil placement into the ruptured aneurysm is under study. (Chapter 28 discusses the management of unruptured intracranial aneurysms.)

VASCULAR MALFORMATIONS

Arteriovenous malformations (AVMs) are the most common type of intracranial vascular malformation causing neurologic symptoms. Other classifications of vascular malformations that may lead to neurologic disease include **cavernous malformations (caver-**

nous hemangiomas), **venous malformations (venous angiomas)**, and **dural-based arteriovenous fistulae.** According to autopsy series, about 63% of supratentorial and 43% of infratentorial vascular malformations are arteriovenous in type. The overall frequency of detection of intracranial vascular malformations is 2.75/100,000 person-years, whereas the prevalence of these lesions in one population-based study was 19.0/100,000 person-years.

AVMs most commonly present with intracranial hemorrhage or seizures. Other manifestations include headaches, which may mimic migraine, progressive neurologic deficit, pulsatile tinnitus, and transient cerebral ischemia. If a lesion is detected before hemorrhage, the risk of hemorrhage is about 2.2%/year, and the case-fatality rate is 15% to 30%. The most frequent site for intracranial hemorrhage is intracerebral, followed by subarachnoid, intraventricular, and subdural. AVMs cause about 5% of all subarachnoid hemorrhages.

Cavernous malformations may also cause significant intracranial hemorrhage, but the hemorrhages are less commonly clinically relevant than AVMs and are typically intracerebral in site. More common presentations include seizures, progressive neurologic deficit, and headache. **Venous malformations** are the most common vascular malformation detected at autopsy, but the clinical importance of these lesions is unclear. They are infrequently associated with intracranial hemorrhage (both intracerebral and subarachnoid) and seizures. **Dural-based arteriovenous fistulae** usually present with pulsatile tinnitus, headache, loss of visual acuity, and diplopia, although intracranial hemorrhage may also occur.

Radiologic imaging studies performed after a patient presents with intracerebral hemorrhage may suggest the presence of an underlying vascular malformation. With AVMs, CT may demonstrate calcification and hypodensity surrounding the lesion. The feeding arteries and draining veins are markedly enhanced after injection of contrast medium. MRI and MRA allow further clarification of the nature of the vascular supply and drainage, but standard arteriography is necessary to better demonstrate the arterial feeding system and venous drainage (Fig. 17-6).

Because AVMs have a lower risk of rebleeding than do saccular aneurysms, conservative management during the immediate posthemorrhage phase is commonly advised to prevent increased intracranial pressure (surgery is usually delayed until 1–2 weeks after the hemorrhage). Generally, relatively young patients with small malformations located superficially in the frontal or temporal area of the nondominant hemisphere are the best candidates for operation; very large malformations (>6 cm in diameter) involving more than one lobe or the posterior fossa and deep areas of the brain may be inoperable or unable to be resected at one sitting. Preceding embolization of feeding vessels may be required. When feasible, early excision of the entire AVM is the preferred therapy. Although newer microsurgical techniques have made safe removal of more malformations possible, many still cannot be totally excised.

Endovascular embolization also should be considered as a preparation for operation in patients with a few major arterial feeders, especially for malformations larger than 3 cm and for treatment of dural AVMs. However, embolization of small feeders is associated with some risk of accidental embolization of a normal artery, which

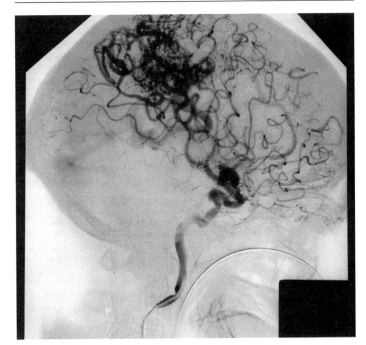

Fig. 17-6. Cerebral arteriogram: left frontoparietal arteriovenous malformation.

results in brain ischemia or infarct, and so this procedure should be avoided. Another possible complication associated with endovascular embolization is intracranial hemorrhage caused by rupture of an arterial feeder. Embolization alone is rarely successful for totally obliterating an AVM and is used infrequently as a sole means of treatment. Other surgical options in the management of AVMs include gamma knife radiosurgery and linear accelerator (LINAC) or Bragg-peak proton beam radiosurgery.

AVMs located deep within the dominant hemisphere, in the brain stem, or in other highly risky areas of the brain such as the internal capsule and the thalamus are often considered to be inoperable because of their inaccessibility or high risk of postoperative severe neurologic deficit and death. Even in the most experienced centers, surgical excision of an AVM with or without embolization is associated with a mortality rate of 1% to 5% and a morbidity rate of 10% to 20%. If surgical excision is not feasible, focused radiotherapy (gamma knife or proton beam radiosurgery) alone or after embolization of the feeders or as an adjunct to embolization and resection may be considered. Radiotherapy (gamma knife) may be especially effective if the nidus is no larger than 3 to 4 cm in diameter (2 cm in the brain stem).

Approximately 40% of lesions are arteriographically obliterated at 1 year after radiosurgery, 80% after 2 years, and about 90% after 3 years. However, intracranial hemorrhage may occur until the lesion is completely obliterated. Other complications of radiosurgery include radionecrosis of normal brain tissue and focal neurologic deficits in approximately 6% of patients (3% transient and 3% permanent). Occasionally, focal seizures occur within the first few days of treatment, usually in patients with a preexisting seizure disorder. Radiotherapy is less satisfactory for treatment of AVMs larger than 3 to 4 cm in the hemispheres or larger than 2 cm in the brain stem. (Chapter 29 discusses the management of unruptured AVMs.)

Cavernous malformations presenting with significant hemorrhage or intractable seizures are typically treated surgically if they are at an accessible site. Rarely, lesions have been treated with gamma knife radiosurgery if surgically inaccessible and presenting with recurrent hemorrhage. **Venous malformations** are usually treated conservatively, although those clearly associated with intracranial hemorrhage are generally excised. **Dural arteriovenous fistulas** may be treated with endovascular occlusive procedures (embolization or coils), surgical excision, or radiosurgery, depending on the size, location, and vascular characteristics.

OTHER CAUSES OF SUBARACHNOID HEMORRHAGE

Other factors that may also be associated with nontraumatic subarachnoid hemorrhage are (1) hypertension; (2) hematologic disorders, such as disseminated intravascular coagulation, often associated with leukemia or thrombocytopenia; (3) anticoagulant therapy; (4) cortical vein and dural sinus thrombosis; (5) primary or metastatic brain tumor; and (6) cerebral vasculitis. Management of these conditions is specific for each underlying pathologic process.

Intracerebral Hemorrhage

The onset of intracerebral hemorrhage is usually rapid, but unlike the acute, sudden onset to maximal deficit of embolism, this process typically evolves during minutes to hours without the stepwise progression of many ischemic strokes. The hemorrhage usually occurs while the patient is up and active, and it frequently presents with a severe headache and decreased level of consciousness, with nonfocal symptoms often predominating over the focal neurologic deficit. Small hemorrhages usually produce restricted focal neurologic deficit accompanied by mild or moderate nonfocal neurologic signs, and those in "silent" regions of the brain may even escape clinical detection, whereas large hemorrhages may produce early coma and signs of herniation.

Rupture of an **intracerebral hematoma** through to the cortical surface may produce associated bleeding **into the subarachnoid space.** When the hemorrhage is in the basal ganglia, thalamus, brain stem, or cerebellum, rupture into the ventricular system may occur. **Intracerebral hemorrhage** occasionally also occurs **within a cerebral infarct** resulting from venous thrombosis or, less commonly, arterial ischemia, together accounting for about 4% of cases.

Hypertension is the most frequently identified predisposing cause of nontraumatic intracerebral hemorrhage in adults. Other common causes are ruptured intracranial saccular aneurysm and vascular malformations such as AVM and cavernous malformations. Causes of intracerebral hemorrhage are reviewed in Table 8-2.

Once the diagnosis of intraparenchymal hemorrhage is established by CT or MRI of the head, one must use the clinical history, physical examination, appearance of the hematoma on CT or MRI (including location and size), and other appropriate laboratory tests to define the underlying cause of the hemorrhage, as delineated in Chapter 15. Decisions regarding diagnostic workup, medical treatment, and timing of operation should be based on both neurologic and neurosurgical criteria. General diagnostic and treatment considerations are outlined in Chapter 15. Management of patients with specifically identified underlying mechanisms for intracerebral hemorrhage is delineated in this chapter.

Primary hypertensive intracerebral hemorrhage is the most common nontraumatic brain hemorrhage and constitutes as much as 60% of all brain hemorrhages. This type of hemorrhage usually occurs with marked hypertension that produces anatomical changes, including microaneurysms and lipohyalinosis in the small intraparenchymal arteries. Less commonly, it occurs with moderate hypertension or even with blood pressure in the normal range. The most common locations of hypertensive intracerebral hemorrhage are the basal ganglia and thalamus (37%; penetrating artery involved); temporal (21%), frontal (15%), or parieto-occipital (15%) lobes; cerebellum (8%); and pons (4%). In pathologic studies, these hemorrhages are described as large (more than 2 cm in diameter), small (1–2 cm in diameter), slit (<1 cm in diameter lying subcortically at the junction of white and gray matter), and petechial. Clinically, with the advent of radiologic imaging studies, the volume of the hemorrhage may be calculated from the maximal diameters of the hemorrhage in three dimensions. The volume and clinical status of the patient at presentation appear to be important predictors of outcome.

Management of patients with hypertensive intracerebral hemorrhage depends on the degree of hypertension; the location, surgical accessibility, and size of the hematoma; and the patient's clinical condition. Efforts should be made to (1) lower the elevated blood pressure that set the stage for the hemorrhage and maintain blood pressure in the appropriate range (see pages 177–178); (2) gradually reduce the mass effect (antiedema agents, see Chapter 15 and Table 11-1); and (3) prevent complications (see Chapters 11 and 15). If the patient's condition is stable and the hemorrhage is not life-threatening, a nonsurgical approach is recommended. In patients with lobar or cerebellar hemorrhage and associated signs of secondary deterioration related to increased intracranial pressure or brain herniation, immediate surgical treatment (evacuation of the hematoma) may be lifesaving and should be strongly considered. Emergency intervention in this setting may begin with maximal medical decompression with mannitol (1 g/kg) and high-dose steroids given intravenously, intubation, and hyperventilation. Blood pressure must be controlled, usually with a beta-adrenergic blocker, calcium channel blocker, or angiotensin-converting enzyme inhibitor. Generally accepted contraindications to operation are massive hemorrhage with loss of brain stem function (such as fixed, dilated pupils and decerebrate posturing) and no response to medical therapy (see pages 176–177).

Nonhypertensive causes of intracerebral hemorrhage include ruptured vascular malformations and aneurysms, complications of anticoagulant or fibrinolytic therapy, hematologic diseases (thrombocytopenia, bleeding diathesis, hemophilia), head trauma, cerebral amyloid angiopathy, primary or metastatic brain tumors, and arteritis affecting the cerebral arteries and veins.

Ruptured vascular malformations (especially arteriovenous and cavernous malformations) cause about 5% of all intracerebral hemorrhages (roughly 1% of all strokes). About 60% of intracranial hemorrhages associated with AVMs are intracerebral in location, whereas subarachnoid hemorrhage occurs in approximately 30% of cases and ventricular hemorrhage in 10%. Headache at the onset of rupture of an AVM, rebleeding, and symptomatic cerebral vasospasm are not as prominent as with a ruptured saccular aneurysm. These intracerebral hemorrhages usually evolve slower than those from hypertension or ruptured saccular aneurysms. The possibility of an underlying vascular malformation should be considered in patients with intracerebral hemorrhage, particularly in patients who have lobar and cortical hemorrhages with associated subarachnoid bleeding of unexplained mechanism, and especially in young adults (15–45 years old). Cerebral arteriography must be considered in young adults with intracerebral hemorrhage of unknown cause and in older patients without a history of hypertension. Other diagnostic and treatment issues regarding vascular malformations are reviewed on pages 216–219.

Intracerebral hemorrhages that are caused by **aneurysmal rupture** are commonly managed with early surgical intervention (within 3 days) to evacuate the hematoma and clip the aneurysm, unless contraindications exist as noted on page 216. For patients in poor medical condition (severe neurologic deficit with altered level of consciousness), operation is usually delayed until the patient's condition improves with conservative management.

Cerebral amyloid angiopathy (congophilic angiopathy) is characterized by the deposition of amyloid protein in media and adventitia of leptomeningeal and cortical small arteries, arterioles, and capillaries, which is not associated with systemic amyloidosis. The amyloid angiopathy predisposes to miliary aneurysm formation or double barreling and fibrinoid necrosis of the affected vessels, which are prone to rupture in response to minor trauma or sudden changes in blood pressure. Although the presence of amyloid seems to be strongly related to advancing age (overall, cerebral amyloid angiopathy causes approximately 15% to 20% of intracerebral hemorrhages in the elderly), the precise mechanism for its development is unknown.

The diagnosis of cerebral amyloid angiopathy should be considered in normotensive patients, primarily those older than 65 years, who have nonhypertensive intracerebral hemorrhage, particularly in a subcortical or lobar location. However, about 30% of patients have coexistent hypertension. Multiple, hyperdense foci of blood on noncontrast CT of the head in lobar locations or multiple punctate hemorrhagic lesions associated with periventricular leukoencephalopathy on MRI suggest the diagnosis of cerebral amyloid angiopathy. Recurrent intracerebral bleeding associated with amyloid angiopathy is common; minor head trauma, anticoagulation, and antiplatelet therapy have been reported as potential precipitants of the bleeding. A definitive diagnosis of cerebral amyloid angiopathy is made by biopsy of the involved brain and leptomeninges, although this is uncommonly indicated.

Because cerebral amyloid angiopathy is a widespread, vascular disease prone to recurrence and because intraoperative hemostasis is difficult, surgical removal of lobar hemorrhage is generally avoided, except in situations of progressive or life-threatening hematomas in patients who are otherwise in relatively good condition. Conservative management consists of close clinical monitoring for signs and symptoms of increased intracranial pressure, maintenance of fluid and electrolyte balance, airway management, treatment of systemic cardiovascular disorders, prevention of secondary complications, and administration of prophylactic anticonvulsants because most hemorrhages involve the cerebral cortex. Anticoagulants and antiplatelet agents should be avoided.

Intracerebral hemorrhages occurring as a **complication of anticoagulant or fibrinolytic therapy** usually evolve more slowly than those caused by hypertension. Intracerebral hemorrhage related to the use of streptokinase or tissue plasminogen activator for myocardial or cerebral infarction tends to occur within 24 hours of infusion of these drugs. In this situation, if possible, appropriate measures (such as protamine for heparin and fresh frozen plasma with or without parenteral vitamin K [25 mg subcutaneously] for warfarin agents) should be taken to reverse coagulation defects.

Intracerebral hemorrhage caused by **thrombocytopenia** is commonly treated with platelet transfusions; for patients who have cerebrovascular disease with a **bleeding diathesis** resulting from low prothrombin, replacement with plasma protein fraction and the administration of vitamin K are recommended. Intracerebral hemorrhage resulting from **hemophilia** (hereditary abnormalities in factor VIII) should be treated with early and aggressive replacement of factor VIII, in the form of cryoprecipitate or commercial factor VIII concentrates.

Head trauma may produce intraparenchymal hemorrhage, often in the form of cortical contusions at the site of impact of a blow to the head (coup injury) or opposite the site of impact (contrecoup injury). Contusion may be associated with petechial hemorrhage or a large area of hemorrhage with more severe injuries, which are typically located along the hemispheric cortical surfaces, the inferior surface of the corpus callosum, the cerebral peduncles, and in the rostral brain stem. In contrast to epidural and subdural hemorrhagic components of traumatic head injury, intraparenchymal hemorrhages are seldom treated surgically unless they are associated with hydrocephalus or evolving mass effect from blood. Efforts are instituted to correct cerebral edema (see pages 139–141 and Table 11-1) and any associated hypocoagulable state.

Bleeding into **brain tumors** is relatively rare and may result from primary brain tumors (for example, glioblastoma, pituitary adenoma, medulloblastoma) or metastases (bronchogenic carcinoma, malignant melanoma, renal cell carcinoma, and choriocarcinoma). Secondary hemorrhage into a previously asymptomatic brain tumor should be suspected in patients with a history of malignant disease or patients presenting with papilledema. Characteristic CT or MRI findings are multiple hemorrhages, ring-like, high-density areas of blood surrounding a low-density center, disproportionate edema and mass effect surrounding the acute hemorrhage, and postcontrast enhancement of nodules at the periphery of the acute hematoma or ring enhancement pattern. Management is based predominantly on neuro-oncologic principles and depends on the precise nature of the underlying tumor, which is usually defined by biopsy of a systemic primary or brain lesion.

Intracerebral hemorrhage resulting from **cerebral arteritis** is usually characterized by preceding chronic headache, progressive intellectual deterioration and altered consciousness, and, often, seizures, recurrent episodes of cerebral infarction, fever, malaise, arthralgias, myalgias, weight loss, and anemia (see page 203). The diagnosis is suggested by elevated erythrocyte sedimentation rate (typical of systemic vasculitides but uncommon in isolated central nervous system angiitis) or cerebrospinal fluid findings, including elevated protein and lymphocytic pleocytosis (occasionally found in isolated central nervous system angiitis). Cerebral arteriography occasionally shows a characteristic beading pattern in multiple intracranial arteries with multiple branch occlusions; in such cases, evacuation of the clot should be considered. The diagnosis can be confirmed with brain biopsy before initiating immunosuppressive treatment (see page 203).

Intraventricular Hemorrhage

Primary intraventricular hemorrhage is relatively rare and usually results from vascular malformation or neoplasm of the choroid plexus. Clinically, primary hemorrhage into the ventricles produces a sudden loss of consciousness without focal neurologic deficit (coma with periodic, generalized tonic seizures may occur in some patients with extensive intraventricular hemorrhage). Most patients with intraventricular hemorrhage are treated medically. However, if indications for surgical treatment (as discussed on page 176 for parenchymal hematoma) exist, immediate evacuation of the clot should be considered. Ventricular drainage is generally of limited value; however, ventriculostomy can be lifesaving for patients who have neurologic deterioration caused by acute hydrocephalus, as shown by CT.

Cerebral Venous Thrombosis

Intracranial venous thrombosis may arise from infectious or non-infectious processes. Since the introduction of antibiotics, the frequency of venous thrombosis has decreased considerably, apparently from the prevention of thrombosis related to local head infections. In recent years, most cases of intracranial venous thrombosis have been aseptic in nature, and most of these are considered idiopathic. Other causes of aseptic intracranial venous thrombosis are polycythemia vera, leukemia, dehydration, cancer, phospholipid antibody syndromes, sickle-cell disease, Behçet's disease and other inflammatory disorders, and other hyperviscosity syndromes.

The clinical presentation of cerebral venous thrombosis varies, depending on the site of the lesion, its rate of progression and extension of thrombosis, and the nature of the underlying disease. Typically, the initial symptom is severe headache, which may precede other signs and symptoms by hours or days. Vomiting and focal seizures also tend to occur early in the course along with weakness and sensory disturbances that are usually progressive and may be unilateral or bilateral. Consciousness is usually altered, and language disturbances occur in about one-fourth of patients. There is a tendency for venous infarcts to become hemorrhagic.

The diagnosis is based on the combination of clinical findings with radiographic documentation of venous occlusion. The patient's pelvis and legs are examined carefully to rule out coexistent peripheral thrombosis. The definitive diagnostic procedure has long been cerebral arteriography, but in recent years computed tomography (CT) and magnetic resonance imaging (MRI) have proved helpful through visualization of hemorrhagic infarcts and thrombosed veins or venous sinuses. Magnetic resonance angiography (MRA) provides excellent visualization of the venous sinuses and is valuable for the early diagnosis of venous thrombosis (Fig. 18-1).

The mortality rate is about 20% (hemorrhagic infarction caused by cerebral venous thrombosis is associated with the worst prognosis), but functional outcome among survivors is usually favorable, with less chance of persistent focal neurologic deficit than that for patients with arterial cerebral infarction. Clinical presentation and underlying causes for venous infarcts vary to some extent with the location of the lesion.

Lateral sinus thrombosis commonly occurs in children and adolescents who have otitis media and may be asymptomatic, but those with propagation of thrombus into the superior sagittal sinus may experience progressive cerebral edema. If the thrombosis extends into the jugular vein, a jugular foramen syndrome may occur (involving cranial nerves IX, X, and XI).

Superior sagittal sinus thrombosis is the most common site of sinus occlusion. Presenting symptoms are variable. Some lesions may be asymptomatic, but significant thrombosis in the posterior segments may lead to increased intracranial pressure, papilledema, headaches, and decreased level of consciousness.

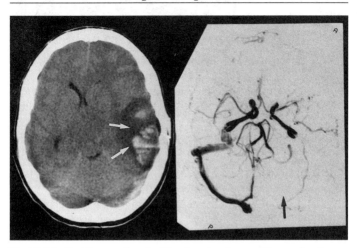

Fig. 18-1. Left. CT scan of head without contrast: area of hemorrhagic venous infarction (arrows). Right. MRA: asymmetry of transverse sinuses, consistent with left transverse sinus occlusion (arrow).

Inferior petrosal sinus or superior petrosal sinus thrombosis may be associated with infections of the middle ear. The former may lead to diplopia caused by involvement of the abducens nerve; the latter may cause facial pain from trigeminal ganglion irritation.

Cavernous sinus thrombosis is usually caused by paranasal sinus infections, facial furuncles, or ear infections and characteristically produces severe headache, ipsilateral proptosis, visual loss, chemosis, and palsies of the third, fourth, or sixth cranial nerves or the first division of the fifth cranial nerve. Ocular signs often become bilateral after a short period, and neck rigidity and hemiparesis may occur. An accompanying palsy of the second and third divisions of the fifth cranial nerve usually indicates superior petrosal sinus involvement. Thrombosis of the jugular vein, lateral sinus, or torcula may produce signs of increased intracranial pressure without ventricular dilatation.

Venous cerebral thrombosis with bland or hemorrhagic infarction should be suspected when focal neurologic symptoms, especially hemiparesis accompanied by severe headache or seizures, develop in the course of meningitis, otitis media, or disseminated malignancy (especially lymphoma, leukemia, or meningeal metastasis), during the postpartum period (pelvic or other deep venous thrombosis is often present), or postoperatively. Thrombosis of cerebral veins can also occur in association with cachexia, dehydration, cardiac failure (especially congenital heart disease), inflammatory disorders such as Behçet's disease, or changes in blood coagulability (for example, primary or secondary polycythemia, use of oral contraceptives, antithrombin III deficiency, disseminated intravascular coagulation, ulcerative colitis, leukemia, polycythemia vera, hemolytic anemia, sickle-cell disease, or antiphospholipid antibody syndrome). Some aseptic thromboses of multiple cerebral veins and sinuses are idiopathic and also involve extracranial veins simultaneously or in succession (thrombophlebitis migrans).

Treatment of intracranial venous occlusions, including those with minor hemorrhagic infarction, generally includes bed rest (the patient's head should be kept elevated at 15 to 30 degrees to improve venous drainage and lessen intracranial pressure), hydration (with half-normal or normal saline to maintain normal fluid status), and heparin anticoagulant therapy for 1 week, followed by warfarin for at least 3 months (longer for specific hypercoagulable states). Antiplatelet agents (such as aspirin) are usually given thereafter. Heparin and warfarin therapy is contraindicated in patients with significant hemorrhage on CT. In these patients, after a delay of 1 to 2 weeks, treatment with antiplatelet agents is often initiated, assuming no new hemorrhage, unless specific hypercoagulable states provide a very compelling case for long-term therapy with anticoagulants.

Antiedema therapy (mannitol or corticosteroids) is indicated only in patients with substantial or persistent papilledema and threatened visual loss (see pages 139–141 and Table 11-1). Thrombolytic therapy of arteriographically proven aseptic cerebral venous thrombosis with intravenous or transjugular infusion of urokinase followed by anticoagulant therapy has been reported but is of unknown efficacy. Hypotension or hypertension also should be corrected.

Treatment of lateral sinus thrombosis caused by otitis media or mastoiditis usually includes removal of the infected bone, administration of antibiotics, and surgical drainage of abscesses. The jugular vein may be ligated if necessary. Antibiotics (with or without anticoagulants) should be administered to patients with septic superior sagittal sinus thrombosis or cavernous sinus thrombosis, and craniotomy with evacuation of subdural or epidural abscess should be performed when these conditions are present.

Patients in whom intracranial venous occlusion develops while they are taking oral contraceptives, antifibrinolytic agents, androgen drugs, or L-asparaginase should be advised to discontinue use of these drugs. If the disease is complicated by seizures, phenytoin or phenobarbital should be given in loading doses as described on pages 160–162.

Other Cerebrovascular Syndromes

Hypertensive Encephalopathy

Acute or sustained elevation of blood pressure may result in failure of cerebral autoregulatory mechanisms, with vasodilatation, hyperperfusion, and exudation of fluid. Increased intracranial pressure, capillary compression, and decreased intraparenchymal blood flow may result in **hypertensive encephalopathy.**

Affected patients have malignant or uncontrolled hypertension from any of various causes, including chronic renal disease, pheochromocytoma, antihypertensive withdrawal syndrome, sympathomimetic drugs, acute toxemia of pregnancy, Cushing's syndrome, aortic dissection, and polyarteritis nodosa. The diagnostic term should be reserved for the few patients who, in addition to extreme increases in blood pressure (diastolic pressure usually >120 mm Hg), have severe hypertensive retinopathy (papilledema, retinal hemorrhages, or exudates, with or without optic nerve infarction) or severe retinal arteriolar spasm and altered consciousness.

The syndrome usually develops during a period of several minutes to several hours and is usually characterized by diffuse, moderate-to-severe headache, nausea, vomiting, and various visual symptoms such as visual blurring or dimming, scintillating scotoma, or cortical blindness, with or without vivid visual hallucinations. Generalized or focal seizures or altered consciousness or behavior (anxiety, agitation, disorientation, drowsiness, confusion, or coma) are common. On examination, generalized hyperreflexia is a common early feature. Focal neurologic findings (which may be postictal) are infrequent and may reflect an underlying intracerebral hemorrhage or infarction. Computed tomography (CT) may reveal evidence of cerebral edema or ischemia (widespread low attenuation primarily involving white matter). Magnetic resonance imaging (MRI) usually demonstrates white matter edema and increased T2-weighted signal bilaterally involving the occipital lobes, the parieto-occipital junction areas, or the superior frontal lobes.

Hypertensive encephalopathy may be complicated by acute congestive heart failure, pulmonary edema, acute anuria, or microangiopathic hemolytic anemia. Prompt reduction in blood pressure is essential and is achieved with sodium nitroprusside (0.3–0.5 µg/kg/minute intravenously, titrated to the desired effect, with the usual dose 1–3 µg/kg/minute), diazoxide (1–2 mg/kg by intravenous bolus, repeated every 10 minutes, not to exceed 150 mg; or 15–30 mg/minute by intravenous infusion), or labetalol hydrochloride (10–20 mg intravenously for 1–2 minutes, repeated or doubled every 10–20 minutes until desired blood pressure is achieved or until a cumulative dose of 300 mg is reached; or 2 mg/minute by intravenous infusion).

The initial aim of antihypertensive therapy should be to reduce the patient's mean arterial blood pressure by approximately 20% within a few hours. Further control of blood pressure is achieved during the next 24 hours with a goal of reducing the diastolic pressure toward, but not less than, 90 mm Hg. This goal can usually be achieved by the administration of direct vasodilators, beta-adrenergic inhibitors, calcium or ganglionic blockers, or sympatholytic agents (see Appendix H). Reduction in blood pressure reverses the pathophysiologic processes responsible for the clinical symptoms.

Vascular Dementia

Vascular or arteriosclerotic dementia constitutes about 10% of all cases of dementia. It is caused by multiple bilateral cerebral infarcts, especially involving regions such as the medial temporal lobes, the medial frontal lobes, the corpus callosum, and the nondominant parietal lobe. A history of one or more strokes preceding the dementia is common, and the first symptoms of dementia commonly appear within 1 year of focal neurologic symptoms or signs. Typical clinical features of the dementia include abrupt onset and a fluctuating course with a stepwise or slowly progressive loss of function (see Chapter 2). Other common neurologic signs include hemiparesis, hemianopia, and pseudobulbar palsy. Associated atherosclerosis, hypertension, diabetes mellitus, and other risk factors for stroke are usually present. The diagnosis should be made on the basis of the historical evaluation (see Chapter 2), examination (see Chapter 5), and diagnostic imaging findings. CT findings include multiple areas of low attenuation in the subcortical white matter or multiple other areas of infarction. MRI demonstrates areas of increased T2 signal diffusely in subcortical regions, although these may be detected in the absence of dementia.

Although effective **specific treatment** of vascular dementia is still lacking, it may be possible to influence the development or progression of this disease by controlling cerebrovascular risk factors, particularly hypertension, sources of emboli, and other risk factors for atherosclerosis (see Chapters 24–27). Palliative **symptomatic treatment** may be useful for abulia or inattention (methylphenidate or dextroamphetamine sulfate, 10–60 mg, divided into two or three doses daily), depression (imipramine, amitriptyline, or desipramine, 75–300 mg, once a day at bedtime), and agitated confusion (lorazepam, 0.5–2 mg, orally or intramuscularly at bedtime; haloperidol, 1–6 mg, orally, divided into two or three doses). One must be careful to avoid overtreatment of hypertension, which may lead to side effects such as orthostatic hypotension.

Vascular dementia should be differentiated from other types of dementia, such as **Alzheimer's disease** (insidious onset, slowly progressive course without focal peripheral neurologic signs or systemic illness at onset, associated with diffuse atrophy of the cortex, especially involving the frontal and temporal lobes, with characteristic neurofibrillary degeneration and senile plaques), **brain tumor or subdural hematoma** (focal neurologic signs often accompanied by symptoms of increased intracranial pressure, history of neoplasm or trauma), **Huntington's disease** (family history, chorea), **normal-pressure hydrocephalus** (gait disturbance and incontinence), **inflammatory disease** (**vasculitis**—evidence of arteritis elsewhere, relatively young age of patient, history of infections that could affect the cerebral vessels, for example, syphilis or tuberculosis), **infectious diseases** (human immunodeficiency virus [HIV] infection, syphilis, meningitis), **nutritional deficiencies** (Wernicke-Korsakoff syndrome, Marchiafava-Bignami disease, pellagra, vitamin B_{12} deficiency), **other syndromes** associated with systemic disorders such as progressive multifocal leukoencephalopathy (systemic illness such as lymphoma or HIV infection, with diffuse, rapidly progressive multifocal neurologic symptoms, sometimes associated with signs of increased intracranial pressure and seizures), **chronic drug intoxication** (alcohol, sedatives), **endocrine-metabolic disorders** (myxedema, Cushing's disease, chronic hepatic or renal encephalopathies), **posttraumatic disease** (history of head trauma), and the **pseudodementia of depression** (see Chapter 2).

Binswanger's Encephalopathy

Binswanger's encephalopathy is a rare disorder that has been associated with diffuse hemispheric demyelination resulting from chronic ischemia in central white matter caused by chronic hypertensive cerebrovascular disease and arteriolar sclerosis. Clinically, this encephalopathy is characterized by progressive dementia and pseudobulbar palsy associated with periventricular low-attenuation areas on CT. There is no specific treatment for Binswanger's encephalopathy, but symptomatic therapy (as discussed above for vascular dementia) and treatment of occult hydrocephalus are recommended in appropriate situations.

Vascular Disease of the Spinal Cord

Spinovascular disease is rare compared with cerebrovascular disease. It includes spinal cord infarction, hemorrhage, transient ischemic attack, and venous disease. The clinical symptoms of spinovascular disease usually begin abruptly and vary in severity and rate of onset, depending on the affected vessel, the level of the lesion (most commonly, lower thoracic cord and conus medullaris), and underlying disease. Spinovascular diseases should be differentiated from **spinal cord compression** (primary or metastatic tumors, acute extradural abscess, spinal tuberculosis, disk prolapse, spinal trauma, and spondylosis), **transverse myelitis** (often occurs with local pain followed by paraparesis or paraplegia, numbness, and urinary retention in association with cerebrospinal fluid lymphocytic pleocytosis and increased protein), **Guillain-Barré syndrome** (progressive weakness during a period of several days or a few weeks, occurring diffusely or beginning in the legs and spreading proximally, involving first the trunk, then arms, neck, respiration, and cranial muscles), **syringomyelia** (typical segmental dysfunction with bilateral and, occasionally, unilateral loss of cutaneous sensation and dissociated sensory loss, but sparing the sense of touch, position, and vibration), **subacute combined degeneration** (often present with gait disorder, lower motor neuron signs with loss of position and vibration, with no motor or sensory level, related to vitamin B_{12} deficiency and pernicious anemia), and **Friedreich's ataxia** (a genetic disorder gradually resulting in ataxia of the limbs and trunk with areflexia and dysarthria, Babinski signs, and, occasionally, pes cavus, optic atrophy, nystagmus, cardiomyopathy, and scoliosis). The diagnosis is suggested by the patient's history and is confirmed by myelography, cerebrospinal fluid analysis, spinal arteriography, computed tomography (CT), or magnetic resonance imaging (MRI).

The general principles outlined for treatment of cerebrovascular disease (see Chapters 11–17) may be applied in cases in which analogies to vascular diseases of the spinal cord can be made, with additional attention to bladder and skin care and physical therapy. For subdural and epidural spinal hemorrhage, immediate operation is often necessary. Although intramedullary hemorrhages from arteriovenous malformations may be removed, followed by successful resection of the malformation, hematomyelia resulting from trauma with no myelographic evidence of an associated compressive lesion is usually treated conservatively.

Spinal Cord Infarction

The common causes of spinal cord infarction are (1) aortic disease (dissecting aneurysm, severe atherosclerosis, thrombosis) or surgical procedures such as aortic aneurysm repair, femoral artery catheterization, and coronary artery bypass grafting; (2) small-vessel disease (polyarteritis nodosa, systemic lupus erythematosus, neurosyphilis, secondary endarteritis resulting from tuberculosis or borreliosis, or isolated central nervous system angiitis); (3) spinal or segmental artery compression or occlusion caused by disk fragments, extradural abscess or tumor, aortic arteriography, or sickle-cell disease; (4) hypotension caused by myocardial infarction or cardiac arrest; and (5) spinal cord arteriovenous malformation.

An ischemic lesion of the spinal cord usually involves the territory of the anterior spinal artery (the ventral two-thirds of the spinal cord, Fig. 20-1) and produces radicular or ascending leg pain at onset; sudden nonprogressive paraplegia or quadriplegia (flaccid legs, which soon become spastic); areflexia (evolving after days or weeks to hyperreflexia with extensor plantar responses); sensory loss to pain and temperature to the level of the lesion with preserved light touch, position, and vibration sense; urinary and fecal incontinence; and, later, focal atrophy and wasting (with cervical or lumbar infarction). Infarction in the territory of the posterior spinal artery (dorsal columns and the posterior horns) may produce loss of joint position and vibration sense below the lesion and deep tendon reflexes at the level of the lesion.

For patients with spinal cord infarction associated with suspected aortic dissection, emergency aortic operation may be indicated after medical and neurologic stabilization. Initial pharmacologic treatment often involves nitroprusside or a beta-adrenergic blocker (see Chapter 11). When the dissection involves the ascending aorta, prompt operation is usually advised. When the dissection originates beyond the origin of the left subclavian artery, pharmacologic therapy can be continued if symptoms are controlled, but surgical resection should be considered. Occasionally, dissection of the ascending thoracic aorta may also compromise cerebral blood flow because of occlusion or stenosis at the origins of the carotid, brachiocephalic, or subclavian artery.

Spinal Cord Hemorrhage

Spinal cord hemorrhage is also rare compared with the frequency of brain hemorrhage. Almost all nontraumatic hemorrhages into the spinal cord are the result of arteriovenous malformations, metastatic tumor, bleeding disorders, and the use of anticoagulants. The invariably sudden onset of symptoms (back or leg pain, paraparesis or quadriparesis, paraplegia or quadriplegia, sensory loss) associated with blood and xanthochromia in the cerebrospinal fluid are the common clinical features of hematomyelia. MRI or myelography may demonstrate the swollen cord, and, additionally, MRI may demonstrate the hemorrhage in the cord.

Bleeding into the epidural or subdural spinal space produces rapidly evolving compressive myelopathy (sudden or gradual onset with severe back pain and a rapidly progressive paraplegia). Most commonly, anticoagulant use is causative, although liver disease is occasionally associated. Spinal subarachnoid hemorrhage is uncommon and is most typically caused by an arteriovenous malformation. Bleeding disorders, use of anticoagulants, and spinal artery aneurysms are less common causes. Clinical features include sudden

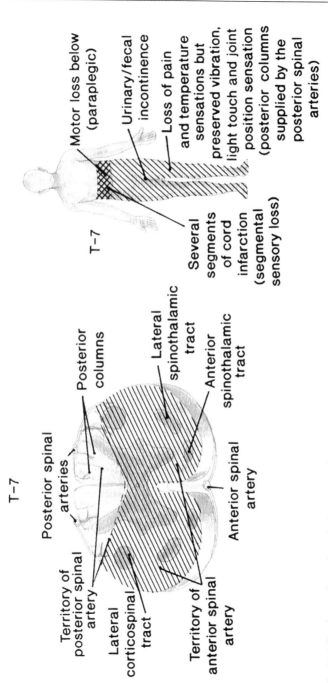

Fig. 20-1. Territory of anterior spinal artery and associated syndromes.

onset of back or leg pain, followed by neck stiffness, but often without headache unless the blood spreads into the cranial subarachnoid space. Symptoms of myelopathy or radiculopathy may occur, helping to localize the process to a spinal cord level.

Transient Spinal Ischemic Attack

Transient spinal ischemic attack is a rare condition resulting from emboli coming from the heart, aorta, or radicular arteries or caused by an arteriovenous malformation or aortic coarctation. Hemodynamic transient spinal ischemic attack is caused by a stenotic arterial lesion, aortic coarctation, or spinal arteriovenous malformation (spinal claudication of Dejerine or aortic "steal" syndrome), usually presenting with transient paraparesis, difficulty walking, and the appearance of Babinski signs induced by exercise because blood is shunted away from the spinal cord, which causes transient ischemia.

Venous Disease of the Spinal Cord

Venous disease of the spinal cord may be caused by coagulopathy with venous thrombosis, venous compression caused by an epidural mass, and spinal vascular malformations. Venous disease of the spinal cord includes hemorrhagic and nonhemorrhagic spinal infarction, which are very rare. Venous hemorrhagic infarctions are characterized by sudden onset of symptoms (back, leg, or abdominal pain, flaccid paraparesis or paraplegia, ascending loss of sensation, disturbances of bowel and bladder function) progressing within 1 to 2 days. Nonhemorrhagic venous infarction may produce the same symptoms but more gradually; the clinical onset may be as long as 1 year, and back pain typically does not occur (there is usually evidence of venous thrombosis elsewhere). The **Foix-Alajouanine syndrome** is characterized by spinal cord necrosis involving the corticospinal tract (anterior horn cells are spared) and evidence of enlarged, tortuous, and thrombosed veins, often found in association with a vascular malformation.

Cerebrovascular Disease in Children and Young Adults

Stroke is uncommon in children younger than 15 years. The annual incidence is about 2.5 cases/100,000 children. Ischemic strokes in young adults (ages 15–40 years) constitute about 4% of all cases. Although the frequency of stroke in children and young adults is far less than that in persons older than 50 years, the causes are more diverse.

The frequency of specific causes of ischemic stroke in patients younger than 40 years depends on age. **Cerebral infarction in children** (ages 1–15 years) most commonly results from cardiac diseases, head and neck trauma with dissection, migraine, hematologic disease, and other large vessel occlusive diseases (Table 21-1). In contrast to arterial thrombosis in adults, arterial thrombosis in children more commonly involves the intracranial internal carotid arterial system. Infarction is more commonly subcortical in children, and particularly involves the striatum and internal capsule.

Clinical Presentation

Because cerebrovascular ischemia in children is uncommonly caused by atherosclerotic occlusive disease, transient ischemic attack before cerebral infarction is relatively uncommon. The clinical features of cerebral ischemia are similar to those noted in adults, but seizures are more common. Aphasias usually have some expressive component even if the lesion is posterior. A less common clinical presentation unique to children includes recurrent or alternating hemiplegia with or without associated headache, which may be caused by hemiplegic migraine, or, less commonly, by bilateral carotid artery thrombosis. The clinical features of craniocervical thrombosis or cerebral embolism vary according to the area involved; the anatomic and pathophysiologic principles are analogous to those described for adults in Chapters 1–7.

Etiology

The differential diagnosis of stroke in children and young adults is outlined in Table 21-1. Many of these disorders are reviewed in the setting of cerebral infarction and intracranial hemorrhage in adults (see Chapters 12–17). Causes of **cerebral ischemia** that occur much more commonly in children include **congenital heart disease,** head and neck **trauma** leading to extracranial carotid or vertebral **dissection,** and distal thromboemboli or hemodynamic events. **Hematologic disorders** such as **sickle-cell disease** are an important cause of infarction in children and lead to cerebrovascular disorders in 6% to 25% of patients (see Chapter 16, Hematologic Disease), and hematologic disorders can cause both ischemic and hemorrhagic stroke. Both ischemic and hemorrhagic events tend to occur

**Table 21-1.   Differential diagnosis
of stroke in children and young adults**

Ischemia
Cardiac disease
   Congenital heart disease
   Rheumatic valve disease
   Mitral valve prolapse
   Patent foramen ovale
   Bacterial or marantic endocarditis
   Atrial myxoma
   Pulmonary arteriovenous fistula
   Rhabdomyoma
   Cardiac or umbilical vein catheterization
   Cardiomyopathies
   Arrhythmias
   Cardiac, thoracic surgery
Large vessel disease
   Premature atherosclerosis
   Dissection
      Traumatic
      Spontaneous
   Inherited metabolic diseases
      Homocystinuria
      Fabry's disease
      Pseudoxanthoma elasticum
      Sulfate oxidase deficiency
      MELAS syndrome
   Fibromuscular dysplasia
   Infection
      Bacterial
      Fungal
      Tuberculosis
      Syphilis
      Lyme disease
   Vasculitis
      Collagen vascular disease
         Systemic lupus erythematosus, rheumatoid arthritis, Sjögren's
            syndrome, polyarteritis nodosa
      Takayasu's disease
      Wegener's disease
      Cryoglobulinemia
      Behçet's disease
      Sarcoidosis
      Churg-Strauss syndrome
      Inflammatory bowel disease
      Isolated central nervous system angiitis
   Moyamoya disease
   Radiation
   Toxic
      Illicit drugs: cocaine, heroin, phencyclidine
      Therapeutic drugs: L-asparaginase, cytosine arabinoside
Small vessel disease
   Vasculopathy
      Infectious
      Noninfectious
      Microangiopathy of brain, ear, and retina
Hematologic disease
   Sickle-cell disease
   Leukemia
   Hypercoagulable states

Antiphospholipid antibody syndromes
Protein C or protein S deficiency
Antithrombin III deficiency
Increased factor VIII
Resistance to activated protein C
Disseminated intravascular coagulation
Thrombocytosis
Polycythemia vera
Thrombotic thrombocytopenic purpura

Venous occlusion
Dehydration
Parameningeal infection (sinusitis, mastoiditis)
Meningitis
Neoplasm
Polycythemia
Leukemia
Inflammatory bowel disease

Hemorrhage

Arteriovenous malformation

Saccular aneurysm

Neoplasm
Primary central nervous system neoplasm
Metastatic neoplasm
Leukemia

Hematologic
Sickle-cell disease
Hemophilia
Neoplasm
Leukemia
Thrombocytopenia

Moyamoya disease

Drug use (especially amphetamines, cocaine, phenylpropanolamine)

MELAS = mitochondrial myopathy, encephalopathy, lactic acidosis, and stroke-like episodes.

---

during a painful crisis and usually are seen in patients with more severe disease that includes frequent crises and decreased hematocrit value. Another cause of stroke occurring more commonly in children than adults is **moyamoya disease**.

The differential diagnosis in young adults mimics closely that noted in children. Important causes include **cardiogenic embolism**, **hematologic diseases**, **large-vessel occlusive disease, and small vessel disorders**. In most series, the most common causes of ischemic stroke in young adults are premature atherosclerosis, cardiogenic embolism, and use of oral contraceptives. Although **migraine** and use of **oral contraceptives** are commonly noted as potential causes of stroke in young adults, it is important to evaluate for other causes of stroke. Other risk factors for arterial occlusive disease are typically present in patients with ischemic events caused by oral contraceptives.

In most young adult patients with **premature atherosclerosis**, prominent risk factors are present, such as familial hypercholesterolemia, severe hypertension, and insulin-dependent diabetes. In addition, early cigarette smoking also has been frequently reported in this subgroup. Less commonly, patients will have premature large-vessel occlusive disease due to Fabry's disease or homocystinuria.

Stroke related to use of **illicit drugs** is also an important consideration in young adults. Ischemia or hemorrhage may result from use or abuse of prescription drugs or illicit drugs, including amphetamines, phenylpropanolamine, heroin, cocaine, phencyclidine, and lysergic acid diethylamide (LSD). Potential mechanisms include direct vascular effects such as vasospasm, vasoconstriction, vasculopathy without inflammation, inflammatory arteritis, prothrombotic state, and cardiac disorders such as cardiac arrhythmia and endocarditis. Intracranial hemorrhage occurs most commonly with use of cocaine, phenylpropanolamine, amphetamines, and heroin; cerebral infarction is often noted with use of heroin and cocaine.

Hypertensive encephalopathy or brain hemorrhage during a **hypertensive crisis** may result when a person receives monoamine oxidase inhibitor antidepressants and then consumes tyramine-rich products such as wine or cheese. Young adults also commonly report a history of trauma, which makes **dissection** an important cause in many series. Although **migraine** is relatively commonly associated with ischemic stroke in young adults, the importance as a causative factor or risk factor for stroke is poorly defined. Most series indicate that 10% to 15% of strokes in this age group are caused by migraine. The concurrent use of **oral contraceptives** may increase the occurrence of stroke in patients with migraine.

Stroke Related to Inherited Syndromes

Inherited syndromes associated with an increased occurrence of stroke include Ehlers-Danlos syndrome, pseudoxanthoma elasticum, Fabry's disease, homocystinuria, and sulfate oxidase deficiency. Although these disorders are relatively uncommon, they more typically become symptomatic in patients younger than 40 years.

Ehlers-Danlos syndrome is an autosomal dominant disorder of unknown cause in which collagen fibers are affected and frequently leads to aneurysmal dilatation or arterial dissection. Clinical features are cutaneous hyperelasticity and fragility, hypermobile joints, and occasionally carotid-cavernous fistula or aneurysmal subarachnoid hemorrhage.

Pseudoxanthoma elasticum is an autosomal recessive disorder in which degeneration and secondary calcification of the elastic tissue lead to vascular disturbances in many organs of the body, including the brain. Clinically, the disorder is characterized by yellowish papules on the neck, face, axilla, inguinal region, and periumbilical area, frequently associated with hypertension, angina pectoris, gastrointestinal bleeding, unequal radial pulses, and progressive, bilateral visual loss caused by retinitis with macular involvement. Ischemic stroke or hemorrhagic stroke as a result of ruptured intracranial aneurysm may occur.

Fabry's disease is an X-linked recessive disorder typically affecting homozygous men in which deficiency of the enzyme alpha-galactosidase A causes accumulation of trihexyl ceramide and a resultant occlusive arteriopathy. Fabry's disease may present with dermal angiokeratomas (reddish or black) in the region of the lower abdomen and the upper thighs and is commonly associated with painful limb paresthesias and generalized hypohydrosis. Chronic renal failure, hypertension, cardiomegaly, myocardial infarction, transient ischemic attacks, or cerebral infarction caused by a narrowing of blood vessel lumina may also occur. Unfortunately, no effective treatment of this disorder exists to prevent cerebrovascular complications.

Clinical features of **homocystinuria** in homozygous patients are characteristic skeletal abnormalities (tall, slender habitus, long limbs, occasional scoliosis and arachnodactyly, kyphosis, and high-arched feet) associated with mental retardation, seizures, ectopia lentis, and multiple cerebral infarctions. Deficiency of the enzyme cystathionine synthetase leads to abnormal conversion of homocysteine to methionine and increased serum homocysteine levels. Endothelial damage with premature atherosclerosis and relative hypercoagulability have been postulated as potential mechanisms.

Whether **heterozygous** patients have sufficient enzyme deficiency to cause similar vascular abnormalities is controversial. In children and young adults with cerebral ischemia of unknown cause, the patient's serum homocysteine level should be checked; if it is high, serum B_{12}, B_6 (pyridoxine), and folate levels should also be evaluated. If none of the vitamin levels is low or low-normal, an assay of fibroblast cystathione synthase activity may be performed, which requires a punch biopsy of the skin. In patients with an elevated homocysteine level, therapy with supplemental B_{12}, B_6, and folate should be considered.

Sulfate oxidase deficiency is a very rare disorder of sulfur metabolism involving increased blood sulfite and S-sulfocysteine levels; it usually manifests clinically during the neonatal period with seizures, multiple cerebral infarcts, decreased responsiveness, generalized spasms, and opisthotonos.

Mitochondrial myopathy, encephalopathy, lactic acidosis, and stroke-like episodes (**MELAS syndrome**) is an uncommon cause of strokes in children and young adults. Presenting symptoms include an abrupt onset of visual dysfunction, motor weakness, ataxia, or sensory abnormalities, often with headache and generalized cognitive decline. Seizures are also common. Imaging studies may reveal multifocal subcortical and cortical abnormalities consistent with infarction, often predominating in the posterior head regions and cerebellum. Abnormal blood test results may include increased serum lactic and pyruvic acid levels; mitochondrial DNA analysis may reveal mutations.

Other Causes of Cerebral Ischemia

Moyamoya disease occurs in a bimodal distribution; children younger than 15 years typically present with episodes of transient ischemic attack or cerebral infarction, whereas those older than 40 years more commonly present with intracranial hemorrhage, particularly in the basal ganglia or thalamus. Children also tend to have more seizures and generalized cognitive impairment. The diagnosis is made on the basis of characteristic arteriographic findings, which include progressive stenosis or occlusion of the intracranial internal carotid arteries and prominent collateral formation appearing as a fine network of vessels deep in the brain, giving the so-called puff-of-smoke appearance, from which the term "moyamoya" arises. The cause of the changes is unknown. Treatment options include extracranial artery-to-intracranial artery bypass and other revascularization procedures.

Hemorrhagic Stroke

The relative frequency of **hemorrhagic stroke** is higher in children and young adults than in patients older than 40 years, and some series have reported that the ratio of hemorrhagic stroke to ischemic stroke is 1:1 to 1.5:1 in the younger age groups. Although **arteriovenous malformations** are a more frequent cause of hemorrhage in younger patients than they are in older patients, **intracranial aneurysms** are still the most common cause of intracranial hemorrhage. In young children, **vein of Galen malformations** (in which the vein of Galen is enlarged, which forms a venous aneurysm or varix) may also cause hemorrhage, although hydrocephalus and congestive heart failure are more common in infants.

Intracranial saccular aneurysms occurring in children may be associated with a genetic disorder such as polycystic kidney disease, Marfan's syndrome, pseudoxanthoma elasticum, coarctation of the aorta, or Ehlers-Danlos syndrome.

In patients older than 15 years, arteriovenous malformations and saccular aneurysms continue to be important causes of intracranial hemorrhage; however, other important causes include drug use, hematologic disorders, and hypertension. Venous occlusive disease is also in the differential diagnosis for hemorrhagic infarction in children and young adults.

Laboratory Evaluation

The evaluation and treatment of ischemic and hemorrhagic disorders in children and young adults are similar to those described earlier (see Chapters 11–17). However, on the basis of the differential considerations presented in this chapter, additional studies evaluating for causes more specific to children and young adults are necessary, with more emphasis on cardiac disorders, hematologic disorders such as hypercoagulable states, infectious and inflammatory causes, and metabolic disorders.

In addition to noninvasive studies to evaluate the extracranial and intracranial arterial system and cardiac imaging studies, detailed hematologic studies should be considered because hematologic disorders play a greater role in stroke occurrence in children and young adults than they do in older groups. Potential types of evaluation may include the sickle-cell preparation; hemoglobin and serum protein electrophoresis; determination of antithrombin III level, partial thromboplastin time, fibrinogen level, protein C and protein S levels;

evaluation for resistance to activated protein C; determination of anticardiolipin antibodies; and lupus anticoagulant testing. If there is a family history of early-onset stroke, or if radiographic or clinical findings suggest the presence of such a disorder, the serum homocysteine level should be determined and evaluation for other hereditary metabolic disorders should be performed.

Treatment

The general principles outlined for treatment of cerebrovascular disease in adults (see Chapters 11–17) may be applied to most cerebrovascular diseases in children and young adults. Some entities described in this chapter are exceedingly rare in patients older than 40 years, and they require treatment of the specific cause, if known.

Treatment issues for intracerebral hemorrhage (see Chapter 17) are also similar to those in adults. Ruptured intracranial aneurysms and arteriovenous malformations in children are usually treated surgically. The preferred procedure for ruptured arteriovenous malformations is excision, but when that is not possible, radiosurgery, embolization, or a combination of both should be considered. For unruptured arteriovenous malformations, rates of future rupture are relatively low—approximately 2% per year—but are persistent over time. Because affected patients otherwise have very long life expectancies, radiosurgery (which may take 2–3 years to obliterate the arteriovenous malformation from the cerebral circulation) becomes more of a consideration for possible first-line therapy, especially for a small arteriovenous malformation in a location that is difficult to access surgically. The management of unruptured intracranial aneurysms is analogous to that described in Chapter 28.

Prognosis

The prognosis for children with ischemic and hemorrhagic stroke is better than that for adults with a comparable lesion. Speech recovery occurs in nearly all children affected by cerebral infarction before the age of 5 years. Children presenting with hemiplegia and seizures before age 2 years have a worse prognosis, and most have persistent behavioral changes, intellectual deficits, hemiplegia, and epilepsy.

Cerebrovascular Disease in Pregnant Patients

Although stroke is the third leading cause of death in the general population in the United States, it is uncommon among women of childbearing age. Pregnancy has long been recognized as a factor that increases the risk of cerebrovascular disease in young women, although the magnitude of the increase in risk has been exaggerated by referral-based studies. Many of the same mechanisms that produce stroke in older age groups are responsible for strokes in pregnant women, but the distribution of mechanisms is different. Furthermore, some mechanisms are unique to pregnancy, particularly in the area of ischemic cerebrovascular disease. Evaluation and management of pregnant patients with cerebrovascular symptoms require an awareness of the differences in underlying pathophysiology between pregnant and nonpregnant patients. The physician must understand the potential adverse effects of diagnostic procedures and medications on the fetus as well as on the patient.

Hemorrhagic Disorders

Hemorrhagic cerebrovascular disorders cause 5% to 10% of all maternal deaths occurring during pregnancy. Most commonly, nontraumatic intracranial hemorrhage in pregnancy occurs within the subarachnoid space (subarachnoid hemorrhage), within the ventricular system (intraventricular hemorrhage), or as a combination of these. Hemorrhage into each of these areas may be produced by various pathophysiologic mechanisms, most commonly (1) rupture of an intracranial aneurysm, which usually produces subarachnoid hemorrhage, occasionally in association with intracerebral hemorrhage or intraventricular hemorrhage; (2) bleeding from an arteriovenous malformation, which frequently produces subarachnoid hemorrhage, intracerebral hemorrhage, or both; and (3) rupture of an intraparenchymal vessel, which results in intracerebral hemorrhage, often with some extension of the bleeding into the subarachnoid space or ventricular system.

INTRACRANIAL ANEURYSM

On the basis of data collected from various referral practices during the past 40 years, the incidence of aneurysmal rupture during pregnancy has been estimated at approximately 1 in 10,000 pregnancies, about 2 to 3 times that of nonpregnant females of the same age group. However, data from the Rochester, Minnesota, population from 1955 to 1979 more recently revealed no instances of intracranial hemorrhage among 26,099 pregnancies, a finding suggesting that previous rates may have been overestimated. Approximately one-half of the patients with ruptured aneurysms during pregnancy have had previous successful pregnancies with no difficulty. As in the general population, there is some tendency toward increasing risk with increased maternal age. During pregnancy, the risk of rupture

**Table 22-1.   Features of intracranial aneurysm
and arteriovenous malformation during pregnancy**

Feature	Aneurysm	Arteriovenous malformation
Age (yr)	25–35	15–25
Peak hemorrhage risk	30–40 wk (3rd trimester)	16–20 wk (2nd trimester)
Parity	Multipara	Primipara
Risk of recurrent hemorrhage		
Same pregnancy	+ +	+ + +
Delivery	+ +	+ + +
Postpartum	+ + +	+
Subsequent pregnancies	+	+ + +

From Wiebers DO: Subarachnoid hemorrhage in pregnancy. *Semin Neurol* 8:226–229, 1988. By permission of Thieme Medical Publishers.

increases with each trimester. Although one might expect the Valsalva maneuver of childbirth to increase the risk of aneurysmal rupture, very few initial ruptures have been reported during labor and delivery. However, rebleeding frequently occurs during labor and the first few weeks postpartum (Table 22-1).

Early investigation and treatment of intracranial aneurysm are important in pregnant patients, particularly when the aneurysm has produced intracranial hemorrhage. Radiographic and surgical procedures should not be delayed or avoided, although special shielding during radiography is required to protect the fetus. The clinical decisions involved in managing these patients vary with the type, size, and location of the aneurysm, the condition of the patient, and whether the aneurysm is symptomatic (see Chapters 14, 15, 17).

If the intracranial aneurysm is successfully obliterated (surgically clipped, trapped, or documented to be obliterated after coil placement) from the circulation before the 35th week of gestation, the rest of pregnancy and delivery can proceed normally. If the ruptured aneurysm cannot be obliterated completely (incompletely clipped, arterial ligation, not obliterated after coil placement, wrapped, or packed), or if operation is not performed, vaginal delivery is generally recommended only if the rupture occurred during the first two trimesters of pregnancy. If the subarachnoid hemorrhage occurred during the third trimester, delivery should be performed by cesarean section at 38 weeks of gestation. Little can be done to avoid the increased postpartum risk of rebleeding in this situation.

INTRACRANIAL ARTERIOVENOUS MALFORMATION

Arteriovenous malformations (AVMs) cause approximately the same number of intracranial hemorrhages during pregnancy as do aneurysms. Although previous data revealed a high incidence of intracranial hemorrhage among patients with arteriovenous malformation, recent data have been conflicting and have shown a minimally increased risk for pregnant patients. AVMs tend to occur in younger pregnant women (ages 15–25 years) and aneurysms in pregnant women aged 25 to 35 years. In contrast to aneurysms, AVMs tend to rupture during the second trimester (peak, 16–20 weeks of gestation), and they are more likely to hemorrhage again in the same pregnancy and in subsequent pregnancies. Rebleeding during delivery may be more common with AVMs than it is with aneurysms. However, the increased risk of AVM hemorrhage during specific trimesters and during delivery was not noted in one study (see Horton reference in Suggested Reading for Part IV). Pregnant patients with AVMs tend to have a lower parity than those with aneurysms (see Table 22-1). A patient with intracranial hemorrhage caused by a ruptured AVM is six times less likely to have had a previous normal pregnancy than a pregnant patient with aneurysmal subarachnoid hemorrhage. Overall, the fetal prognosis is worse when there is known maternal intracranial AVM compared with the prognosis with intracranial aneurysm.

The mechanism for the somewhat increased risk of rupture of AVMs during pregnancy is unknown. Many investigators have suggested that the periods of greatest risk of rupture (16–20 weeks of gestation and at the time of labor and delivery) correlate with the greatest increases in cardiac output. Shunting through intracranial AVMs presumably increases during pregnancy. No direct measurements are available, but analogies have been made to visible cutaneous spider nevi and vascular tumors of the skin and gums. These tumors increase in size as pregnancy progresses (particularly during times of increased cardiac output) and decrease in size or disappear after delivery. Increased shunting is thought by some physicians to predispose to rupture and to focal ischemic events from the AVM. The latter condition has been noted only rarely during pregnancy.

Some pregnant patients with AVMs also present with periodic throbbing headache that appears in the same location with each episode and is indistinguishable from classic migraine. Others present with progressive neurologic deficits or seizures without evidence of associated cerebral hemorrhage or infarction. However, during pregnancy, initial presentation with subarachnoid hemorrhage is approximately 5 to 10 times more likely than is any other type of presentation.

As noted with intracranial aneurysms, early investigation and treatment of intracranial AVMs are important in pregnant patients, particularly in the setting of intracranial hemorrhage. Radiographic and surgical procedures should not be delayed or avoided, although special shielding during radiography is required to protect the fetus. The clinical decisions involved in managing these patients vary with the type of vascular malformation and whether it is symptomatic (see Chapters 14, 15, 17).

If the AVM can be totally excised before the 35th week of gestation, the rest of pregnancy and delivery can proceed normally. If the lesion is not operable or only partially resectable and has bled during the pregnancy, elective cesarean section at 38 weeks of gestation is usually recommended, especially in a nulliparous patient. If the patient is multiparous with a proven adequate pelvis, some investigators have advocated vaginal delivery in which Valsalva maneuver is minimized by administering regional lumbar epidural anesthesia or by having the patient learn breathing techniques to be used during delivery to obviate the cardiovascular stresses that would otherwise occur.

RUPTURE OF INTRAPARENCHYMAL VESSELS

Rupture of an artery, capillary, or vein within the brain parenchyma commonly results in intracerebral hemorrhage and sometimes subarachnoid or intraventricular bleeding. In both pregnant and nonpregnant women, certain underlying conditions may predispose to nontraumatic rupture of the intraparenchymal vessel. **Hypertension** is the most frequently identified predisposing cause of intracerebral hemorrhage in nonpregnant women and has been implicated in some cases of intracerebral hemorrhage in pregnant women, particularly in the setting of eclampsia. In both situations, the basal ganglia area seems to be the most common site of hemorrhage, although there are very few well-documented cases in pregnant patients.

Other conditions that have been associated with nontraumatic intracerebral bleeding in pregnancy are (1) **hematologic disorders** such as disseminated intravascular coagulation, often associated with placental abruption, leukemia, thrombocytopenia, or carcinoma; (2) **anticoagulant therapy**; (3) **cortical vein and dural sinus thrombosis;** and (4) **metastatic choriocarcinoma.** Patients with angiopathies such as systemic lupus erythematosus might also be expected to have intracranial hemorrhage because this disorder is often exacerbated by pregnancy, but a relationship has not yet been documented.

If the pregnant patient with intraparenchymal hemorrhage survives to the time of delivery and an underlying structural lesion has been found and repaired, labor and delivery can proceed normally. The remainder of survivors should undergo either elective cesarean section at 38 weeks of gestation or vaginal delivery with epidural lumbar anesthesia, depending on the individual circumstance.

Ischemic Cerebrovascular Disease

Pregnancy appears to increase the risk of focal ischemic cerebrovascular events. However, recent population-based data from Rochester, Minnesota, indicated only one cerebral infarction among 26,099 pregnancies during a period of 25 years (5.1/100,000 patient-years of observation), a finding suggesting that previous estimates of risk (5–15 times the expected risk) were probably exaggerated. Until recently, cerebral venous thrombosis was thought to be the cause of most focal cerebral ischemic lesions in pregnancy. However, during the past 20 years, available data in the Western literature suggest that arterial occlusions cause approximately 60% to 80% of these lesions. Arterial occlusions tend to occur during the second and third trimesters of pregnancy and during the puerperium; venous occlusions tend to occur 1 to 4 weeks after childbirth.

When the various possible causes of ischemic cerebrovascular events in pregnancy are considered, it is useful to categorize the various pathophysiologic mechanisms according to which part of the vascular system is most prominently involved: cardiac disease, large- or small-vessel arterial disease, hematologic disorders, venous occlusions, and other uncommon disorders.

CARDIAC DISEASE

In pregnancy, cardiac disease may produce symptoms of focal cerebral ischemia through various mechanisms. Cardiac ischemic sources cause a higher percentage of focal ischemic neurologic deficits in pregnant patients than they do in the rest of the adult population. This is at least partially a result of the lower prevalence of advanced atherosclerosis in the younger age group. In addition, pregnancy may aggravate preexisting maternal heart disease (such as rheumatic fever, subacute bacterial endocarditis) or may cause maternal heart disease (such as peripartum cardiomyopathy).

Valve-Related Emboli

Cerebral embolization occurs in about 20% of patients with infective endocarditis and may be the presenting symptom. During pregnancy, streptococcus viridans is the most common infective agent, particularly with preexisting rheumatic heart disease. Among cases of **subacute bacterial endocarditis** during pregnancy, 8% are enterococcal, which is particularly common after delivery, abortion, or insertion of an intrauterine device. Staphylococcal subacute bacterial endocarditis is more common among narcotic addicts and is associated with an increased risk of cerebral abscess formation and a higher fatality rate. Four distinct clinical and pathologic syndromes occur: (1) focal cerebral infarction resulting from embolic occlusion of large arteries (the most common), (2) multiple small areas of cerebral infarction producing diffuse encephalopathy, (3) meningitis from small infected emboli lodging in meningeal arteries, and (4) mycotic aneurysm formation with subsequent intracranial hemorrhage caused by septic embolization and vessel wall rupture.

There is some evidence that **rheumatic fever** is more likely to recur during pregnancy, and this occasionally causes serious maternal cardiac decompensation and death. Cerebral embolization in rheumatic heart disease may occur either during the acute illness when inflammatory vegetations on the heart valve may detach and embolize or, more commonly, during the chronic phase of the disease, when valvular deformity, atrial enlargement, and abnormal cardiac rhythm develop. Atrial fibrillation, congestive heart failure, atrial enlargement, or associated mitral insufficiency also increase the risk of cerebral embolization.

Mitral valve prolapse occurs in approximately 5% of otherwise healthy young women. During the past decade, cerebral ischemic events unrelated to other recognized risk factors have been noted in patients with this condition. However, an increased risk of cerebral embolization during pregnancy in patients with mitral valve prolapse has not yet been documented. Some have advocated close observation for the appearance of arrhythmias as well as the utilization of antibiotic prophylaxis and aspirin, particularly when associated mitral regurgitation is present. These recommendations, however, are not based on strong scientific evidence.

Intracardiac Thrombi

In the childbearing years, the cardiac arrhythmia most frequently associated with embolic brain infarction is **atrial fibrillation,** which predisposes to blood stagnation and the formation of intracardiac thrombi. During pregnancy, the risk of systemic embolism from the arrhythmia has been estimated at 10% to 23%, including a 2% to 10% risk of symptomatic brain embolism.

Also known as **peripartum cardiomyopathy, cardiomyopathy of pregnancy** is a syndrome that resembles other congestive cardiomyopathies, occurring during late pregnancy or the puerperium in the absence of any of the well-recognized causes of heart disease. There is still no unanimity of opinion about whether this syndrome is a specific entity caused by pregnancy or whether pregnancy unmasks preexisting latent myocardial disease. Like other congestive cardiomyopathies, this condition predisposes to blood stagnation with consequent mural thrombi, which may embolize to the cerebrum, especially from the left ventricle. Multiparous black women older than 30 years are at the highest risk for development of this condition. In most patients, the heart returns to normal soon after delivery, but chronic congestive heart failure develops in some women.

Acute myocardial infarction occurs in about 1 in 10,000 pregnancies, and the overall maternal mortality rate is approximately 30%. When the infarction occurs during the last month of pregnancy, the maternal mortality rate is considerably higher (approximately 50%). The frequency of cerebral embolization with acute myocardial infarction during pregnancy is unknown.

The foramen ovale is anatomically patent in 15% of persons and retains the functional capacity of patency in an additional 15%. In these situations, venous emboli can enter the cerebral circulation **(paradoxical embolism),** especially after pulmonary embolization with associated increases in pulmonary arterial and right atrial pressures. The risk of paradoxical embolism increases with pregnancy because of the increased risk of thrombophlebitis in the pelvis and lower extremities, especially during early puerperium after cesarean section, forceps rotation, or manual removal of the uterus.

LARGE- OR SMALL-VESSEL ARTERIAL DISEASE

Atherosclerosis

In the general population, **atherosclerosis** is the most common identifiable disease process producing cerebral ischemia. Among females of childbearing age and even more so among pregnant females, atherosclerosis plays a smaller role in the pathogenesis of cerebral ischemic events. The number of well-studied cases is too small to allow definitive percentages, but roughly 10% of all cerebral infarctions during pregnancy are related to atherosclerosis. Young women with long-standing hypertension, diabetes mellitus, hyperlipidemia, cigarette abuse, and radiation therapy to the neck may be predisposed to the development of atherosclerosis (accelerated atherosclerosis).

In pregnancy, **hypotensive episodes** may result from acute blood loss, vasovagal-induced syncope, or epidural or spinal anesthesia. Such episodes may produce transient or permanent cerebral ischemic lesions with or without underlying atherosclerosis. The terminal branches (watershed areas) of the anterior, middle, and posterior cerebral arteries are most frequently involved. Severe intrapartum hypotension also may result in Sheehan's syndrome (pituitary necrosis) as a result of infarction in the distribution of the inferior hypophyseal artery.

Arteritis

A pregnant patient is as subject to pyogenic central nervous system infections as any other person but is not unusually predisposed to them. **Leptomeningitis** produced by meningococcus is the most common, but the frequency of cerebrovascular complications in pregnant patients with this condition is unknown. **Tuberculous meningitis** in pregnant women is rare in Western countries, but it occurs frequently in less industrialized nations. **Tertiary syphilis,** once a common cause of ischemic stroke in young patients, is now rare.

The presumably noninfectious inflammatory angiopathies include those that primarily affect the arterioles and capillaries **(systemic lupus erythematosus),** those that primarily affect small or medium-sized arteries **(polyarteritis nodosa, isolated central nervous system angiitis),** and those that primarily affect medium-sized to large arteries **(temporal arteritis, Takayasu's disease).** Systemic lupus erythematosus and Takayasu's disease tend to occur in women of childbearing age.

Exacerbations of **systemic lupus erythematosus** often occur during pregnancy, and the risk of abortion and stillbirth is significantly increased. Because the cerebral vessel arteriopathy primarily affects small vessels diffusely, the central nervous system findings are usually those of a diffuse encephalopathy with delirium, seizures, acute cyanosis, and increased intracranial pressure. Focal or multifocal cerebral and brain stem infarcts occur, but they rarely produce recognizable arterial syndromes.

Takayasu's disease (pulseless disease) is a chronic inflammatory arteriopathy of unknown origin which results in narrowing of major-vessel ostia involving the aortic arch and its branches. Clinically, the ischemic symptoms include Takayasu's retinopathy and thromboembolic or hemodynamic focal or multifocal cerebral ischemia. There may be reduction or absence of subclavian, carotid, brachial, and radial pulses with bruits over affected or collateral vessels; secondary hypertension; aortic regurgitation; and aortic aneurysm. The course of the disease during pregnancy is variable. Approximately half the patients will notice some increase in symptoms during pregnancy, possibly explained by the increased blood volume and cardiac output during pregnancy in conjunction with the variability of venous return caused by impingement of the enlarging uterus on the inferior vena cava. Vaginal delivery is generally preferred in these patients unless cesarean section is indicated for obstetric reasons (regional anesthesia should be used with caution because of the danger of hypotension).

Hypertension

No data are available regarding the occurrence of hypertensive lacunar infarction in pregnancy. In contrast, **hypertensive encephalopathy** frequently has been described in association with eclampsia in the second half of pregnancy. Affected patients have accelerated severe hypertension with severe hypertensive retinopathy or retinal arteriolar spasm and alteration of consciousness. Seizures and cortical blindness are often present, but focal neurologic findings are infrequent and may reflect an underlying intracerebral hemorrhage or infarction.

INTRACRANIAL VENOUS OCCLUSION

Intracranial venous thrombosis has long been recognized as a cause of cerebral infarction in pregnancy and the puerperium. Such thromboses may arise from infectious or noninfectious processes and should be diagnosed and treated as discussed in Chapter 18. The vast majority of venous thromboses occur 3 days to 4 weeks after childbirth, and 80% occur in the second or third postpartum week. Venous occlusion probably causes between 20% and 40% of cerebral infarctions during pregnancy. The overall average mortality rate of pregnant patients with cerebral venous thromboses is approximately 25%. For patients who survive, the outlook is usually good, and they have less chance of persistent focal neurologic deficit than do patients with cerebral infarction from arterial lesions.

HEMATOLOGIC DISORDERS

In a normal pregnancy, increases in plasma fibrinogen and clotting factors VII, IX, and XI, along with decreased blood coagulation factor inactivation, produce a mild hypercoagulable state, especially during the third trimester. Similar effects have been noted with the use of birth control pills. In addition, other abnormalities in blood cell constituents and plasma proteins may result in a hypercoagulable state, with increased blood viscosity and stasis, which predispose the patient to cerebral ischemia.

The most commonly described of these disorders in pregnancy is **sickle-cell disease.** The structure of red blood cells containing hemoglobin SS or SC is altered when these cells are exposed to low oxygen tension, which increases blood viscosity and predisposes to diffuse small vessel wall ischemia from occlusion of nutrient arteries. Sickle-cell crisis is relatively common in pregnancy in the setting of SS and SC disease. Rarely, pregnant patients with sickle-cell trait have suffered brain infarction or sudden death.

Thrombotic thrombocytopenic purpura is a rare syndrome that likely is a multicentric vasculitis. It occurs about three times as often in pregnant and puerperal women as in other women of the same age group. The hematologic and cerebrovascular manifestations are the result of secondary mechanical damage to erythrocytes. The damage causes increased use of platelets to form diffuse microthrombi, which in turn occlude terminal arterioles in the brain and produce multiple small infarcts and a fluctuating encephalopathy. Many pregnant women with thrombotic thrombocytopenic purpura are admitted to the hospital during the final weeks of pregnancy, at which time petechiae, ecchymoses, and purpuric patches may be present.

OTHER UNCOMMON CONDITIONS ASSOCIATED WITH PREGNANCY

Particles from amniotic fluid embolize to the brain and other parts of the body. These emboli tend to occur most frequently in multiparous women who are older than 30 years and who have uterine, cervical, or vaginal tears as portals for amniotic fluid to enter the systemic circulation. The clinical picture that has been described includes convulsions, sudden dyspnea, cyanosis, disseminated intravascular coagulation, shock, and death. Antemortem diagnosis is made by finding fetal epithelial cells just above the buffy coat layer of settled blood (which may be withdrawn from the right atrium while a central venous pressure catheter is placed).

Air emboli during pregnancy and the puerperium have been associated with abortion, complicated vaginal delivery, cesarean section, vaginal air insufflation, and puerperal knee-chest exercises. The symptoms are similar to those of amniotic fluid emboli. Cardiac examination may reveal a gurgling, churning heart sound that results from frothy blood.

Fat emboli have rarely been reported in pregnancy, but they occur in the setting of sickle-cell crisis, in association with amniotic fluid embolization, and, independently, in obese women.

Rarely, **metastatic choriocarcinoma** may present with cerebral infarction or hemorrhagic cerebral infarction as a result of vessel occlusion by embolic chorioepithelioma cells. Once these cells lodge in blood vessels, they tend to lead to destruction and rupture of the walls of the artery. Early diagnosis is facilitated by measurement of human chorionic gonadotropin levels in the serum.

Although some authors have associated **spontaneous carotid artery dissection** with use of oral contraceptives, only one case has been described in association with pregnancy. In that case, a cerebral infarction occurred 6 days after a cesarean section that had been done after 14 hours of strenuous, unsuccessful labor.

EVALUATION AND MANAGEMENT OF ISCHEMIC CEREBROVASCULAR DISEASE IN PREGNANCY

Focal ischemic cerebrovascular disease may arise from any one of the described pathologic processes through hemodynamic and thromboembolic mechanisms. Whenever possible, management should be based on a precise definition of the underlying pathophysiologic mechanism and its appropriate treatment (as outlined above and in Chapters 16 and 17).

In the general population, patients with recent onset or an increase in the frequency of transient ischemic attack and minor cerebral infarction are at high risk for cerebral infarction. Among women of childbearing age, the risk is substantially reduced. For patients with a single transient ischemic attack and no source identified from noninvasive examinations, arteriography is usually deferred and medical treatment with low-dose aspirin is recommended. In patients with multiple transient ischemic attacks or increasing frequency or duration of transient ischemic attacks in the carotid system, treatment with intravenously administered heparin is suggested. These patients are hospitalized and usually undergo evaluation, including noninvasive vascular studies, echocardiography, hematologic evaluation, and other studies, such as cerebral arteriography, as indicated (see Chapter 12).

Patients with multiple or crescendo transient ischemic attacks of the carotid system and pressure-significant atherosclerotic stenosis or severe ulceration in a surgically accessible ipsilateral carotid lesion are considered for carotid endarterectomy if there is a surgeon available whose operative morbidity and mortality results are very favorable.

For patients who are not candidates for operation, treatment with intravenously administered heparin is suggested during the first 1 to 2 weeks after the most recent transient ischemic attack. Subcutaneous heparin can be self-administered for 2 to 6 weeks thereafter. Arteriography is generally not performed in pregnant patients with vertebrobasilar transient ischemic attack because of the availability of noninvasive studies such as magnetic resonance angiography and transcranial Doppler ultrasonography. In these patients, medical treatment is instituted on the basis of the results of the evaluations (see Chapter 12).

In general, warfarin is avoided during pregnancy, particularly during the first trimester, because of the increased risk of teratogenic complications and fetal wastage with this therapy. Most of the evidence for this approach is based on sporadic case reports. The teratogenic complications have included one or more of the following:

1. Skeletal abnormalities such as stippling of bone epiphyses, nasal hypoplasia (saddle nose), hypertelorism, frontal bossing, short neck, short stature, and high arched palate
2. Psychomotor retardation
3. Optic atrophy or cataracts

Increased fetal wastage has been well documented only for women receiving warfarin therapy at conception and during the first trimester of pregnancy. Therefore, when anticoagulants are indicated in pregnancy, it has been suggested that heparin be given subcutaneously during the first trimester followed by warfarin during the second trimester and up to 37 weeks of gestation. Heparin is again instituted from week 37 to delivery with resumption of warfarin therapy postpartum. Recently, some investigators have advocated the use of subcutaneously administered heparin instead of warfarin throughout pregnancy and for 6 weeks postpartum.

Heparin has not been associated with a high frequency of fetal wastage or with congenital abnormalities. With a molecular weight of approximately 20,000, heparin does not cross the placental barrier to a significant degree, but warfarin, with a molecular weight of approximately 1000, crosses the placental barrier and hence predisposes to fetal hemorrhagic complications.

There have been a few isolated reports of congenital anomalies in babies born of mothers taking aspirin. However, a prospective study by Heinonen and colleagues under the auspices of the National Institute of Neurological and Communicative Disorders and Stroke (NINCDS) (see Suggested Reading for Part IV) of more than 50,000 pregnancies indicated that use of aspirin did not cause any congenital malformations. No definitive data are available regarding the use of ticlopidine or dipyridamole in pregnancy.

Management of patients with major ischemic stroke and progressing infarction is based on the principles outlined in this chapter and in Chapters 11, 13, and 16. For pregnant women with progressing infarction, mannitol should be avoided because of its relative lack of usefulness to the mother and because of the significant risk of fetal dehydration.

Suggested Reading for Part IV

Adams HP Jr: Calcium antagonists in the management of patients with aneurysmal subarachnoid hemorrhage: A review. Angiology 41:1010–1016, 1990.

Antiplatelet Trialists' Collaboration: Secondary prevention of vascular disease by prolonged antiplatelet treatment. BMJ (Clin Res Ed) 296:320–331, 1988.

Asplund K: Hemodilution in acute stroke. Cerebrovasc Dis 1(Suppl 1):129–138, 1991.

Atrial Fibrillation Investigators: Risk factors for stroke and efficacy of antithrombotic therapy in atrial fibrillation: Analysis of pooled data from five randomized controlled trials. Arch Intern Med 154:1449–1457, 1994.

Auger RG, Wiebers DO: Management of unruptured intracranial aneurysms: A decision analysis. J Stroke Cerebrovascular Dis 1:174–181, 1991.

Auger RG, Wiebers DO: Management of unruptured intracranial arteriovenous malformations: A decision analysis. Neurosurgery 30:561–569, 1992.

Barnett HJ: Stroke prevention by surgery for symptomatic disease in carotid territory. Neurol Clin 10:281–292, 1992.

Barnwell SL, Higashida RT, Halbach VV, et al: Direct endovascular thrombolytic therapy for dural sinus thrombosis. Neurosurgery 28:135–142, 1991.

Ben-Yehuda D, Rose M, Michaeli Y, et al: Permanent neurological complications in patients with thrombotic thrombocytopenic purpura. Am J Hematol 29:74–78, 1988.

Bick RL: Disseminated intravascular coagulation: Objective criteria for diagnosis and management. Med Clin North Am 78:511–543, 1994.

Biller J: Medical management of acute cerebral ischemia. Neurol Clin 10:63–85, 1992.

Biller J, Mathews KD, Love BB, eds: Stroke in Children and Young Adults. Boston: Butterworth-Heinemann, 1994.

The Boston Area Anticoagulation Trial for Atrial Fibrillation Investigators: The effect of low-dose warfarin on the risk of stroke in patients with nonrheumatic atrial fibrillation. N Engl J Med 323:1505–1511, 1990.

Broderick J, Talbot GT, Prenger E, et al: Stroke in children within a major metropolitan area: The surprising importance of intracerebral hemorrhage. J Child Neurol 8:250–255, 1993.

Brown RD Jr, Evans BA, Wiebers DO, et al: Transient ischemic attack and minor ischemic stroke: An algorithm for evaluation and treatment. Mayo Clin Proc 69:1027–1039, 1994.

Buchbinder R, Detsky AS: Management of suspected giant cell arteritis: A decision analysis. J Rheumatol 19:1220–1228, 1992.

Butler RN, Ahronheim J, Fillitt H, et al: Vascular dementia: An updated approach to patient management. A roundtable discussion: Part 3. Geriatrics 49:39–40, 43–46, 1994.

Chakravarty K, Elgabani SH, Scott DG, et al: A district audit on the management of polymyalgia rheumatica and giant cell arteritis. Br J Rheumatol 33:152–156, 1994.

Collins R, Baigent C, Sandercock P, et al: Antiplatelet therapy for thromboprophylaxis: The need for careful consideration of the evidence from randomised trials. Antiplatelet Trialists' Collaboration. BMJ 309: 1215–1217, 1994.

Connolly SJ, Laupacis A, Gent M, et al: Canadian Atrial Fibrillation Anticoagulation (CAFA) Study. J Am Coll Cardiol 18:349–355, 1991.

Coull BM, Levine SR, Brey RL: The role of antiphospholipid antibodies in stroke. Neurol Clin 10:125–143, 1992.

Croce MA, Dent DL, Menke PG, et al: Acute subdural hematoma: nonsurgical management of selected patients. J Trauma 36:820–826, 1994.

Crowell RM, Ojemann RG, Ogilvy CS: Spontaneous brain hemorrhage: Surgical considerations. In: Barnett HMJ, Stein BM, Mohr JP, Yatsu FM, eds. Stroke: Pathophysiology, Diagnosis, and Management (2nd ed). New York: Churchill Livingstone, 1992, pp 1169–1187.

Davis WD, Hart RG: Cardiogenic stroke in the elderly. Clin Geriatr Med 7:429–442, 1991.

Donnan GA: Investigation of patients with stroke and transient ischaemic attacks. Lancet 339:473–477, 1992.

The Dutch TIA Trial Study Group: A comparison of two doses of aspirin (30 mg vs. 283 mg a day) in patients after a transient ischemic attack or minor ischemic stroke. N Engl J Med 325:1261–1266, 1991.

EAFT (European Atrial Fibrillation Trial) Study Group: Secondary prevention in non-rheumatic atrial fibrillation after transient ischaemic attack or minor stroke. Lancet 342:1255–1262, 1993.

The EC/IC Bypass Study Group: Failure of extracranial-intracranial arterial bypass to reduce the risk of ischemic stroke: Results of an international randomized trial. N Engl J Med 313:1191–1200, 1985.

Eden OB, Lilleyman JS: Guidelines for management of idiopathic thrombocytopenic purpura. Arch Dis Child 67:1056–1058, 1992.

Einhäupl KM, Villringer A, Meister W, et al: Heparin treatment in sinus venous thrombosis. Lancet 338:597–600, 1991.

Erbguth F, Brenner P, Schuierer G, et al: Diagnosis and treatment of deep cerebral vein thrombosis. Neurosurg Rev 14:145–148, 1991.

European Carotid Surgery Trialists' Collaborative Group: MRC European Carotid Surgery Trial: Interim results for symptomatic patients with severe (70–99%) or with mild (0–29%) carotid stenosis. Lancet 337:1235–1243, 1991.

Executive Committee for the Asymptomatic Carotid Atherosclerosis Study: Endarterectomy for asymptomatic carotid artery stenosis. JAMA 273:1421–1428, 1995.

Farrell B, Godwin J, Richards S, et al: The United Kingdom transient ischemic attack (UK-TIA) aspirin trial: Final results. J Neurol Neurosurg Psychiatry 54:1044–1054, 1991.

Feldmann E, Tornabene J: Diagnosis and treatment of cerebral amyloid angiopathy. Clin Geriatr Med 7:617–630, 1991.

Fletcher AE, Bulpitt CJ: How far should blood pressure be lowered? N Engl J Med 326:251–254, 1992.

Gent M, Blakely JA, Easton JD, et al: The Canadian American Ticlopidine Study (CATS) in thromboembolic stroke. Lancet 1:1215–1220, 1989.

Hacke W, Kaste M, Fleschi C, et al: Intravenous thrombolysis with recombinant tissue plasminogen activator for acute hemispheric stroke: The European Cooperative Acute Stroke Study (ECASS). JAMA 274:1017–1025, 1995.

Haley EC Jr, Brott TG, Sheppard GL, et al: Pilot randomized trial of tissue plasminogen activator in acute ischemic stroke: The TPA Bridging Study Group. Stroke 24:1000–1004, 1993.

Haley EC Jr, Kassell NF, Torner JC: The International Cooperative Study on the Timing of Aneurysm Surgery: The North American experience. Stroke 23:205–214, 1992.

Haley EC Jr, Kassell NF, Torner JC, et al: A randomized trial of two doses of nicardipine in aneurysmal subarachnoid hemorrhage: A report of the Cooperative Aneurysm Study. J Neurosurg 80:788–796, 1994.

Hart RG, Kanter MC: Hematologic disorders and ischemic stroke: A selective review. Stroke 21:1111–1121, 1990.

Hass WK, Easton JD, Adams HP Jr, et al: A randomized trial comparing ticlopidine hydrochloride with aspirin for the prevention of stroke in high-risk patients: Ticlopidine Aspirin Stroke Study Group. N Engl J Med 321:501–507, 1989.

Haynes RB, Taylor DW, Sackett DL, et al: Prevention of functional impairment by endarterectomy for symptomatic high-grade carotid stenosis. North American Symptomatic Carotid Endarterectomy Trial Collaborators. JAMA 271:1256–1259, 1994.

Heinonen OP, Slone D, Shapiro S: Birth Defects and Drugs in Pregnancy. Littleton, MA: Publishing Sciences Group, 1977.

Hobson RW II, Weiss DG, Fields WS, et al: Efficacy of carotid endarterectomy for asymptomatic carotid stenosis. The Veterans Affairs Cooperative Study Group. N Engl J Med 328:221–227, 1993.

Horton JC, Chambers WA, Lyons SL, et al: Pregnancy and the risk of hemorrhage from cerebral arteriovenous malformations. Neurosurgery 27:867–871, 1990.

Jonas S: Anticoagulant therapy in cerebrovascular disease: Review and meta-analysis. Stroke 19:1043–1048, 1988.

Kaku DA, Lowenstein DH: Emergence of recreational drug abuse as a major risk factor for stroke in young adults. Ann Intern Med 113:821–827, 1990.

Komsuoglu SS, Komsuoglu B, Ozmenoglu M, et al: Oral nifedipine in the treatment of hypertensive crises in patients with hypertensive encephalopathy. Int J Cardiol 34:277–282, 1992.

Martin N, Khanna R, Rodts G: The intensive care management of patients with subarachnoid hemorrhage. In: Andrews BT, ed. Neurosurgical Intensive Care. New York: McGraw-Hill, 1993, pp 291–310.

Mascio RD, Marchioli R, Tognoni G: From pharmacological promises to controlled clinical trials to meta-analysis and back: The case of nimodipine in cerebrovascular disorders. Clin Trials Metaanal 29:57–79, 1994.

Mayo Asymptomatic Carotid Endarterectomy Study Group: Results of a randomized controlled trial of carotid endarterectomy for asymptomatic carotid stenosis. Mayo Clin Proc 67:513–518, 1992.

Meyer FB, ed: Sundt's Occlusive Cerebrovascular Disease (2nd ed). Philadelphia: WB Saunders, 1994.

National Institute of Neurological Disorders and Stroke rt-PA Stroke Study Group: Tissue plasminogen activator for acute ischemic stroke. N Engl J Med 333:1581–1587, 1995.

North American Symptomatic Carotid Endarterectomy Trial Collaborators: Beneficial effect of carotid endarterectomy in symptomatic patients with high-grade carotid stenosis. N Engl J Med 325:445–453, 1991.

Petersen P, Boysen G, Godtfredsen J, et al: Placebo-controlled, randomised trial of warfarin and aspirin for prevention of thromboembolic complications in chronic atrial fibrillation: The Copenhagen AFASAK study. Lancet 1:175–179, 1989.

Pickard JD, Murray GD, Illingworth R, et al: Effect of oral nimodipine on cerebral infarction and outcome after subarachnoid haemorrhage: British aneurysm nimodipine trial. BMJ 298:636–642, 1989.

Poungvarin N, Bhoopat W, Viriyavejakul A, et al: Effects of dexamethasone in primary supratentorial intracerebral hemorrhage. N Engl J Med 316:1229–1233, 1987.

Ramsey RG: Neuroradiology (3rd ed). Philadelphia: WB Saunders, 1994, pp 174–224.

Riela AR, Roach ES: Etiology of stroke in children. J Child Neurol 8:201–220, 1993.

Rogvi-Hansen, Boysen G: Intravenous glycerol treatment of acute stroke: A statistical review. Cerebrovasc Dis 2:11–13, 1992.

Rothrock JF, Hart RG: Antithrombotic therapy in cerebrovascular disease. Ann Intern Med 115:885–895, 1991.

The SALT Collaborative Group: Swedish Aspirin Low-Dose Trial (SALT) of 75 mg aspirin as secondary prophylaxis after cerebrovascular ischaemic events. Lancet 338:1345–1349, 1991.

Sherman DG, Dyken ML Jr, Fisher M, et al: Antithrombotic therapy for cerebrovascular disorders. Chest 102(Suppl 4):529S–537S, 1992.

Shuaib A: Alteration of blood pressure regulation and cerebrovascular disorders in the elderly. Cerebrovasc Brain Metab Rev 4:329–345, 1992.

Stein BM: Surgical decisions in vascular malformations of the brain. In: Barnett HJM, Stein BM, Mohr JP, Yatsu FM, eds. Stroke: Pathophysiology, Diagnosis, and Management (2nd ed). New York: Churchill Livingstone, 1992, pp 1093–1133.

Steinberg MH: Sickle cell anemia: Pathophysiology, management, and prospects for the future. J Clin Apheresis 6:221–223, 1991.

Stroke Prevention in Atrial Fibrillation Investigators: Stroke Prevention in Atrial Fibrillation Study: Final results. Circulation 84:527–539, 1991.

Tefferi A, Hoagland HC: Issues in the diagnosis and management of essential thrombocythemia. Mayo Clin Proc 69:651–655, 1994.

Viñuela F, Halbach VV, Dion JE, eds: Interventional Neuroradiology: Endovascular Therapy of the Central Nervous System. New York: Raven, 1992.

Wiebers DO: Ischemic cerebrovascular complications of pregnancy. Arch Neurol 42:1106–1113, 1985.

Wiebers DO: Subarachnoid hemorrhage in pregnancy. Semin Neurol 8: 226–229, 1988.

Wiebers DO: Intracranial aneurysm. Curr Ther Neurol Dis 3:192–194, 1990.

V

Primary Prevention of Cerebrovascular Disorders

As medicine moves into the twenty-first century with the added pressure of increasing costs and limited resources, successful diminution of the impact of stroke on the population will require shifting emphasis from treatment of end stages of generalized atherosclerosis and other underlying diseases to primary prevention of underlying diseases and stroke. This approach will, in many cases, require more sophisticated and more definitive studies to identify, verify, and better explain the relative importance of known risk factors, the interactions of various risk factors, and the existence of currently unknown or unverified risk factors.

Successful primary prevention of stroke is now becoming possible with the identification of important risk factors such as hypertension, cardiac disease, transient ischemic attack, asymptomatic and symptomatic carotid artery stenosis or occlusion, cigarette smoking, and diabetes mellitus, which may be modified by treatment or other means. Other factors that are not as strongly correlated with an increased risk of stroke but are amenable to treatment or to some kind of modification include hypercoagulable state (including increased concentration of fibrinogen), sickle-cell disease, migraine, contraceptive use, drug abuse, low body and environmental temperature in the cold season, and dyslipidemia (including a high ratio of total cholesterol to high-density lipoprotein cholesterol). A family history of stroke, advanced age, sex, and race are untreatable risk factors, but they may be useful for identifying persons at higher risk of stroke who might then be more motivated to address other risk factors. Stroke is often a preventable catastrophic event. It can be prevented by identifying persons at high risk (see Appendix I) and initiating a cost-effective approach addressing the reversible risk factors.

23

Modifiable Lifestyle and Environmental Factors

Much of the desirable reduction in risk factors requires modification of environmental factors and maintenance of an appropriate lifestyle, including cessation of cigarette smoking, dietary adjustment, weight control, physical activity, cessation of drug abuse, modification of oral contraceptive use, and maintenance of adequate personal and environmental temperatures during the cold season.

Cigarette Smoking

Smoking increases the risk of stroke by approximately 40% in men and 60% in women. Cigarette smoking raises the blood fibrinogen concentration, enhances platelet aggregation, and increases hematocrit level and blood viscosity. It is one of the most powerful risk factors contributing to the development of carotid atherosclerosis and also appears to contribute significantly to the development of intracranial aneurysms. Smoking cessation substantially decreases the risk of subsequent stroke in a remarkably short time and is particularly vital for patients who present with cerebral or retinal ischemic events. The risk of stroke decreases substantially each year after cessation of cigarette smoking, and by the end of 5 years the risk is nearly that of a person who never smoked. The physician should review with the patient who smokes the benefits of quitting and the risk of continuing. Nicotine patches or nicotine-replacement gum (initial dose depends on number of cigarettes smoked per day) or clonidine may be useful smoking cessation aids unless contraindications exist.

Diet

In coronary atherosclerosis, preliminary evidence suggests that to stabilize or reverse atheroma, dietary intake of fat (especially saturated fat) must be reduced to less than 10% of the total caloric intake and cholesterol to less than 5 mg/day (major sources of saturated fatty acids and cholesterol are meat, eggs, and dairy products) through a very low-fat vegetarian diet. The same principles may also apply to carotid and other large-vessel atherosclerosis. However, randomized, controlled trials have not yet been reported, except with respect to coronary artherosclerosis. There is also some evidence that eating fish more than two times/month and using reduced-fat milk (along with other appropriate dietary modifications) may reduce the risk of stroke. Restriction of dietary salt (to about 6 g/day) or sodium intake (to about 2.3 g/day) helps in the prevention and management of hypertension. In hot, humid climates, the reduction in dietary sodium should be modified to accommodate for the loss of sodium in such extreme conditions. In general, patients should be discouraged from consuming salt-rich foods or adding salt to already prepared foods.

In the typical American diet, approximately 40% to 45% of the dietary caloric intake is in the form of fat (most of which is saturated fat) and the cholesterol intake is approximately 400 mg/day. The standard low-fat diet (see Appendix K-1) seeks to reduce fat consumption to approximately 30% of the dietary caloric intake and cholesterol consumption to approximately 300 mg. This diet is recommended as a minimal modification for general health reasons, even for persons without atherosclerosis.

An even more healthful alternative for prevention of atherosclerosis in the general population and the diet strongly recommended for persons with symptomatic or asymptomatic coronary or craniocervical atherosclerosis is a very low-fat diet (see Appendix K-2) because coronary atherosclerosis appears to progress with the typical American diet and standard low-fat diets. A very low-fat diet is aimed at reducing fat intake to 10% or less of the total calories and cholesterol intake to 5 mg/day.

Calorie restriction to achieve and maintain ideal body weight is recommended to control obesity, particularly because appropriate weight reduction enhances the regulation of hypertension and type II diabetes mellitus. Ideal body weight determinations based on height and weight (see Appendix K-3) are appropriate for some people but should not be considered necessary for everyone. In general, a healthy adult needs approximately 30 to 35 kcal/kg of body weight. With any type of restrictive diet, it is generally recommended that patients take a multivitamin and mineral supplement to ensure adequate intake of various nutrients such as iron, vitamin B_{12}, vitamin D, magnesium, and calcium, particularly if patients are likely to avoid certain food groups.

Dietary recommendations are most effective when they are specific. Therefore, a dietitian or similarly trained physician should interview each patient and characterize the eating patterns and daily calorie intake to design the most appropriate and comfortable diet. In some patients, adherence to the modified diet should be monitored under medical supervision.

Physical Exercise

Increased relative weight (body mass index, ≥ 24 kg/m²) or obesity (body weight > 10% above ideal weight) is associated with increased blood pressure, cholesterol, blood glucose, uric acid, and relative risk of death from cardiovascular disease. Weight loss of 5 to 10 kg in patients who are obese usually leads to a substantial reduction of blood pressure. In most cases, appropriate weight reduction may be achieved by dietary modification in association with physical exercise. Medical supervision, especially in the early stages of a weight control program, is desirable. A sedentary lifestyle predisposes to obesity, hypertension, glucose intolerance, hypertriglyceridemia, and reduced high-density lipoprotein cholesterol levels.

Regular moderate physical activity helps to control weight and elevated triglyceride levels, reduce blood pressure (particularly, systolic), increase high-density lipoprotein cholesterol levels, and reduce the risk of myocardial infarction and stroke. In general, exercise can be obtained by (1) altering daily lifestyle to incorporate appropriate levels of physical exertion into an overall routine or (2) undertaking regular aerobic recreational or sporting activities (as a rule, patients with moderate-to-severe hypertension or coronary artery disease should avoid isometric or static exercise) at least three times a week or frequent brisk walking from 30 to 45 minutes as often as six times/week. To facilitate the aerobic aspect of the program, the patient should warm up slowly to lessen anaerobic exercise, which may lead to early fatigue.

Exercise regimens should be prescribed individually on the basis of results of a baseline treadmill electrocardiographic test. The target heart rate should be 50% to 75% of the maximal heart rate during the treadmill exercise study or the calculated maximal pulse rate for the patient's age (220 − age). In general, the patient should be asked to walk briskly for approximately 15 minutes/session (2 times a day) for the first week, 20 minutes/session (2 times a day) for the second week, 25 minutes/day in a single session for the third week, 30 minutes/day in a single session for the fourth week, and thereafter 40 to 60 minutes six times weekly; the pulse rate should be recorded and any symptoms or complications reported at each exercise session. Preliminary evidence indicates that this type of regular exercise in combination with a strict vegetarian diet and various stress reduction techniques (without medication) may reverse coronary atherosclerosis.

Oral Contraceptives

Oral contraceptives (especially when used by someone who smokes cigarettes or is hypertensive) can cause systemic thromboembolism and result in ischemic stroke and cerebral vein thrombosis in women of childbearing age. Replacement of high-estrogen contraceptives with low-estrogen compounds or an alternative contraceptive strategy should be considered for women with ischemic cerebrovascular disease without other identifiable cause. Special precautions should be taken by women who have other stroke risk factors, particularly hypertension and cigarette smoking.

Alcohol

There is no convincing evidence that occasional or modest use of alcohol is either a risk factor or a protective factor for stroke. However, alcohol abuse (habitual drinking of > 2 oz ethanol daily or binge drinking) increases blood pressure, platelet aggregability, blood coagulation, triglyceride levels, paroxysmal atrial fibrillation, and cardiomyopathy and is associated with an increased risk of stroke (especially hemorrhagic stroke) and deaths from stroke.

Drug Abuse

Alcohol, heroin, amphetamines, cocaine, phencyclidine, and other recreational drugs may produce cerebral infarction or hemorrhage caused by vasculitis, vasospasm, noninflammatory vasculopathy, cardiac dysfunction including arrhythmias, hypercoagulability and hypocoagulability, or acute circulatory abnormalities (such as hypertensive crisis). Cessation of drug abuse and recreational drug use may prevent stroke in many young adults.

Ambient Temperature

Avoidance of low body and environmental temperatures in the cold season is recommended because they are associated with increased blood pressure, fibrinogen level, and cholesterol concentration and may increase the risk of stroke, particularly hemorrhagic subtypes.

Asymptomatic Carotid and Vertebral Stenosis

Asymptomatic Carotid Stenosis

The management of patients with asymptomatic carotid disease (bruit, stenosis, or occlusion) continues to be somewhat controversial, although recent data have clarified some aspects. It is generally accepted that all patients with asymptomatic carotid bruits should be evaluated with a complete neurologic examination, including ophthalmoscopy and one or more of the noninvasive carotid artery techniques, including oculopneumoplethysmography or carotid duplex ultrasonography. If abnormalities suggest relatively high-grade lesions (stenosis of $\geq 60\%$) or there is evidence of cholesterol or fibrin platelet retinal emboli, antiplatelet therapy is generally used with or without carotid endarterectomy, which appears to benefit some of these patients. Although the effectiveness of antiplatelet agents for reducing stroke in these patients has not been proven, these agents may also be beneficial for reducing the risk of myocardial infarction. Antiplatelet therapy is also generally recommended for patients with lesser degrees of carotid stenosis (nonpressure-significant lesions) who have other direct evidence for or risk factors associated with generalized atherosclerosis.

Data from the Asymptomatic Carotid Atherosclerosis Study (ACAS) indicate that selected patients with reduction in the diameter of the carotid artery of more than 60% may benefit from endarterectomy in addition to use of aspirin and management of risk factors. Participating surgical investigators performed carotid endarterectomy with a combined perioperative morbidity and mortality rate of less than 3%. The risk during 5 years for the primary outcome (any stroke or death within 30 days postoperatively or any **ipsilateral stroke** or death from stroke thereafter) was 5.1% (approximately 1%/year) for patients treated surgically and 11.0% (approximately 2%/year) for those treated without operation. The relative risk reduction was 53%, with a 66% reduction in men (statistically significant) and 17% in women (not statistically significant). The perioperative morbidity and mortality were higher in women, contributing to the lack of clear benefit in women. Evaluation of secondary end points revealed that the differences between the operation and nonoperation groups with respect to **total stroke and ipsilateral major stroke and death** were not statistically significant, although there was a trend in favor of operation.

These data suggest that carotid endarterectomy, performed in centers with low (less than 3%) perioperative morbidity and mortality, may be considered for high-grade asymptomatic carotid stenosis in selected patients with a life expectancy of at least 5 years. In patients with significant medical problems that may preclude general anesthesia, surgical management is contraindicated and management with antiplatelet agents is more appropriate. Additional features that make operation more compelling are progressing stenosis despite risk factor management, very high-grade lesions, and relatively localized rather than diffuse atherosclerotic disease (see Appendix J-6).

Asymptomatic Vertebral Stenosis

In the presence of stenosis or occlusion of the proximal vertebral arteries, the cervical anastomotic network usually provides efficient alternative blood flow. The natural history of vertebrobasilar ischemia resulting from asymptomatic vertebral artery occlusive disease is relatively benign, and corrective operation in the proximal or distal portions of the artery is relatively risky; thus, medical management (antiplatelet agents) is the treatment of choice. Alternative treatment approaches, such as anticoagulants, endovascular procedures, and open operation, are considerations in patients with symptomatic vertebrobasilar stenosis, as outlined in Chapters 12, 13, and 16. In both asymptomatic and symptomatic vertebrobasilar stenosis, aggressive management of modifiable risk factors is indicated.

Hypertension

Hypertension (systolic or diastolic) is an important risk factor for ischemic and hemorrhagic stroke in males and females at all ages. **Definite hypertension** (blood pressure more than 160/95 mm Hg) increases the risk of stroke to about four times that of normotensive persons (blood pressure < 140/90 mm Hg). **Borderline hypertension** (blood pressure 140–159/90–94 mm Hg) increases the risk of stroke to about two times that of normotensive persons. Atherosclerosis occurs with increased frequency and severity in patients with chronic hypertension. However, the more specific nonatherosclerotic cerebrovascular abnormality in patients with sustained hypertension consists of lipohyalinosis and fibrinoid necrosis with microaneurysm formation in penetrating arterioles. Such lesions may lead to lacunar infarction or intracerebral hemorrhage.

Hypertension is also a highly prevalent abnormality. As many as 50 million Americans have elevated blood pressure (systolic pressure ≥140 mm Hg or diastolic pressure ≥90 mm Hg) or are taking antihypertensive drugs. Reducing blood pressure to a normal range produces a corresponding decline in the occurrence of stroke. A currently used classification (Joint National Committee on Detection, Evaluation and Treatment of High Blood Pressure, 1993) categorizes hypertension into four groups: stage 1 (mild hypertension), systolic pressure 140 to 159 mm Hg or diastolic pressure 90 to 99 mm Hg; stage 2 (moderate hypertension), systolic pressure 160 to 179 mm Hg or diastolic pressure 100 to 109 mm Hg; stage 3 (severe hypertension), systolic pressure 180 to 209 mm Hg or diastolic pressure 110 to 119 mm Hg; and stage 4 (very severe hypertension), systolic pressure 210 mm Hg or more or diastolic pressure 120 mm Hg or more. For most people, a reasonable goal of treatment to lower blood pressure involves stabilization of systolic pressure at 130 to 140 mm Hg and diastolic pressure at 80 to 90 mm Hg.

In selecting drugs and providing long-term drug therapy, the physician should try to prescribe the fewest number of drugs in the smallest effective amount and lowest frequency. In this respect, monotherapy (especially for initial treatment) is desirable, but if monotherapy proves ineffective even after the dose is increased to or near maximal levels (usually after 1–3 months), combination therapy may help (if a diuretic is not chosen as the first drug, it may be useful as a second-step agent). Initial pharmacologic therapy of patients with primary hypertension without target-organ changes or with cardiovascular disorders usually includes beta-adrenergic blocking drugs, angiotensin-converting enzyme inhibitors, calcium antagonists, or diuretics. The initial therapy of patients with bilateral renal arterial disease, stenosis in an artery to a solitary kidney, or renal insufficiency may be loop diuretics. In other clinical situations, centrally acting alpha$_2$-agonists, peripheral-acting adrenergic antagonists, or direct vasodilators may be used as initial agents (see Appendix G).

In some patients with mild hypertension (diastolic pressure in the range 90–94 mm Hg and systolic pressure in the range 140–149 mm Hg) that has been successfully treated for at least 2 years, treatment may be gradually discontinued for 2 months. During that period, if the patient's blood pressure increases to above normal, treatment should be reinstituted. If the patient remains normotensive, evaluation (blood pressure measurement, electrocardiography, measurement of serum creatinine level) should be performed every 6 months and no pharmacologic therapy given (maintenance of recommended lifestyle modifications is important). However, complete cessation of antihypertensive treatment is seldom indicated, especially in patients with more severe hypertension or other risk factors.

Beta-adrenergic blockers are common first-line agents that are well tolerated and available in many forms (see Appendix G). They are especially indicated in young patients with "hyperkinetic" circulations, but they are relatively or absolutely contraindicated in patients with congestive heart failure, asthma, chronic bronchitis, bronchospasm, bradycardia (sinus rate <60 beats/minute), heart block, sick sinus syndrome, insulin-dependent diabetes mellitus, administration of monoamine oxidase inhibitors, and dyslipidemia. (In patients with hyperlipidemia, labetalol or cardioselective $beta_1$-blockers such as atenolol, metoprolol, and acebutolol may be used.) The most common side effects of beta-adrenergic blockers are heart failure, bronchospasm, Raynaud's phenomenon (episodic vasoconstriction of arteries and arterioles of the fingers, toes, and sometimes the face brought on by cold or emotional stimuli), depression, fatigue, and hypotension.

Angiotensin-converting enzyme inhibitors (benazepril, captopril, cilazapril, enalapril, fosinopril, lisinopril, perindopril, quinapril, ramipril, and spirapril) are relatively contraindicated in patients with renal failure (reduction of dose is required) and may cause hyperkalemia in patients with renal impairment or in those receiving potassium-sparing agents (see Appendix G). Side effects (chronic cough, urticarial rash, loss of taste, angioedema, proteinuria, fever, leukopenia, pancytopenia, and acute renal failure in bilateral renal artery stenosis) are uncommon. Captopril is especially indicated for the treatment of resistant hypertension and hypertension associated with renal artery stenosis.

Some **calcium channel blockers** are available in extended-release forms, allowing once-daily therapy (see Appendix G) (diltiazem, verapamil, amlodipine, felodipine, and nifedipine), whereas others are generally taken twice daily (isradipine) or thrice daily (nicardipine and nifedipine). Among these drugs, dihydropyridines (amlodipine, felodipine, isradipine, nicardipine, nifedipine) may cause dizziness, headache, flushing, peripheral edema, and tachycardia, whereas the side effects of others (diltiazem, verapamil) are symptomatic reduction in heart rate and heart block.

Distal potassium-losing diuretics (hydrochlorothiazide, chlorthalidone, metolazone), **loop diuretics** (furosemide, bumetanide, ethacrynic acid), and **distal potassium-sparing diuretics** (spironolactone, amiloride, and triamterene) are particularly effective in elderly patients (see Appendix G). Among these diuretics, thiazides (hydrochlorothiazide, chlorthalidone, metolazone) have the longest duration of action and so are preferable over the others, but they also may cause hypokalemia, hyperglycemia, and hyperuricemia, which restrict the use of high doses in some patients. Distal potassium-losing diuretics are contraindicated in patients with diabetes mellitus, hyperuricemia, and primary aldosteronism; adverse effects include potassium depletion, hyperglycemia, hyperuricemia, dermatitis, and purpura. Contraindications for loop diuretics are hyperuricemia and primary aldosteronism; they also may produce potassium depletion, hyperuricemia, nausea, vomiting, and diarrhea. Distal potassium-sparing diuretics should be avoided in patients with renal failure. Among the side effects of spironolactone are hyperkalemia, diarrhea, gynecomastia, and menstrual irregularities; amiloride and triamterene may produce hyperkalemia, nausea, vomiting, leg cramps, nephrolithiasis, and gastrointestinal disturbances.

Other widely used antihypertensive drugs include **centrally acting alpha$_2$-agonists** (clonidine, guanabenz, methyldopa, guanfacine, clonidine patch), **peripheral-acting adrenergic antagonists** (guanadrel, guanethidine, rauwolfia serpentina, and reserpine), and **direct vasodilators** (hydralazine and minoxidil). None of the **centrally acting alpha$_2$-agonists** should be withdrawn abruptly because of possible rebound hypertension, and they should be avoided in patients who may not comply with treatment. Among these agents, only methyldopa is contraindicated in patients with pheochromocytoma or active hepatic disease (intravenous infusion) and during administration of monoamine oxidase inhibitors; however, all these agents may cause postural hypotension. In addition, clonidine and guanabenz may produce drowsiness, insomnia, or lupus-like syndrome. Side effects of methyldopa include sedation, fatigue, diarrhea, impaired ejaculation, fever, chronic hepatitis, acute ulcerative colitis, gynecomastia, and lactation. Adverse reactions of guanfacine include dry mouth, sedation, asthenia, dizziness, constipation, and impotence.

Peripheral-acting adrenergic antagonists may cause serious orthostatic and exercise-induced hypotension and are contraindicated in patients with pheochromocytoma and during administration of monoamine oxidase inhibitors. Also, rauwolfia alkaloids should be avoided in patients with peptic ulcer or depression, and guanethidine and guanadrel should not be used for patients with severe coronary artery disease or cerebrovascular insufficiency.

Direct vasodilators should be taken with diuretics and beta-adrenergic blockers because of their side effects of fluid retention and reflex tachycardia. Hydralazine may cause headache, anorexia, vomiting, diarrhea, and lupus-like syndrome, and minoxidil may produce hair growth on the face and body, coarsening of facial features, and pericardial effusion.

Treatment of malignant hypertension (very severe hypertension but without severe symptoms or progressive target-organ complications and severe perioperative hypertension) must be provided within 24 hours and usually includes intravenous or intramuscular administration of rapidly acting antihypertensive drugs such as direct vasodilators, adrenergic inhibitors, calcium or ganglionic blockers, or sympatholytic agents (see Appendix G).

26

Dyslipidemia

To illustrate the heterogeneity that exists among various dyslipidemias, some of the different primary (inherited) and secondary disorders associated with each lipoprotein phenotype are outlined in Table 26-1. Major apolipoproteins associated with chylomicrons and very low-density lipoproteins (VLDL) are B, C, and E; with low-density lipoproteins (LDL), B; and with high-density lipoproteins (HDL), A-I and A-II.

Causes of secondary hyperlipidemia must be sought and treated. **Secondary hypercholesterolemia** may be associated with hypothyroidism, nephrotic syndrome, obstructive liver disease, acute intermittent porphyria, pregnancy, anorexia nervosa, and certain drugs (such as thiazide diuretics, retinoids, glucocorticoids, cyclosporine, progestins, and androgens). **Secondary hypertriglyceridemia** may result from diabetes mellitus, obesity, alcohol intake, excess intake of refined sugars, chronic renal failure, myocardial infarction, infections (bacterial, viral), systemic lupus erythematosus, dysglobulinemia, glycogen storage disease (type I), lipodystrophy, nephrotic syndrome, bulimia, autoimmune disorders, pregnancy, and certain drugs (such as beta-adrenergic blockers, retinoids, and estrogens). The most common causes of **secondary combined hyperlipidemia** include hypothyroidism, nephrotic syndrome, chronic renal failure, liver disease, Werner's syndrome, acromegaly, and certain drugs such as thiazide diuretics, glucocorticoids, and retinoids.

Blood lipid abnormalities (particularly elevated levels of LDL cholesterol, low levels of HDL, HDL_2, and HDL_3 cholesterol, and high levels of fasting triglycerides), contributing to craniocervical atherosclerosis, are important risk factors for ischemic stroke (more so in Western societies than in Asian populations). There is also some evidence of an inverse association between serum cholesterol values and the risk of intracerebral hemorrhage. Correction of these and other lipid abnormalities leading to atherosclerosis is expected to be beneficial for the prevention of stroke.

Therapy for lipid disorders must be individualized and includes dietary changes (the basic initial step for most patients), maintenance of ideal body weight, aerobic exercise, and pharmacologic agents. A decade or two ago, many cardiologists and other clinicians accepted a total cholesterol value of less than 240 mg/dl as a reasonable target for patients with or without symptomatic atherosclerosis. More recently, standard medical recommendations have changed to advocate target total cholesterol levels of 200 mg/dl or less and a daily cholesterol intake of 300 mg or less. However, the most recent evidence suggests that coronary atherosclerosis may continue to progress at such levels and that coronary atherosclerotic lesions may be stabilized or regressed by maintaining a total cholesterol level of 150 mg/dl or less and a daily cholesterol intake of less than 5 mg (see Appendix K).

Therefore, for general health purposes in persons who do not have symptomatic or asymptomatic coronary or craniocervical atherosclerosis, it is recommended that, at a minimum, patients follow a

Table 26-1.   Classification of primary and secondary blood lipid disorders

Group (Fredrickson phenotype)	Lipoprotein in excess	Primary dyslipidemias Typical lipid range Total cholesterol (mg/dl)	Total triglyceride (mg/dl)	Most common causes	Secondary dyslipidemias Typical lipid range Total cholesterol (mg/dl)	Total triglyceride (mg/dl)	Most common causes
I	Chylomicrons	300–500	5000–6000	LPL or apoprotein C-II deficiency	300–400	3000–6000	Systemic lupus erythematosus
IIA	LDL	350–400	<250	Familial (heterozygote) hypercholesterolemia, familial defective apoprotein B, familial combined hyperlipidemia	300–400	100	Obesity, hypothyroidism, nephrotic syndrome, hepatoma
		250–325		Polygenic hypercholesterolemia			
		400–800	<250	Familial (homozygote) hypercholesterolemia			
IIB	LDL	240–350		Familial combined hyperlipidemia Polygenic hypercholesterolemia or familial hypercholesterolemia plus	300–400	250–500	Cushing's syndrome, dysglobulinemia, acute intermittent porphyria, anorexia nervosa, Werner's

Type	Lipoprotein			Genetic disorder			Secondary causes
				familial hypertriglyceridemia			syndrome
III	Beta-VLDL	300–450	300–1000	Familial dysbetalipoproteinemia	300–500	300–800	Dysglobulinemia
IV	VLDL	200–240	300–700	Familial combined hyperlipidemia, familial hypertriglyceridemia	200–250	300–700	Obesity, diabetes mellitus, estrogen therapy, acromegaly
V (mild)	Chylomicrons VLDL	200–300	500–1000	Familial combined hyperlipidemia plus LPL deficiency			Cushing's syndrome, acute viral hepatitis, dysglobulinemia, alcoholic hyperlipidemia, third-trimester pregnancy
V (severe)	Chylomicrons VLDL	300–1000	2000–6000	LPL deficiency Apoprotein C-II deficiency	600–800	2000–6000	Poorly controlled diabetes mellitus, estrogen therapy, alcoholic hyperlipidemia

LDL = low-density lipoprotein; LPL = lipoprotein lipase; VLDL = very low-density lipoprotein.

low-fat diet aimed at lowering total fat and saturated fat in the diet to 30% and 10% of total calories, respectively, and restricting total cholesterol intake to less than 300 mg/day (see Appendix K-1). An even more healthful approach to prevention of atherosclerosis is to adopt the stricter, very low-fat diet, an approach that is strongly recommended for patients with known symptomatic or asymptomatic coronary or craniocervical atherosclerosis (see Appendix K-2). This diet is aimed at restricting total fat intake to 10% of total calories and cholesterol intake to less than 5 mg/day.

The approach for increasing a low HDL cholesterol value includes smoking cessation, weight loss, dietary measures, and exercise. There is evidence that regular aerobic exercise done for 20 to 30 minutes three to five times per week may increase HDL cholesterol levels and improve the blood lipid profile.

Patients with isolated increases in VLDL levels usually respond well to weight reduction, avoidance of large amounts of fructose and sucrose, and restriction of ethanol. Increasing the intake of omega-9 monounsaturated fatty acids such as oleic acid (olive oils, rapeseed oil) and omega-3 fatty acids (fish oils) also may help to lower triglyceride and LDL cholesterol levels in these patients. Patients with increases in both VLDL and LDL levels should be advised to restrict the intake of cholesterol and saturated fats and to increase the intake of fiber and complex carbohydrates (beans, oat bran, and other forms of soluble fiber).

Patients with elevated LDL cholesterol levels ($\geq$130 mg/dl) should receive appropriate dietary therapy administered by a nutritionist. Patients with isolated increases in LDL levels (especially patients with familial hypercholesterolemia) often have a less dramatic response to weight loss and dietary changes. If the LDL goal is not reached after 6 months of dietary therapy, lipid-lowering drug therapy should be considered (see Appendix F).

Other Host Factors

Transient Ischemic Attack

Because transient ischemic attack (TIA) predisposes to stroke, its prevention (modification of lifestyle as outlined in Chapter 23 and therapy for hypertension, atherosclerosis, cardiac disease, or other cerebrovascular risk factors) and treatment (surgical, medical, or lifestyle modification) reduces the risk of subsequent cerebrovascular events. Patients must be aware that it is important to get immediate medical consultation whenever the **warning signs** of acute ischemic cerebrovascular disease occur (see Appendix J-1 and Chapter 12). Warning signs include sudden weakness or numbness of the face, arm, and leg, especially on one side of the body; sudden darkening or loss of vision, particularly in one eye; loss of speech or trouble talking or understanding speech; sudden, severe headache with no apparent cause; and sudden unexplained dizziness, unsteadiness, double vision, or sudden fall, especially along with any of the other symptoms.

The evaluation and treatment of transient ischemic attack are outlined in Chapters 12 and 16.

Cardiac Disease

Because cardiac diseases (particularly congestive heart failure, coronary artery disease, valvular disease, arrhythmias, and left ventricular hypertrophy seen by electrocardiography) predispose to stroke, prevention and specialized treatment of these cardiovascular contributors can be anticipated to reduce the occurrence of stroke. (The specific treatment of patients with cardiac disorders already causing transient ischemic attack or stroke is outlined in Chapter 16.) Regarding primary prevention, smoking cessation, dietary adjustment and weight control, physical exercise, and control of hypertension and blood lipid abnormalities (in particular, reducing elevated levels of total and low-density lipoprotein cholesterol and increasing the high-density lipoprotein cholesterol fraction) may be beneficial. Aspirin, 325 mg daily, may reduce the risk of ischemic heart disease (prophylactic use of aspirin is not advisable in persons with poorly controlled hypertension because of possible increased risk of hemorrhagic stroke). Individual decisions are required regarding therapy for specific cardiac diseases.

To prevent stroke in patients with **recent myocardial infarction** (especially if the infarct is large, if it involves the anterior/septal ventricular wall, or if it is associated with atrial fibrillation, congestive heart failure, thrombi, or cerebral or retinal ischemic events), anticoagulant therapy is recommended. Therapy should begin with heparin during the first week followed by oral anticoagulant therapy (warfarin) alone (International Normalized Ratio [INR], 2.0–3.0). The most efficacious duration of therapy is not known. Recent data indicate that after acute myocardial infarction, patients treated with warfarin (INR, 2.8–4.8) compared with those who received placebo had reductions in recurrent myocardial infarction and cerebrovascular events. The mortality was not different in the two groups (see ASPECT reference in Suggested Reading for Part V). Further studies in one European country indicated the cost-effectiveness of oral anticoagulant therapy (see Asplund reference in Suggested Reading for Part V).

Among **cardiac arrhythmias**, atrial fibrillation is the most powerful risk factor for embolic brain infarction. Therefore, every attempt should be made to restore sinus rhythm in appropriate cases, preferably with cardioversion. Many issues must be considered before performing cardioversion, such as the potential for maintaining sinus rhythm after the procedure, the benefit of cardioversion, and risk of adverse complications, including risk of systemic embolic events. The best candidates for long-term successful cardioversion are patients who have short-term atrial fibrillation with no significant atrial enlargement and with minimal coronary artery disease. Conversion of atrial fibrillation to a normal rhythm is associated with risk of embolization, which often occurs within 48 hours after conversion. Anticoagulant therapy with heparin should precede cardioversion, especially in patients with associated mitral valve disease, cardiac enlargement, congestive heart failure, or previous embolization. If sinus rhythm is not restored, long-term stroke prevention through anticoagulation with warfarin or aspirin should be considered.

The decision should be made on the basis of data available from clinical trials, although some questions persist in regard to safety of anticoagulation in patients older than 75 years and in regard to the efficacy of aspirin in some subgroups. Lone atrial fibrillation indicates patients without any associated clinical risk factors such as previous stroke or transient ischemic attack, diabetes, hypertension, congestive heart failure, coronary artery disease, or valvular disease such as mitral valve disease or prosthetic valves. Patients younger than 60 years without clinical risk factors have a low risk of stroke and require no treatment or treatment with aspirin. In patients aged 60 to 75 years, those with lone atrial fibrillation may be treated with aspirin; for those older than 75 years, anticoagulation should be used (warfarin; INR, 2.0–3.0), unless contraindications exist, with close monitoring of INR. In patients with atrial fibrillation and any risk factors, chronic anticoagulation with warfarin (INR, 2.0–3.0) should be used, although, again, warfarin must be used cautiously in patients older than 75 years.

In pregnant patients, subcutaneously administered heparin is often given throughout pregnancy or, alternatively, warfarin is administered only during the second and third trimesters up until gestation week 37, at which time heparin should again be given (see Chapter 22).

Cardiac surgery of many types also is associated with an increased risk of cerebral ischemia. Improvements in the pump oxygenator and surgical techniques have helped reduce the occurrence of multifocal ischemic syndromes. Anticoagulant therapy may reduce the frequency of postoperative embolization, particularly in patients with prosthetic mitral valves. The protective value of alternative or supplemental treatment with antiplatelet agents has also been suggested.

In patients with **rheumatic fever**, treatment with salicylates, corticosteroids, and antibiotics (benzathine penicillin G, intramuscularly or orally, or erythromycin orally) should be instituted. Antibiotic prophylaxis (usually with 1 monthly intramuscular injection of 1.2 million U benzathine penicillin G or oral penicillin, 200,000 units, twice daily) is generally advocated for children with one or more episodes of acute rheumatic fever and should be given through the school years until the patient is 18 years of age. For persons with onset of rheumatic fever after the age of 18, antibiotic prophylaxis is suggested for a minimum of 5 years after the episode. Antibiotic prophylaxis is also generally recommended for patients with a history of rheumatic heart disease, especially pregnant patients, to prevent **infective endocarditis**.

In patients with **aortic stenosis or regurgitation**, or in patients with **mitral stenosis or regurgitation**, an appropriate surgical procedure (aortic balloon valvuloplasty or valve replacement) should be considered. The most efficacious treatment to prevent stroke in patients with **mitral valve prolapse** associated with ischemic cerebral or retinal events is controversial. Asymptomatic mitral valve prolapse occurs in about 5% of the population, with a marked preponderance in women. Thus, it is difficult to define the etiologic relationship of mitral valve prolapse with stroke of unknown cause. In general, in patients with no other cause despite a comprehensive evaluation for a cerebral ischemic event that may be embolic in nature, mitral valve prolapse may be managed with at least short-term warfarin anticoagulation followed by antiplatelet therapy. Patients with more severe mitral regurgitation may require valve replacement.

For prevention of ischemic stroke in patients with **prosthetic heart valves**, warfarin anticoagulation is typically used, and dipyridamole may be added for patients who have ongoing thromboembolic events while receiving warfarin. A combination of warfarin and aspirin is typically not recommended because it prolongs bleeding time and increases hemorrhage risk, although the combination is sometimes necessary for patients with recurrent symptoms, despite an increase in INR and additional treatment with dipyridamole.

Although the benefit of antibiotic prophylaxis against **infective endocarditis** has not been clearly proved, most cardiologists recommend prophylaxis with parenteral aqueous penicillin G or gentamicin for patients with significant valvular disease, particularly patients with prosthetic valves. To prevent ischemic stroke in patients with **cardiomyopathy**, treatment that includes bed rest, digitalis, diuretics, and sodium restriction is recommended. Anticoagulants should be used if any embolic complications have occurred, if definite mural thrombi are seen on echocardiography, or if ejection fraction decreases to less than 30%.

Diabetes Mellitus

Typically, patients have more than one risk factor for cardiac disease. Clustering of risk factors is usually manifested as hypertension, truncal (central) obesity, dyslipidemia, and insulin resistance. Several factors have an impact on insulin resistance, including weight, a sedentary lifestyle, hyperglycemia, and multiple medications.

There are two major types of diabetes. In type I diabetes (insulin-dependent diabetes mellitus), onset typically occurs before the person is 30 years old, and the diabetes may be associated with ketoacidosis, which often occurs in lean persons with a dependence on exogenous insulin. In type II diabetes (non-insulin-dependent diabetes mellitus), persons are typically older, most are obese, and ketoacidosis usually does not develop in the absence of exogenous insulin. Diagnosis is usually made on the basis of a fasting glucose level ($\geq$140 mg/dl) and typical clinical symptoms such as polyuria, polyphagia, and polydipsia, often with weight loss. Treatment may include oral hypoglycemic agents and insulin.

Vascular complications include accelerated atherosclerosis in large vessels and microangiopathy, most commonly involving retinal and renal vasculature. Diabetes mellitus is a risk factor for stroke and, in particular, for ischemic stroke (cerebral infarction). Because diabetes is often associated with other risk factors for atherosclerosis, such as hypertension and dyslipidemia, patients with diabetes must be followed closely for co-occurring processes and treated aggressively. Treatment of the diabetes to bring the glucose level into a normal range may also decrease the occurrence of stroke.

28

Unruptured Intracranial Aneurysms

Unruptured intracranial aneurysms (UIAs) constitute a significant public health problem. Several large autopsy studies have reported a wide range in the overall frequency of intracranial aneurysms, varying from 0.2% to 9.9% (mean, approximately 5%), which suggests that among the U.S. population, approximately 12 million persons have or will have intracranial aneurysms.

The magnitude of the problem of UIAs is increasing. The change is at least partly a result of the increasing age of the population, in that these lesions develop with increasing age. In addition, in recent years, the widespread use of computed tomography (CT) and magnetic resonance scanning has greatly increased the numbers of aneurysms discovered incidentally. The quality of these techniques has also improved, particularly magnetic resonance imaging (MRI) and magnetic resonance angiography (MRA) studies.

Besides the fortuitous discovery of UIAs on CT, MRI, or MRA studies done for unrelated reasons, UIAs may also be discovered when a physician investigates subarachnoid hemorrhage from a different source such as an aneurysm or arteriovenous malformation, or investigates aneurysmal symptoms other than rupture. These symptoms include the following:

1. Cranial nerve palsies (most commonly cranial nerves II, III, IV, and VI)
2. Compression of other central nervous system structures (including the brain stem and pituitary)
3. Persistent and often focal vascular headaches that are usually of relatively recent onset and new character
4. Focal ischemic symptoms from distal embolization of aneurysmal clot
5. Seizure foci resulting from impingement on supratentorial brain structures

Headache may be caused by a sudden dilatation of the aneurysm or by chronic compression of pain-sensitive structures, such as the ophthalmic and maxillary divisions of the trigeminal nerve. Such headaches are usually persistent and focal, corresponding to the location of the aneurysm. They may also be associated with cranial nerve palsies. However, sudden and unusually severe headache associated with nausea or vomiting is always suspicious for a warning leak (or minor subarachnoid hemorrhage) from an intracranial aneurysm. In these cases, CT should be obtained, and if this study is negative and there are no signs of mass effect, lumbar puncture should be performed.

When decisions about management of UIAs need to be made, it is very important to recognize potential differences in behavior between these lesions and previously ruptured intracranial aneurysms. Among patients with UIAs, there should be a distinction between patients without a history of subarachnoid hemorrhage and those with a history of subarachnoid hemorrhage from a different source, most commonly another aneurysm that was successfully repaired.

Previously ruptured intracranial aneurysms have a much greater likelihood of subsequent growth and rupture than do those that are previously unruptured.

Among patients with UIAs and no history of previous subarachnoid hemorrhage from a different source, natural history studies indicate that size of the aneurysm at the time of discovery is by far the most important individual variable for predicting rupture. However, in analyses of combinations of variables, the combination of size of the aneurysm and age of the patient was a better predictor of future rupture. When the product of aneurysm size (in mm) times the patient's age (in years) exceeds 1000, the risk is particularly high.

The mean frequency of intracranial aneurysms in autopsy studies (approximately 5%) combined with a population-based incidence of aneurysmal subarachnoid hemorrhage (approximately 10/100,000/year) suggests that most aneurysms that form never rupture. In view of this, the selection of patients for surgical treatment ideally should depend on predicting which patients have unruptured aneurysms that will subsequently rupture. If one were to take the approach of attempting to identify and repair all UIAs, the direct surgical cost among today's U.S. population would exceed $275 billion. The cost of screening the population with magnetic resonance studies and performing subsequent cerebral arteriography for patients with positive or suspicious magnetic resonance scans would exceed direct surgical costs.

For unruptured aneurysms 10 mm or more in diameter in patients without previous subarachnoid hemorrhage, the risk of subsequent rupture is fairly high. Current knowledge suggests that for patients with unruptured aneurysms of this size, particularly those more than 25 mm in diameter, an intracranial procedure should be considered by a neurosurgeon and an interventional radiologist (preferably working as a team with experience in both conventional open procedures and endovascular operation) to isolate the aneurysm from the circulation as soon as possible. Patients with aneurysms 10 to 25 mm in diameter should also be considered for operation, which seems to be particularly justifiable for women younger than 75 years and for men younger than 69 years.

Patients who have UIAs less than 10 mm in diameter and who have no previous subarachnoid hemorrhage from a different source appear to have a very low risk of subsequent rupture (almost certainly less than 0.5%/year). Even if one considers a rupture rate of 0.5%/year for these patients, a decision analysis indicates that elective surgery would, at best, be of marginal value. Consequently, it is difficult to recommend surgical intervention for these patients, particularly those with aneurysms 5 mm or less in diameter.

It is certainly possible that patients with an unruptured aneurysm who have a history of subarachnoid hemorrhage from a different source have a different prognosis than patients who have never had subarachnoid hemorrhage. Whatever caused the initial rupture may make it more likely for such patients to have rupture of a second or third aneurysm, and the risk associated with size may be different or conceivably irrelevant in these patients. There are several case reports involving subsequent rupture of unruptured aneurysms less than 10 mm in diameter (particularly aneurysms 6–9 mm in diameter), almost all of which have occurred in patients with a history of subarachnoid hemorrhage from a different source. Consequently, in this group of patients, it is more compelling to consider surgical intervention and prophylactic repair for patients with unruptured aneurysms of 6 mm or more in diameter.

If compressive or embolic symptoms of an aneurysm develop after the original diagnosis, the aneurysm probably has enlarged and thus has a higher probability of rupture. In this circumstance, the patient should be restudied with cerebral arteriography and considered for neurologic surgery if the aneurysm has enlarged.

Operative morbidity and mortality for unruptured aneurysms vary with the individual surgeon, the size and location of the aneurysm, and whether recent subarachnoid hemorrhage from a separate aneurysm has occurred. Recent North American series involving conventional surgical clipping have reported no operative mortality and permanent neurologic morbidity rates of 3.6% to 6.5%. A meta-analysis including case series from 1970 to 1993 reported an operative mortality of 1% and an operative morbidity of 4.1% (see King reference in Suggested Reading for Part V). However, in a large survey from Japan constituting the largest series to date (217 patients), the operative mortality rate was 7%; operative morbidity, which usually exceeds mortality, was not reported (see Nishimoto reference in Suggested Reading for Part V).

In recent years, ruptured and unruptured aneurysms have been repaired with endovascular surgical techniques, including the placement of metallic coils within aneurysms. Such techniques are evolving over time and their uses are increasing, but their precise role in the management of UIAs has not been well defined.

In regard to the issue of **screening** for unruptured aneurysms, general screening of the population is unlikely to be beneficial. The yield would be extremely low because aneurysms generally develop with increasing age, and most aneurysms that are going to rupture probably will do so at the time of or soon after formation. In addition, the economic costs would be prohibitive. At this point, it seems reasonable to restrict screening for UIAs to patients with one or more conditions associated with intracranial aneurysms (such as autosomal dominant polycystic kidney disease) who also have a family history of intracranial aneurysm or subarachnoid hemorrhage (particularly those with several affected family members). For patients with **either** a condition associated with intracranial aneurysms **or** positive family history (for intracranial aneurysm or subarachnoid hemorrhage), some screening may also be reasonable, especially for those who will be undergoing major elective surgery in whom hemodynamic instability is anticipated, those who have indeterminate symptoms that might suggest intracranial aneurysms, those who have high-risk occupations (for instance, airline pilots), and those who want to be screened for purposes of reassurance. The most reliable noninvasive studies for screening asymptomatic patients for UIAs are MRA and high-resolution CT scanning, including helical and dynamic multiplane CT.

In patients with **UIAs associated with unruptured arteriovenous malformations,** aneurysms are likely to be located within the feeding system of the arteriovenous malformation. The probability of future subarachnoid hemorrhage in these patients is considerably higher than that in patients with UIAs or unruptured arteriovenous malformations alone. When operation is contemplated, many (but not all) experts believe it is generally wise to clip the aneurysm before addressing the arteriovenous malformation, if individual circumstances allow this, especially in patients with large aneurysms, because sudden changes in the hemodynamics of the feeding system may predispose to aneurysmal rupture and because aneurysmal rupture is associated with a higher morbidity and mortality than rupture of arteriovenous malformation.

When **carotid endarterectomy** is performed in patients with UIAs, the sudden change of hemodynamics in the distal carotid system as a result of correcting a pressure-significant stenosis may predispose to enlargement or rupture of a previously unruptured aneurysm. Even endarterectomy for non-pressure-significant stenosis could cause substantial pressure alterations in the distal carotid system with clamping and unclamping. Thus, carotid endarterectomy should be approached with increased caution in patients with UIAs, particularly for aneurysms that are more than 5 mm in diameter in the ipsilateral carotid system.

Unruptured Intracranial Vascular Malformations

Intracranial vascular malformations such as arteriovenous malformation (AVM), cavernous malformation, telangiectasia, venous malformation, and vein of Galen malformation are congenital developmental abnormalities (most dural and extracerebral AVMs may be acquired) and usually take many years before they become clinically apparent. Most commonly, AVMs present with intracerebral or subarachnoid hemorrhage or with a seizure disorder.

AVMs are the most commonly clinically recognized form of intracranial vascular malformation. Symptoms of unruptured AVMs often appear in adolescence or later (most frequently in the third and fourth decades of life), and usually produce intracranial hemorrhage, recurrent unilateral headache (which may resemble migraine), focal or generalized seizures (also characteristic of cavernous and venous malformations), dizziness or syncope, fleeting neurologic symptoms resembling transient ischemic attacks, or progressing neurologic deficits. AVMs are occasionally associated with a cranial or orbital bruit. The clinical diagnosis is documented by computed tomography (CT) with contrast enhancement, magnetic resonance imaging (MRI), magnetic resonance angiography (MRA), or cerebral arteriography (an oval or pyramidal heterogeneous nidus with typical serpentine channels and poorly defined margins is common).

Cavernous malformations are frequently associated with focal or generalized seizures, focal neurologic deficits, or nonspecific headache. Symptoms are caused by small hemorrhages occurring within the lesion or at the periphery, although significant intraparenchymal hemorrhage is rare. CT with contrast enhancement may demonstrate a characteristic mulberry-shaped lesion with calcification, although MRI is typically necessary to detect these angiographically occult lesions.

Telangiectasias are anomalies of capillary-sized vessels, which characteristically are located in the brain stem or cerebellum. They are usually asymptomatic (when associated with the syndrome of Rendu-Osler-Weber they may be clinically recognized elsewhere in the body) and have little risk of hemorrhagic complications.

Unruptured **venous malformations** are usually asymptomatic but occasionally may produce headaches, seizures, and intracranial hemorrhage. On arteriography (venous phase) they are represented by a deep prominent vein of varying size associated with finger-like projections (caput medusa). Asymptomatic venous malformations have a benign prognosis.

Vein of Galen malformations usually manifest with cyanosis and respiratory distress in the neonatal period, seizures and hydrocephalus in infancy, and headache and subarachnoid hemorrhage in older children and adults. Scalp or face veins may be enlarged.

In view of this background information, doubts continue about the optimal management of patients with unruptured vascular malformations, and dogmatic statements cannot be made on the basis of current scientific knowledge. However, certain guidelines seem reasonable. All patients who have indeterminate symptoms that might suggest an intracranial vascular malformation should undergo noninvasive tests such as CT with contrast enhancement, MRI, or MRA, if available. Conventional arteriography should be considered for the definitive diagnosis and characterization of the lesion in patients who are appropriate candidates for surgery.

The decision regarding conservative or surgical treatment (including radiosurgery and endovascular embolization) of an AVM must be made individually on the basis of the following factors: (1) the clinical presentation and type of malformation; (2) the location, size, and anatomy of the malformation; (3) the patient's age and overall health; (4) the patient's and the physician's thorough awareness of the potential problems associated with suggested aggressive treatment; and (5) the availability of a vascular and stereotactic neurosurgeon, neuroradiologist, and radiotherapist who are experienced in the treatment of vascular malformations.

In reference to age, older patients with AVM seem to have a lower natural history risk of hemorrhage but a poorer tolerance to surgical excision. Overall health also has to be considered in establishing the appropriate management. Although the natural history of asymptomatic AVMs, including those with headache or seizures alone, is still not known with certainty, the risk of hemorrhage is about 2.5%/year, and this risk does not appear to decrease over time. Multiple potential predictors of intracranial hemorrhage have been evaluated. Some have reported small size as a risk factor for hemorrhage. Arterial factors including presence of a nidal aneurysm may increase the risk of intracranial hemorrhage. Characteristics of venous drainage, including deep venous drainage, dilatation of a draining vein, and a single draining vein, all may be important in predicting future hemorrhage. Elective surgical resection should be considered before rupture, particularly in young patients who are otherwise healthy, with AVMs whose size, venous drainage, arterial supply, and location allow relatively safe excision. Patients with untreatable vascular malformations should be observed with recommendations to avoid taking antiplatelet or anticoagulant drugs.

The natural history of clinically unruptured telangiectasias is usually benign. The natural history of clinically unruptured venous malformations is also typically benign, and conservative management is usually indicated, unless hemorrhage, seizure disorder resistant to medical management, or progressive neurologic deficit occurs. Similarly, although the natural course of cavernous malformations has not been defined with certainty, the annual risk of significant hemorrhage is likely less than 1%/year. However, intractable seizures and progressive neurologic deficit from small hemorrhages may lead to consideration of surgery.

Periodic assessment of patients, with timely intervention to prevent complications, is important for prolonging survival. If a previously asymptomatic unruptured AVM hemorrhages, if seizures associated with the lesion are medically intractable, if there is evidence of progressive neurologic deficit associated with an unruptured vascular malformation, or if the patient wants the reassurance of taking the risk of treatment, appropriate intervention should be considered.

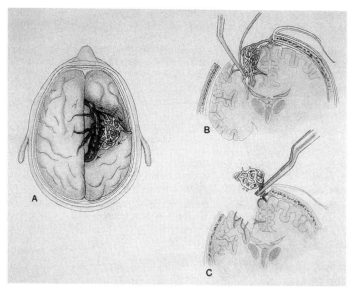

Fig. 29-1. Technique for removal of arteriovenous malformation.

Patients with hypertension should be strictly advised to control their blood pressure within the normal range. Women of childbearing age should be aware that the risk of intracranial hemorrhage may be somewhat higher during a pregnancy, although most women complete the pregnancy without significant problem. Patients with vascular malformations who have seizures should be treated with anticonvulsants (such as phenytoin, 300 mg/day).

When possible, a **surgical total removal** of an AVM with or without preceding embolization is the preferred approach to treatment, especially for patients who have had recent rupture (Fig. 29-1). Generally, relatively young patients with a small AVM in the nondominant hemisphere located superficially in the frontal or temporal area are the best candidates for operation. Very large AVMs (more than 6 cm in diameter) involving more than one lobe or the posterior fossa and deep areas of the brain may be inoperable or cannot be resected at one sitting (preceding embolization of the feeders is usually required).

AVMs located deep within the dominant hemisphere, in the brain stem, or in other high-risk areas of the brain such as the internal capsule and the thalamus are usually considered to be inoperable because of their inaccessibility or high risk of postoperative severe neurologic deficit and death. Even in the most experienced centers, surgical excision of these AVMs with or without embolization is associated with a mortality rate of 1% to 5% and a morbidity rate of 10% to 20%. In this case, **focused radiotherapy** (gamma knife radiosurgery) or **proton beam radiation** alone or after embolization of the feeders or as an adjunct to embolization and resection may be considered. Gamma knife radiotherapy may be especially effective if the nidus is no larger than 2 cm in diameter. Approximately 40% of patients have arteriographic obliteration of the lesion at 1 year after radiosurgery, 84% after 2 years, and about 97% after 3 years. However, intracranial bleeding may occur before obliteration of the AVM. Radiotherapy alone is less optimal for treatment of large AVMs (more than 3 cm in every dimension) and may result in radionecrosis of normal brain tissue with associated neurologic deficit or hydrocephalus.

Endovascular embolization, balloon or coil placement, should also be considered as a preparation for operation in patients who have a few major feeders supplying the AVM, especially for AVMs larger than 2 cm, and for treatment of dural AVMs (usually excluding those involving the tentorium). Possible complications associated with endovascular procedures include intracranial hemorrhage caused by rupture of an arterial feeder and cerebral ischemia; the risk of a permanent complication is about 10%.

Symptomatic cavernous malformations requiring treatment are typically surgically excised, if possible. Some brain stem or subcortical lesions presenting with recurrent hemorrhage that cannot be approached surgically may be treated with gamma knife radiosurgery, although the efficacy of this treatment approach in arteriographically occult lesions is uncertain.

The natural course of a vein of Galen malformation presenting with severe cardiac failure in the first few weeks of life is invariably fatal and therapeutic measures generally have been futile, but for older children who present with mild or none of the major complications (cardiac failure or progressive hydrocephalus) of this lesion, shunting procedures and interruption of feeding arteries may be considered.

Hematologic Disease

Stroke is a major complication of **sickle-cell disease,** which typically develops when a person is between the ages of 9 and 15 years. Cerebral infarction in sickle-cell disease is associated with an occlusive vasculopathy involving the distal intracranial segments of the cerebral arteries, with documented thrombosis formation in some cases. To decrease the risk of stroke in sickle-cell disease, patients should be advised to avoid excesses of unaccustomed physical exertion, hypoxia (as occurs in high altitude or with climbing), exposure to excessive heat, stress, and acute infection.

Management of **other hematologic diseases** (such as polycythemia, thrombotic thrombocytopenic purpura, dysproteinemia, thrombocythemia, leukemia) and conditions and circumstances that result in **hypercoagulable state** (such as cancer, pregnancy, trauma, postoperative period, postpartum period, disseminated intravascular coagulation), which increases the risk for stroke, is specific to each underlying cause. (A more complete discussion of hematologic disease can be found in Chapters 16 and 17.)

Suggested Reading for Part V

Albers GW, Sherman DG, Gress DR, et al: Stroke prevention in nonvalvular atrial fibrillation: A review of prospective randomized trials. Ann Neurol 30:511–518, 1991.

American College of Physicians: Guidelines for medical treatment for stroke prevention. Ann Intern Med 121:54–55, 1994.

Anticoagulants in the Secondary Prevention of Events in Coronary Thrombosis (ASPECT) Research Group: Effect of long-term oral anticoagulant treatment on mortality and cardiovascular morbidity after myocardial infarction. Lancet 343:499–503, 1994.

Asplund K, Marké LA, Terént A, et al: Costs and gains in stroke prevention: European perspective. Cerebrovasc Dis 3(Suppl 1):34–42, 1993.

Atrial Fibrillation Investigators: Risk factors for stroke and efficacy of antithrombotic therapy in atrial fibrillation. Analysis of pooled data from five randomized controlled trials. Arch Intern Med 154:1449–1457, 1994.

Auger RG, Wiebers DO: Management of unruptured intracranial aneurysms: A decision analysis. J Stroke Cerebrovasc Dis 1:174–181, 1991.

Auger RG, Wiebers DO: Management of unruptured intracranial arteriovenous malformations: A decision analysis. Neurosurgery 30:561–569, 1992.

Brown RD Jr, Wiebers DO, Forbes G, et al: The natural history of unruptured intracranial arteriovenous malformations. J Neurosurg 68:352–357, 1988.

Executive Committee for the Asymptomatic Carotid Atherosclerosis Study: Endarterectomy for asymptomatic carotid artery stenosis. JAMA 273:1421–1428, 1995.

Feigin VL, Wiebers DO, Whisnant JP: Update on stroke risk factors. J Stroke Cerebrovasc Dis 4:207–215, 1994.

Fletcher AE, Bulpitt CJ: How far should blood pressure be lowered? N Engl J Med 326:251–254, 1992.

Gorelick PB: Stroke prevention. An opportunity for efficient utilization of health care resources during the coming decade. Stroke 25:220–224, 1994.

Gould KL: Reversal of coronary atherosclerosis. Clinical promise as the basis for noninvasive management of coronary artery disease. Circulation 90:1558–1571, 1994.

Grundy SM, Greenland P, Herd A, et al: Cardiovascular and risk factor evaluation of healthy American adults: A statement for physicians by an ad hoc committee appointed by the Steering Committee, American Heart Association. Circulation 75:1340A–1362A, 1987.

Hobson RW II, Weiss DG, Fields WS, et al: Efficacy of carotid endarterectomy for asymptomatic carotid stenosis. The Veterans Affairs Cooperative Study Group. N Engl J Med 328:221–227, 1993.

Juvela S, Porras M, Heiskanen O: Natural history of unruptured intracranial aneurysms: A long-term follow-up study. J Neurosurg 79:174–182, 1993.

King JT Jr, Berlin JA, Flamm ES: Morbidity and mortality from elective surgery for asymptomatic, unruptured, intracranial aneurysms: A meta-analysis. J Neurosurg 81:837–842, 1994.

Lavie CJ, Gau GT, Squires RW, et al: Management of lipids in primary and secondary prevention of cardiovascular diseases. Mayo Clin Proc 63:605–621, 1988.

Marmot MG, Poulter NR: Primary prevention of stroke. Lancet 339:344–347, 1992.

Matchar DB, McCrory DC, Barnett HJ, et al: Medical treatment for stroke prevention. Ann Intern Med 121:41–53, 1994.

Nishimoto A, Ueta K, Onbe H, et al: Nationwide co-operative study of intracranial aneurysm surgery in Japan. Stroke 16:48–52, 1985.

Ornish D, Brown SE, Scherwitz LW, et al: Can lifestyle changes reverse coronary heart disease? The Lifestyle Heart Trial. Lancet 336:129–133, 1990.

Stroke Prevention in Atrial Fibrillation Investigators: Stroke Prevention in Atrial Fibrillation Study. Final results. Circulation 84:527–539, 1991.

Wiebers DO, Torres VE: Screening for unruptured intracranial aneurysms in autosomal dominant polycystic kidney disease. N Engl J Med 327:953–955, 1992.

Wiebers DO, Whisnant JP, Sundt TM Jr, et al: The significance of unruptured intracranial saccular aneurysms. J Neurosurg 66:23–29, 1987.

Wolf PA, Belanger AJ, D'Agostino RB: Management of risk factors. Neurol Clin 10:177–191, 1992.

VI

Assessing and Discussing Prognosis and Natural History of Cerebrovascular Disorders

Carotid or Vertebral Artery Occlusive Disease

Carotid or vertebral artery disease may be asymptomatic or symptomatic. Factors associated with an increased risk of ischemic stroke related to carotid or vertebral artery occlusive disease include age, cigarette smoking, hypertension, ischemic heart disease, diabetes, hyperlipidemia, and hypercoagulable states.

Asymptomatic Carotid Artery Disease

Carotid bruit occurs in 4% to 5% of the population aged 45 to 80 years. However, a carotid bruit is merely a reflection of turbulence in the artery and a relatively poor predictor of underlying internal carotid stenosis in asymptomatic patients. Bruits are noted in about 40% of patients with 50% or more linear carotid stenosis (≥75% cross-sectional area stenosis) and 10% of those with less than 50% linear stenosis. Patients with carotid bruit who have asymptomatic pressure-significant occlusive lesions of the carotid system (abnormal ocular pneumoplethysmography) are at greater risk for stroke than patients with bruit who have normal ocular pneumoplethysmography (twofold) and the general population (sevenfold). In one study, the annual stroke rate during a period of 3 years among patients with carotid bruit was 3.4% in those with pressure-significant stenosis on ocular pneumoplethysmography, 1.5% in those with normal ocular pneumoplethysmography, and 0.5% in a normal age- and sex-matched population. Similar figures have been documented for patients with high-grade asymptomatic carotid stenoses diagnosed on carotid ultrasonography.

Various characteristics of the bruit, including location, loudness, or pitch, are relatively poor predictors of underlying stenosis. Bruits with a diastolic component in addition to the usual systolic component generally have an associated underlying high-grade stenosis. An ocular bruit is a relatively good predictor of some degree of underlying internal carotid artery siphon stenosis, although the stenosis may not be severe.

Patients with asymptomatic carotid bruits are at greater risk than the general population for all forms of atherosclerotic vascular disease. The risk of myocardial infarction is also increased (about 2.5 times) in patients with asymptomatic carotid bruit, and myocardial infarction is the leading cause of death. However, these patients are at far less risk for ischemic stroke than are patients with symptomatic bruits or stenoses (see below). The risk of stroke in elderly persons with asymptomatic carotid bruit is relatively small, but it increases significantly in patients of all ages when associated with hypertension.

The **degree of stenosis** in the carotid artery is a better predictor of stroke risk. In one study of asymptomatic patients, Doppler ultrasonographic evidence of more than 75% stenosis was associated with a 5.5% (during a mean of 28 months) annual risk of stroke. The range of stroke risk reported for patients with asymptomatic high-grade (≥75% cross-sectional stenosis) carotid stenosis was 2% to 5.5% during the first year, but the risk after the first year decreased, particularly if the stenosis was stable. Stroke risk depends on the percentage of stenosis, progression of stenosis between noninvasive examinations, and the presence or absence of ulceration. In another study, stroke risk among asymptomatic patients with 60% or more carotid stenosis was 11% during a mean of about 5 years; these patients were treated with aspirin and correction of risk factors.

The presence of **ulceration** appears to increase the risk for subsequent stroke, depending on the size and extent of the ulceration. However, these lesions are difficult to define in many cases, even with conventional arteriography. When ulcers are identified on conventional cut-film arteriography, their size can be defined by multiplying the length and width of the ulcer in millimeters. The presence of small "A" ulcers (<10 mm^2) is not associated with an increased risk of stroke, but the presence of "B" ulcers (10–40 mm^2) or "C" ulcers (>40 mm^2) has been associated with stroke rates of 4.5% and 7.5%/year, respectively (in "C" ulcers, the rate of stroke may be somewhat independent of associated carotid stenosis).

Data from the Asymptomatic Carotid Atherosclerosis Study indicate that there may be a select group of otherwise relatively healthy patients with 60% or more carotid stenosis (diameter reduction) who have a lower risk of ipsilateral stroke and death with carotid endarterectomy than do patients treated with aspirin and reduction of risk factors, when carotid endarterectomy is performed with less than 3% surgical morbidity and mortality. The risk of any stroke or death within 30 days postoperatively or any ipsilateral stroke or death after 30 days was 5.1% for surgical patients and 11.0% for those treated medically for 5 years. The resultant 66% relative risk reduction in men was statistically significant, but the reduction was not statistically significant in women (17%). Perioperative morbidity and mortality were higher in women and contributed to the lack of clear benefit in women. With respect to overall stroke rates and ipsilateral major stroke and death, the difference between the groups that had surgery and the groups that did not have surgery was not statistically significant, although there was a trend favoring surgery.

Anesthesia and operation do not appear to pose substantial additional risks of stroke for patients with carotid bruits, although some have suggested that a subgroup of patients with bruit and asymptomatic, hemodynamically significant stenosis (as defined by abnormal oculopneumoplethysmography) may be at increased risk of stroke during peripheral vascular or cardiac surgery.

Symptomatic Carotid Artery Disease

Symptomatic carotid artery disease includes symptoms related to transient or persistent monocular visual loss, hemispheric transient ischemic attack (TIA), and ischemic stroke. In patients with symptoms of carotid system cerebral ischemia, a localized or diffuse carotid bruit is approximately 75% predictive of ipsilateral moderate or high-grade carotid stenosis. When both carotid arteries are assessed together, a carotid bruit is 85% predictive of moderate-to-severe stenosis at any extracranial carotid site. Patients who present with TIA or minor stroke related to severe carotid stenotic lesions ($\geq$70% linear stenosis) are at risk of stroke at the rate of 13%/year for 2 years after onset of symptoms. Patients who present with hemispheric TIA, recent TIA, increasing frequency of TIA, or high-grade stenosis have stroke rates that are higher than those in patients with transient monocular blindness, a remote event, a single event, or less stenosis.

The risk of stroke is lower among patients presenting with amaurosis fugax than the risk in patients with hemispheric TIA. In one study, the risk of stroke in patients presenting with amaurosis fugax was one-half that of patients presenting with hemispheric TIA in the setting of 70% or more ipsilateral carotid stenosis. The risk in both groups increased with increasing degrees of stenosis. Patients seen early after the onset of symptoms, particularly patients with multiple TIAs, are at increased risk of stroke. In another study, patients with five or more TIAs within 14 days before medical attention had a higher risk of subsequent stroke than did those with less than four spells. Increasing frequency or severity of ischemic cerebrovascular events also likely indicates a high risk of stroke, although definitive data are unavailable. Patients who have had an ischemic stroke continue to be at risk for subsequent strokes at the rate of 5% to 9%/year; approximately 25% to 45% of patients have another stroke within 5 years of the original event.

Plaque characteristics may have an important effect on subsequent ischemic events. Echolucent and heterogeneous plaques are present in about 70% of symptomatic patients (compared with 20%–30% of asymptomatic patients). These types of plaques generally have a high content of lipid or intraplaque hemorrhage, which may lead to plaque ulceration and a greater embolic potential. Patients with echolucent or heterogeneous plaques appear to have a neurologic event rate 2 to 4 times that of patients with echogenic plaques. Patients presenting with TIA or minor stroke with high-grade carotid artery stenosis in the absence of arteriographic evidence of ulceration have a 2-year stroke rate of 17%, in contrast to a 2-year stroke rate of 30% when ulceration is present with similar degrees of stenosis.

In symptomatic patients with carotid stenosis, the combined morbidity and mortality with carotid endarterectomy is 2% to 6% in centers experienced and expert in performing the procedure. Patients presenting with TIA are at somewhat lower operative risk than patients with stroke. After endarterectomy, the risk of ipsilateral hemispheric stroke is 1% to 2%/year in patients presenting with TIA and 2% to 3%/year for those with previous stroke.

Vertebrobasilar System Occlusive Disease

Although atherosclerotic occlusive disease of the vertebral arteries is less common than it is in the carotid system, the development of disease in both is associated with the same or similar risk factors. About 90% of stenoses in the vertebral system involve the origins of the vertebral arteries. Natural history data are sparse regarding patients with asymptomatic vertebral stenosis. In the small studies available, the risk of brain stem stroke is less than 1% to 2%/year, but it is higher if associated with basilar stenosis. The risk of any stroke or myocardial infarction is much higher than that in the general population because of co-occurring anterior circulation atheromatous occlusive disease and coronary artery disease. Hemodynamic compromise of distal flow in the basilar artery also does not occur in unilateral proximal vertebral artery stenosis.

Cervical portions of the vertebral arteries are uncommonly affected by atherosclerosis. The frequency of cerebral infarction in this subgroup is unknown, although it is likely higher than that in patients with lesions at the origin. The basilar artery is typically affected by atherosclerosis in the proximal portion. Natural history data are also somewhat lacking for this entity. Symptomatic basilar artery stenosis or occlusion is associated with a high rate of recurrent stroke (approximately 10%–20%) within 1 year. The risk in asymptomatic patients is uncertain.

Overall, both referral-based and population-based studies indicate that stroke rates after TIA or minor stroke do not differ substantially according to whether the initial symptoms were localized to the anterior or posterior circulation.

32

Transient Ischemic Attack

About one-third of patients with transient ischemic attack (TIA) (including all underlying mechanisms) have a stroke within 5 years of the first attack. More than 20% of these strokes occur within 1 month of the initial attack, and about 50% occur within 1 year, irrespective of the territory involved (carotid or vertebrobasilar system). The causes of death after carotid or vertebrobasilar TIA are similar (approximately 45% cardiac and 30% hemorrhagic or ischemic stroke). Survival is nearly 90% at 1 year after the first TIA and approximately 70% at 5 years, 50% at 8 years, and 40% at 10 years. After a TIA, women who are older than 70 years have a worse survival rate than do men who are older than age 70, but women younger than 70 years have a better survival rate than that of their male counterparts.

The probability of stroke after TIA strongly correlates with the patient's age at onset (the relative risk of subsequent stroke is 1.45 for each 10 years of increasing age) and a high frequency of TIAs in a short time after the initial event (≥ five TIAs within 2 weeks is associated with a subsequent ischemic stroke rate of approximately 20% in the first 3 months and 30% in the first 6 months). Amaurosis fugax alone is associated with a better prognosis than that of hemispheric TIAs, especially in the setting of severe ipsilateral carotid artery stenosis. In patients with more than 70% extracranial carotid stenosis, the risk of stroke within 2 years after diagnosis is 12% in persons presenting with retinal ischemia and 28% in those with hemispheric ischemic events. Sex does not predict the risk for stroke in individual cases, but women generally have a more benign prognosis after TIA than do men. The natural history and prognosis of TIA specifically associated with carotid stenosis are discussed in Chapter 31.

33

Reversible Ischemic Neurologic Deficit

A neurologic deficit caused by focal cerebral ischemia that persists for more than 24 hours but clears in less than 3 weeks is a cerebral infarction subtype called a reversible ischemic neurologic deficit (RIND). Survival rates in patients with RIND are similar to those of patients with transient ischemic attack (TIA) and better than those of patients with major cerebral infarction (ischemic stroke). The most common cause of death is coronary artery disease, followed by cerebral infarction, cancer, and respiratory disease.

Approximately 25% of patients with RIND have an ischemic stroke or another RIND within 5 years of the initial event. Patients with RIND whose symptoms resolve within 7 days have a probability of subsequent ischemic stroke or RIND analogous to that of patients with TIA, which is higher than that of patients with RIND whose symptoms resolve in 8 to 21 days. This difference is especially apparent in the first year after the initial RIND. In patients with a carotid-distribution RIND and subsequent cerebral infarction, less than 50% of subsequent RINDs occur in the same distribution as the first RIND, but more than 75% of patients with vertebrobasilar RIND who have subsequent events have involvement in the same distribution.

The natural history and prognosis of patients with RIND specifically associated with carotid stenosis appear to be very similar to those of patients with TIA associated with carotid stenosis. This finding is based on data from the North American Symptomatic Carotid Endarterectomy Study, which provided some subanalyses regarding patients with minor cerebral infarction (including patients with RIND) compared with patients with TIA. Surgical morbidity and mortality were comparable in the patients with minor cerebral infarction who had carotid endarterectomy and the patients presenting with TIA.

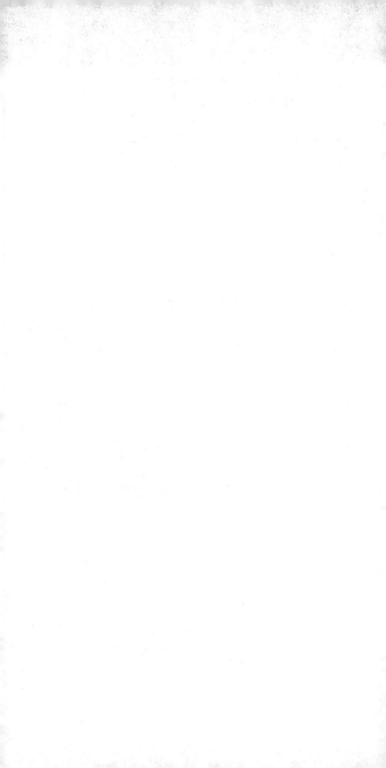

34

Cerebral Infarction

After a person has had cerebral infarction, the 30-day **case fatality rate** is about 20%. **Survival** after the first cerebral infarction is about 65% at 1 year, approximately 50% at 5 years, 30% at 8 years, and about 25% at 10 years. The most common **causes of death** after cerebral infarction are transtentorial herniation, pneumonia, cardiac disorders, pulmonary embolus, and septicemia. Patients presenting with altered sensorium and hemiplegia frequently die of herniation. Death from herniation occurs more commonly on day 1 or 2 after the onset of infarct than on any other days and considerably less frequently after day 7. Overall, nearly 40% of deaths from any cause occur within 48 hours. Other causes of death within the first month include pneumonia, cardiac disease, pulmonary embolus, and septicemia.

Significant independent **predictors of death** within 5 years after cerebral infarction are age (increased age is associated with a decreased survival rate), previous myocardial infarction, atrial fibrillation present at the time of stroke, and congestive heart failure anytime before stroke. In patients with multi-infarct dementia, the mortality rate is about 50% during the 5 years after presentation, and nocturnal confusional state is a sign of a poor prognosis.

Recurrent cerebral infarction occurs in about 30% of patients within 5 years, although symptoms of coronary artery disease or peripheral vascular disease also may ensue. **Myocardial infarction** occurs in patients presenting with cerebral infarction at a rate of about 5%/year. Significant independent predictors of recurrent stroke after cerebral infarction are cardiac valve disease (including replacement) and congestive heart failure. The probability of recurrent stroke among patients with a probable cardiac source of emboli is 2% at 1 month, 5% at 1 year, and 32% at 5 years. These data do not significantly differ from those for patients without a probable cardiac source of embolus (26% at 5 years) or from those with lacunar infarcts (27% at 5 years).

In general, about 60% to 70% of patients have early functional disability after a stroke. This rate usually improves to about 40% in 6 months and 30% in 1 year. Although some late improvement may occur for up to 2 years after the event, most improvement occurs within 6 months. Severe neurologic deficits with no return of motor function within 1 month, marked cognitive-perceptual dysfunction, apraxia, or impairment in construction ability (especially with lesions in the dominant hemisphere or the frontal lobes), and urinary incontinence 2 weeks after a stroke are indicators of a poor functional prognosis and identify patients who are likely to need long-term care.

In addition to these prognostic indicators, previous stroke, symptomatic systemic diseases (such as cardiac or pulmonary insufficiency or frequent angina pectoris), severe mental abnormalities, lack of spouse or family members, and a duration of more than 30 days from onset of stroke to rehabilitation are other factors that may deter recovery. In general, patients with lacunar infarction have a better recovery rate than that of patients with nonlacunar ischemic stroke.

In the first days after a stroke, the patient's paralyzed muscles are usually flaccid, and the deep tendon reflexes are depressed. However, spasticity gradually develops, and deep tendon reflexes increase. Early development of spasticity in the arm generally is considered a favorable sign for a better outcome. Motor recovery tends to occur in the first 2 to 3 months, and leg improvement is usually better than arm improvement. In patients with hemiparesis, only about 20% have persistent severe hemiparesis at 6 months after the event, and at 1 year 50% have perceptible weakness. Arm function improves partially or completely in 40% of patients presenting with severe weakness. Complete arm paralysis at onset and minimal improvement at 4 weeks are predictive of poor outcome.

Hemineglect or sensory deficits causing impaired proprioception usually improve. Aphasia may continue to improve for a year or more after onset of symptoms, and global aphasia may improve more in the second 6 months than in the first 6 months. Aphasia in left-handed patients, regardless of the hemisphere involved, tends to be milder and resolves more rapidly than that in right-handed patients with a left hemisphere lesion.

Intracerebral Hemorrhage

For persons with intracerebral hemorrhage, the reported 30-day survival rate ranges from 40% to 70%; immediate functional prognosis with intracerebral hemorrhage is usually better than that with cerebral infarction because of differences in the amount of brain tissue damaged. The prognosis for persons with **lobar hematomas** is usually better than that for persons with other forms of intracerebral hemorrhages. The overall mortality rate is about 15% to 30%; approximately 50% of survivors have full functional recovery. Predictors of poor outcome after lobar hemorrhage include hemorrhage of more than 40 ml, intraventricular extension of the hemorrhage, and degree of midline shift. The outcome of **caudate hemorrhage** is usually benign, and patients typically have full recovery without permanent neurologic deficit. Even with intraventricular extension, which is common, the prognosis is still relatively good.

For persons with **putaminal hemorrhage,** the mortality rate is about 40%, although the range of clinical presentations is marked and typically depends on the volume of hemorrhage. Progressive neurologic deficit with hemiplegia and coma at admission correlate with poor functional outcome among survivors, whereas a normal level of consciousness, normal extraocular movements, and partial hemiparesis portend a better functional level among survivors. Radiologic imaging characteristics predictive of a poor prognosis include large hemorrhage size and intraventricular extension.

The outlook for functional status for patients with **thalamic hemorrhage** is usually poor, directly depending on the size of the lesion; hemorrhages more than 3 cm in diameter are almost always fatal. Intraventricular extension is common in thalamic hemorrhage but is not necessarily associated with a poor prognosis unless hydrocephalus occurs. Level of consciousness at presentation is also a good predictor of survival.

In **brain stem hemorrhage,** death usually occurs within a few hours, but, occasionally, patients with a small hemorrhagic lesion may survive, with functional level dependent on the site and size of hemorrhage and on the severity of symptoms at onset.

The clinical course in **cerebellar hemorrhage** is unpredictable; as the hours pass, some patients who are alert or drowsy on admission can suddenly become stuporous and then comatose as a result of progressive brain stem compression, whereas others with a similar clinical status at admission have complete functional recovery (vermis hemorrhage is associated with relatively poor survival rates). Patients who have progression have a much better prognosis with surgery if they are still arousable when taken to the operating room than do patients in coma. Computed tomography findings showing hydrocephalus, intraventricular hemorrhage, and hemorrhage of 3 cm or more are also associated with a poor prognosis. Overall, survivors of cerebellar hemorrhage typically have a good functional prognosis.

Primary intraventricular hemorrhage often has a benign clinical course with full recovery, but significant hemorrhage may cause death from progressive hydrocephalus.

Recurrent cerebral hemorrhage is uncommon, in part because of the high 30-day mortality rate. Nevertheless, recurrent hemorrhage represents about 4% of all cases of intracerebral hemorrhage.

Overall, **unfavorable prognostic signs** of intracerebral hemorrhage are (1) decreased level of consciousness after the ictus (especially comatose state), (2) large hematoma (≥60 ml), (3) midline shift on computed tomography or magnetic resonance imaging, (4) intraventricular blood volume of 20 ml or more, (5) advanced age (especially patients >70 years), (6) limb plegia, and (7) early hyperglycemia.

Much of the natural history data refers to all cases of intracerebral hemorrhage or to cases unassociated with underlying vascular malformation or intracranial aneurysm, the majority of which are caused by hypertensive vascular disease. However, the natural history risk differs if a specific cause is detected. About 10% to 25% of patients with intracerebral hemorrhage from an **arteriovenous malformation** die within 30 days, and 25% of survivors have persistent, long-term morbidity. The risk of recurrent hemorrhage during the first year after the initial bleed is 6% to 16%, during the second year it is 2% to 6%, and then it returns to a long-term, persistent risk of 2% to 3%/year. Clinical and radiologic predictors of an increased risk of hemorrhage are not known with certainty. Some have reported an increased risk of hemorrhage with small lesions, whereas others have noted the character of the venous drainage system (such as a single draining vein, deep drainage, or impairment in venous outflow) to be important predictors. Patients with co-occurring **arteriovenous malformations and aneurysms** have a higher risk of intracranial hemorrhage, about 7%/year.

Dural arteriovenous malformations may also cause intracranial hemorrhage, although the risk is not known with certainty. Some hemorrhages can be fatal, although the mortality rate is probably lower than that associated with intraparenchymal arteriovenous malformation.

Cavernous malformations have a lower risk of clinically significant hemorrhage, about 0.1% to 0.25%/person-year. Complete recovery occurs in most cases, although the natural history data are incomplete. Fatal hemorrhage is extremely rare. The risk of recurrent, clinically apparent hemorrhage is also uncertain, and location and size of cavernous malformations have not been found to be predictors of hemorrhage. Patients presenting with hemorrhage are more likely to have another hemorrhage than are patients presenting with seizure. Women may be at increased risk of hemorrhage.

The risk of hemorrhage from a **venous malformation** is also uncertain, although this lesion is generally thought to be much more benign than an arteriovenous malformation. Some investigators have reported that if a hemorrhage occurs with radiologic demonstration of a venous malformation, there will likely be a different vascular malformation subtype detected underlying the hemorrhage. Others believe that venous malformations, particularly those in the cerebellum, may cause intracranial hemorrhage, although the risk is unknown.

Intracranial aneurysms may also cause intracerebral hemorrhage with relatively little subarachnoid hemorrhage. The overall prognosis is similar to that of aneurysmal subarachnoid hemorrhage (see Chapter 36) but may be somewhat better if there is minimal subarachnoid blood.

36

Subarachnoid Hemorrhage

The 30-day case-fatality rate in patients with subarachnoid hemorrhage is about 40%. If the patient is seen at 24 hours after subarachnoid hemorrhage, the mortality rate at 30 days is decreased to approximately 35%, at 48 hours to about 30%, at 1 week to about 25%, and at 2 weeks to 10%. Approximately 10% of patients die before they receive medical attention. Mortality after 30 days declines substantially, leveling off between 30 and 60 days. Significant predictors of outcome are the patient's level of consciousness and clinical grade at admission. The probability of survival is better for patients with no neurologic deficit other than cranial nerve palsy (Hunt and Hess clinical grade 1 or 2) and worse for patients presenting with coma, decerebrate rigidity, and moribund appearance (Hunt and Hess clinical grade 3, 4, or 5). The 30-day probability of survival is less than 20% for persons with clinical grades 4 and 5 and approximately 70% with grades 1 and 2. In addition, intracerebral hematoma or a history of hypertension increases the probability of death in patients with subarachnoid hemorrhage.

One of the major causes of mortality after initial subarachnoid hemorrhage is rebleeding. The rebleeding rate is approximately 2%/day during the first 10 days (total, approximately 20%). The occurrence of rebleeding is a little less than 30% at 30 days and about 1.5%/year after 30 days. In patients with clinical grade 1, 2, or 3, the probability of having isolated cranial nerve palsies or an altered level of consciousness in the first 30 days after subarachnoid hemorrhage is nearly 50%.

Patients with subarachnoid hemorrhage of unknown origin in whom cerebral arteriography and other laboratory studies do not show an aneurysm or other cause of the hemorrhage (such as vascular malformation or tumor) have a relatively good prognosis, with a rate of recurrent hemorrhage of about 2% to 10% within a follow-up period as long as 15 years.

In general, subarachnoid hemorrhage caused by an arteriovenous malformation is associated with a much lower 30-day case-fatality rate (10%–20%) than that caused by saccular aneurysm. Vasospasm and delayed ischemic neurologic deficit are also uncommon and contribute to a lower occurrence of long-term morbidity and mortality in the arteriovenous malformation subgroup.

Patients with subarachnoid hemorrhage localized to the perimesencephalic region without extension into the sylvian fissures or interhemispheric fissure have a very benign prognosis if their cerebral arteriograms are normal. The risk of rebleed is extremely low, although some patients may have early deterioration after presentation because of hydrocephalus. Delayed cerebral ischemia is also extremely uncommon.

Suggested Reading for Part VI

Bamford J, Sandercock P, Jones L, et al: The natural history of lacunar infarction: The Oxfordshire Community Stroke Project. Stroke 18: 545–551, 1987.

Bounds JV, Wiebers DO, Whisnant JP, et al: Mechanisms and timing of deaths from cerebral infarction. Stroke 12:474–477, 1981.

Broderick JP, Phillips SJ, O'Fallon WM, et al: Relationship of cardiac disease to stroke occurrence, recurrence, and mortality. Stroke 23:1250–1256, 1992.

Chambers BR, Norris JW: Outcome in patients with asymptomatic neck bruits. N Engl J Med 315:860–865, 1986.

European Carotid Surgery Trialists' Collaborative Group: MRC European Carotid Surgery Trial: Interim results for symptomatic patients with severe (70–99%) or with mild (0–29%) carotid stenosis. Lancet 337:1235–1243, 1991.

Evans BA, Wiebers DO, Barrett HJM: Natural history of patients with TIA and minor ischemic stroke. In: Moore WS, ed. Vascular Surgery (5th ed). Philadelphia: WB Saunders, 1995.

Executive Committee for the Asymptomatic Carotid Atherosclerosis Study: Endarterectomy for asymptomatic carotid artery stenosis. JAMA 273:1421–1428, 1995.

Ingall TJ, Whisnant JP, Wiebers DO, et al: Has there been a decline in subarachnoid hemorrhage mortality? Stroke 20:718–724, 1989.

Kappelle LJ, Adams HP Jr, Heffner ML, et al: Prognosis of young adults with ischemic stroke. A long-term follow-up study assessing recurrent vascular events and functional outcome in the Iowa Registry of Stroke in Young Adults. Stroke 25:1360–1365, 1994.

Meissner I, Wiebers DO, Whisnant JP, et al: The natural history of asymptomatic carotid artery occlusive lesions. JAMA 258:2704–2707, 1987.

North American Symptomatic Carotid Endarterectomy Trial Collaborators: Beneficial effect of carotid endarterectomy in symptomatic patients with high-grade carotid stenosis. N Engl J Med 325:445–453, 1991.

Whisnant JP, ed: Stroke: Populations, Cohorts, and Clinical Trials. Oxford: Butterworth-Heinemann, 1993.

Wiebers DO, Whisnant JP, O'Fallon WM: Reversible ischemic neurologic deficit (RIND) in a community: Rochester, Minnesota, 1955–1974. Neurology 32:459–465, 1982.

VII

Management and Rehabilitation After Stroke

Physical Therapy

Available data support the usefulness of a coordinated rehabilitation program for treating functional impairment resulting from a stroke. The rehabilitation program should provide an environment of high motivation to help achieve the patient's maximal physical and psychological functional capacity and should be tailored to meet the needs of each patient and family. To plan and implement this program most effectively, a coordinated, interdisciplinary team approach is required. Besides a physician knowledgeable in stroke rehabilitation, the composition of the team varies but often includes rehabilitation nurses, physical therapists, occupational therapists, speech therapists, psychologists, and social workers.

Rehabilitation should be started with early, systematic, and realistic increases in the patient's activities and should be advanced in stages in a local hospital, in an outpatient clinic, at home, or in a specialized rehabilitation unit. The program must include rehabilitation that is specific to the deficit. For productive rehabilitation, the patient must willingly participate and have the cognitive ability to follow at least one-step commands and the memory to remember the lessons learned in therapy. For patients who have cerebrovascular disease and who have significant cardiac dysfunction (such as angina, arrhythmia, or myocardial infarction), the rehabilitation program should be combined with a cardiac rehabilitation program.

The **frequency of rehabilitation treatment** sessions varies with the setting and timing after a stroke and with the patient's response to therapy. Generally, therapy is provided twice daily in an inpatient setting, three times/week in an outpatient setting, and daily, when requested by a physician, in a nursing home setting. On the basis of the Mayo Clinic experience, about 50% of patients who survive ischemic stroke for 1 week are good candidates to benefit from physical therapy (the median number of sessions is 16); 40% benefit from occupational therapy (the median number of sessions is 8); and 13% benefit from speech therapy. Approximately 15% of patients eventually are transferred to a rehabilitation unit, in which the median duration of stay is about 32 days. About half the patients who survive for 6 months after stroke are partially or totally dependent in activities of daily living such as bathing, dressing, feeding, and mobility (including 10% of survivors who need long-term nursing care). About one-third of patients surviving stroke for 1 year are unable to remain independent, and this proportion remains relatively unchanged in survivors followed as long as 5 years.

Although the **duration of rehabilitation** therapy is generally determined by the patient's rate of functional recovery, the probability of improvement of movement in paralyzed limbs is maximal during the first month after stroke and decreases significantly after 6 months, whereas considerable improvement of speech, domestic and working skills, and steadiness can continue as long as 2 years. Recovery of arm movement is usually less complete than that of leg movement, and complete lack of any movement at onset of stroke or no measurable grip strength by 4 weeks is associated with a poor prognosis for return of useful arm function. However, functional recovery

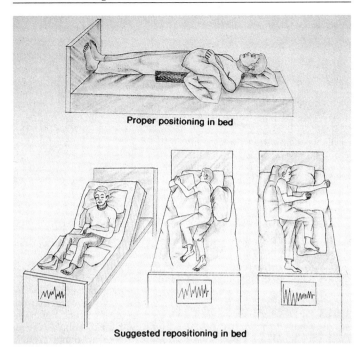

Proper positioning in bed

Suggested repositioning in bed

Fig. 37-1. *Top:* **Positioning in bed for a patient who has had a stroke.**
Bottom: **Suggested repositioning in bed.**

(lessening of disability or handicap), depending on both intrinsic neuronal recovery and adaptive recovery (the use of alternative strategies or adaptive equipment to perform an activity), often continues long after specific neurologic deficits have ceased to change. No established guidelines yet exist to help select patients for specific rehabilitation interventions.

Proper **positioning** in bed and repositioning (patients with hemiplegia should be turned every 1–2 hours, and side rails should be provided to prevent the patient from falling out of bed) help prevent contractures and decubitus ulcers and should begin as soon as the patient has been admitted and the diagnosis made (Fig. 37-1). For alert patients, a trapeze should be put over the bed to enable them to change their own position.

Physiotherapy in the form of passive exercises should begin as soon as the deficit is stable (a full, passive range of motion of paretic and nonparetic limbs should be performed for approximately 15 minutes at least three times a day, with special attention to the shoulders, elbows, hips, and ankles), and active exercises and ambulation should be attempted as soon as the patient can tolerate them. These measures are important not only for maintaining and increasing limb function and mobility but also for preventing deep vein thromboses, especially in patients who are not receiving an anticoagulant (or antiplatelet) agent.

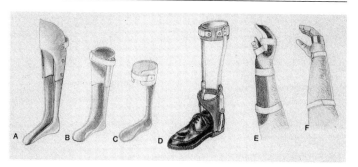

Fig. 37-2. Types of orthoses (A–D). Plastic positioning splint (E). Dorsal wrist cock-up positioning splint (F).

Patients who are alert and have a stable cardiovascular system should **sit up** in bed as soon as the neurologic deficit is stable (usually within the first or second day after onset of symptoms), except for conservatively treated patients with aneurysmal subarachnoid hemorrhage, in whom bed rest until definitive treatment or for at least 2 to 3 weeks is usually recommended. Patients who tolerate sitting up in bed may sit in a chair and then should be aided or instructed in a stepwise fashion about how to **stand,** transfer to and from a wheelchair, **walk** (or push a wheelchair), and **perform other regular activities** of daily living, including eating, brushing teeth, washing, shaving, dressing, and undressing, as their neurologic status permits (sudden or intense activity should be avoided). During the early part of the exercise program, patients should be monitored closely, and special attention should be given to changes in blood pressure and heart function. For hemiplegic patients, the occupational therapist should cooperate closely with the physiotherapist, nursing staff, speech therapist, and the patient's spouse or family to provide retraining in basic self-care activities (such as feeding, dressing, and washing). The occupational therapist can individualize various types of upper extremity splints that can assist patients to increase their functional capabilities.

For prevention of **ulnar nerve compression palsy** and **shoulder-hand syndrome** (decreased mobility of the affected shoulder joint and edema over the hand and fingers with local tenderness over the shoulder and hand), the patient's weak arm should not be left to hang without support. (The treatment of shoulder-hand syndrome is discussed in Chapter 39). For patients with equinovarus deformity of the foot or flexion contracture of the paretic wrist and fingers, a foot-ankle plastic orthosis (a short or long leg brace) or a wrist-finger extension splint is commonly used (Fig. 37-2).

Selective gymnastic therapy in conjunction with point massage and autogenous training, heat therapy, cryotherapy, and acupuncture also may be instituted to **reduce spasticity**. Coordination exercises and frequent practice of standing and walking between parallel bars are required for patients with **poor coordination** (ataxia without paralysis) and **dysequilibrium.** If cognitive function is preserved in a patient with hemiparesis, instructions in the use of various special devices (such as handrails along walls, quad canes, bedside table, specially designed card holders, typewriters, telephones, and other specific activity aids) can assist the patient in becoming more independent in the activities of daily living.

Speech Therapy

A speech pathologist normally evaluates patients with deficits in swallowing, communicating, or thinking who are alert enough to participate. Intensive speech therapy is commonly indicated for motivated patients with dysphasia. The therapy to establish an effective means of communication is begun when the patient with dysphasia or dysarthria is awake, alert, and stable (the involvement of a speech therapist is generally very helpful). Communication techniques, alternatives, and therapies can be provided to the patient to enhance communication skills and to avoid the frustration that occurs when patients cannot adequately communicate their needs. The therapist may use verbal or nonverbal techniques, and communication may be facilitated by using a word board or by combining written and spoken language.

To be effective, auditory stimulation must be combined with visual stimulation, which should be sufficiently intense, clear, repetitive, and slow to assist the learning process according to the patient's functional status. Stimuli should be further tailored to be consistent with and use the patient's background, education, work history, and hobbies. The patient should hear speech frequently from conversation, radio, or television and be encouraged to respond (with adequate intervals of rest). Motivation by encouragement and other positive reinforcement is important. Drawing, copying, tracing letters and geometric designs, and various occupational therapies also are helpful.

Other Chronic Complications of Stroke

Common secondary impairments in patients who survive cerebral infarction or intracerebral hemorrhage are pain and edema in the hemiplegic arm, also known as **shoulder-hand syndrome** (5%–10% of patients) or, less commonly, pain and edema in the leg. Edema in the paralyzed limb(s) may be relieved by elevation, pneumatic compression, or compression gloves. Treatment of painful joints in paralyzed limbs includes maintenance of appropriate passive range of motion within a pain-free arc(s) and proper positioning (cold or superficial heat should precede passive stretching). A paralyzed shoulder should be positioned in external rotation (forearm with supination and finger extension with abduction) and the hip in internal rotation and flexion with the knee and ankle in flexion.

Treatment with corticosteroids or nonsteroidal analgesics and a low-dose antidepressant (such as amitriptyline, 50–75 mg, in divided doses or at bedtime, especially for chronic pain associated with depression) or anticonvulsant agents (such as phenytoin, 100 mg daily; carbamazepine, 400 mg daily; or clonazepam, 0.5 mg daily) may also be considered. Local anesthetic agents (0.5% lidocaine hydrochloride given percutaneously, to 60 ml, or regional intravenous routes, 10–50 ml), stellate ganglion blocks (as many as 7–10 treatments if the patient responds within 3–4 blocks), heat treatment of poststroke arthropathy, transcutaneous nerve stimulation, and acupuncture also may be effective, especially for localized pain.

In patients who have **swallowing problems** that place them at risk for aspiration pneumonia and choking, short-term (to 4–6 weeks) use of nasogastric tube feedings until function returns or long-term use of a percutaneous feeding tube should be considered. Percutaneous placement of a feeding tube into the stomach or small bowel is particularly advisable for patients who have persistent, profound impairment of swallowing associated with bilateral hemispheric strokes or brain stem strokes.

Diplopia usually improves over time, and subtle deficits can be managed with prism glasses. For persistent diplopia that has been stable for more than 6 months, surgical correction may be considered.

Seizures can complicate cerebrovascular disorders beginning during the acute phase or many months after the event. Chronic convulsions are more often associated with lobar hemorrhagic stroke, cortical ischemic stroke, and subarachnoid hemorrhage. Treatment of seizure disorders in patients who survive stroke is similar to that for patients with epilepsy resulting from other causes. Carbamazepine, 600 to 1600 mg/day in divided doses, or phenytoin, 100 mg three times daily, is usually recommended initially. If neither of these agents is effective, treatment with phenobarbital or valproic acid should be considered.

Spasticity and contractures may be controlled by standard physiotherapy techniques of repetitive muscle stretching through range-of-motion exercises, positioning, and handling (with splints). Either heat or ice massage may lead to a short-term reduction in spasticity. Although no medication has been uniformly useful in the treatment of spasticity, if physiotherapeutic measures are ineffective and the spasticity is marked, medical therapy that may be considered includes baclofen (starting with 5 mg twice daily and increasing, as tolerated, to 80 mg daily in 2–4 divided doses), diazepam (starting with 2–5 mg twice a day and increasing gradually, as tolerated), dantrolene sodium (starting with 25 mg and increasing, as tolerated, to 400 mg/day), and tizanidine in doses to 36 mg/day (not yet available in the United States). However, all these drugs have potential side effects, including weakness or apparent weakness, which often develops as spasticity is lessened because the stiffness associated with spasticity may help support weak extremities, particularly the legs. Other possible side effects include drowsiness, gastric distress, and nausea with baclofen, sedation and cognitive clouding with diazepam, and nausea, drowsiness, and hepatotoxicity with dantrolene. Tizanidine may also produce systemic hypotension. If all these measures fail, other potential therapeutic approaches include intrathecal administration of baclofen or morphine, peripheral nerve or spinal cord electrical stimulation (dorsal column stimulation), botulinum toxin injections, and various surgical procedures (such as cutting, lengthening, or transplanting tendons).

Patients with **urinary incontinence** should be evaluated for urinary tract infection. If no infection is present, or if treatment does not resolve the incontinence, postvoid residual urine volumes should be measured. Anticholinergic agents may be administered in patients with sterile urine and postvoid residual urine volumes less than 100 ml. If the urine is sterile and postvoid volumes are more than 100 ml, intermittent catheterization followed by a complete urologic evaluation is usually indicated. Urinary tract infections should be treated appropriately.

Cognitive deficits and depression are frequent complications of stroke and affect approximately 64% and 70% of all survivors, respectively. Cognitive deficits caused by stroke lead to 15% to 20% of dementias in the elderly, and severe depression occurs in approximately 33% of all patients after stroke (the risk of depression is particularly high in patients with damage in the dominant frontal hemisphere). Sexual dysfunction after stroke may result from depression, medication, paralysis, or fear. Reactive depression can often be helped substantially by encouraging verbalization of the patient's fears and anger. It is important for recovering persons and their families to realize that most behavioral problems that develop as a direct result of stroke (such as inappropriate laughing, crying, or irritation with little provocation) usually do not last very long and often do not express the person's true feelings.

Psychotherapeutic agents and formal psychotherapy may be necessary for some patients (such as patients with considerable apathy, depression, indifference, or opposition to treatment). Agents used include nortriptyline hydrochloride (initially 25 mg once a day, as tolerated, and increased, as needed, gradually to 100 mg/day in divided doses) or trazodone hydrochloride (initially 50 mg two to three times daily, as tolerated, and increased, as needed, by 50 mg/day every 3–4 days to 200–400 mg/day in divided doses) for depression; levodopa (0.5–1 g daily in divided doses with food) or amantadine hydrochloride (100 mg/day) for behavioral problems such as inappropriate laughing or crying; and low doses of haloperidol (0.5 mg once or twice daily) for poststroke delirium.

Family and Patient Education

Psychosocial therapy should be started with the patient's family at the time of the patient's hospitalization and begin with the patient as soon as feasible. Family members should be given realistic, straightforward information and instructions to provide support for the patient and to develop a partnership for solutions to problems as early as possible. The family member closest to the patient should observe health personnel assisting the patient and practice under the supervision of a nurse or physical therapist. The physician should provide information and dispel myths regarding stroke to help provide the most positive yet realistic psychosocial environment for motivating, energizing, and inspiring the patient to move forward to return to a productive, useful life. Accurate and simply explained facts about the cause of the cerebrovascular event are essential for both the patient and the family, and both should understand that recovery from a stroke is often a slow process.

Family involvement becomes even more important when the patient is cared for at home after dismissal. Family members should provide encouragement, show confidence in improvement, and permit the recovering person to do as much as he or she can and to be as independent and vigorous as possible. It is important that the patient not become overly discouraged by failures. Patients need to be reassured that they are wanted and needed and that they are still important to the family and part of the social picture. They need to understand that many others have recovered from strokes and have been able to return to normal activities or continue to do very useful work. Giving the recovering person certain reasonable tasks (such as encouraging him or her to assume some household duties) is often helpful. It may also be very useful to assist the patient to develop new outside interests within his or her given capacities, particularly if the person is unable to return to gainful employment. Family counseling and education in the form of individual sessions or through regional family support groups are important to help the family overcome the stresses associated with new responsibilities and, sometimes, the depression that may occur in family members.

The physician should also be familiar with local driving guidelines and share this information with the patient and family. Generally, ongoing seizures and significant visual field deficit are considered to be absolute contraindications to driving; marked memory problems, poor concentration, and severe aphasia are relative contraindications to driving.

A treatment program that reduces the likelihood of further morbidity or mortality of patients after acute cerebrovascular events depends on (1) the pathophysiologic mechanism responsible for the event, (2) the degree of functional deficit (the degree of aggressiveness in the use of specific therapies varies inversely with the degree of residual functional deficit), and (3) the potential benefits and risks of the therapeutic method being considered. If specific therapy for the underlying mechanism is available, appropriate measures should be provided, as outlined in Chapters 16 and 17. Correction of associated cerebrovascular risk factors with appropriate monitoring may also help reduce the risk of a subsequent cerebrovascular event (see Chapters 23–30).

RESOURCES FOR PATIENTS

National Stroke Association
1420 Ogden Street
Denver, Colorado 80218
Telephone: (303) 839-1992

American Heart Association
7320 Greenville Avenue
Dallas, Texas 75231
Telephone: (214) 373-6300

Suggested Reading for Part VII

Dombovy ML, Basford JR, Whisnant JP, et al: Disability and use of rehabilitation services following stroke in Rochester, Minnesota, 1975–1979. Stroke 18:830–836, 1987.

Dromerick A, Reding M: Medical and neurological complications during inpatient stroke rehabilitation. Stroke 25:358–361, 1994.

Ernst E: A review of stroke rehabilitation and physiotherapy. Stroke 21:1081–1085, 1990.

Evans RL, Hendricks RD, Haselkorn JK, et al: The family's role in stroke rehabilitation: A review of the literature. Am J Phys Med Rehabil 71:135–139, 1992.

Feder M, Ring H, Rozenthul N, et al: Assessment chart for inpatient rehabilitation following stroke. Int J Rehabil Res 14:223–229, 1991.

Gibbons B: Stroke and rehabilitation. Nurs Stand 8:49–54, 1994.

Gladman J, Whynes D, Lincoln N: Cost comparison of domiciliary and hospital-based stroke rehabilitation. DOMINO Study Group. Age Ageing 23:241–245, 1994.

Hamilton BB, Granger CV: Disability outcomes following inpatient rehabilitation for stroke. Phys Ther 74:494–503, 1994.

Intiso D, Santilli V, Grasso MG, et al: Rehabilitation of walking with electromyographic biofeedback in foot-drop after stroke. Stroke 25:1189–1192, 1994.

Kalra L: Does age affect benefits of stroke unit rehabilitation? Stroke 25:346–351, 1994.

Kalra L: The influence of stroke unit rehabilitation on functional recovery from stroke. Stroke 25:821–825, 1994.

Noll SF, Roth EJ: Stroke rehabilitation. 1. Epidemiologic aspects and acute management. Arch Phys Med Rehabil 75:S38–S41, 1994.

Oczkowski WJ, Ginsberg JS, Shin A, et al: Venous thromboembolism in patients undergoing rehabilitation for stroke. Arch Phys Med Rehabil 73:712–716, 1992.

Reding MJ, McDowell F: Stroke rehabilitation. Neurol Clin 5:601–630, 1987.

Reding MJ, McDowell FH: Focused stroke rehabilitation programs improve outcome. Arch Neurol 46:700–701, 1989.

Roth EJ: Heart disease in patients with stroke. Part II: Impact and implications for rehabilitation. Arch Phys Med Rehabil 75:94–101, 1994.

Sandin KJ, Cifu DX, Noll SF: Stroke rehabilitation. 4. Psychologic and social implications. Arch Phys Med Rehabil 75:S52–S55, 1994.

Shah S, Vanclay F, Cooper B: Efficiency, effectiveness, and duration of stroke rehabilitation. Stroke 21:241–246, 1990.

Teasdale TW, Christensen AL, Pinner EM: Psychosocial rehabilitation of cranial trauma and stroke patients. Brain Inj 7:535–542, 1993.

Teraoka J, Burgard R: Family support and stroke rehabilitation. West J Med 157:665–666, 1992.

Wade DT: Stroke: Rehabilitation and long-term care. Lancet 339:791–793, 1992.

Wild D: Stroke focus. Stroke: A nursing rehabilitation role. Nurs Stand 8:36–39, 1994.

Wolfe CD, Taub NA, Woodrow EJ, et al: Assessment of scales of disability and handicap for stroke patients. Stroke 22:1242–1244, 1991.

Appendixes

A

Clinical Anatomy of the Brain and Spinal Cord Vascular System

A-1.   Brain and spinal cord vascular anatomy and syndromes

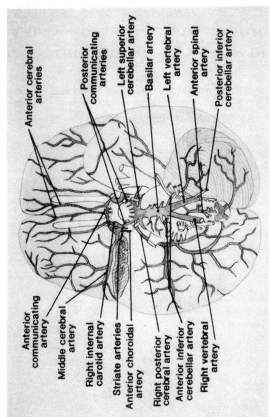

Fig. A-1-1.   Blood supply of the brain.

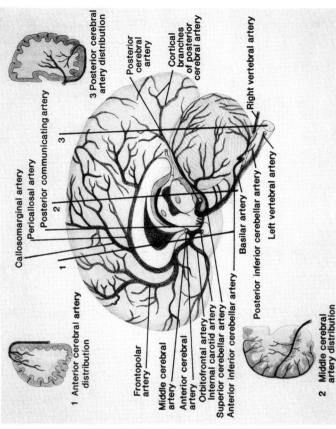

Callosomarginal artery
Pericallosal artery
Posterior communicating artery

3 Posterior cerebral artery distribution

Posterior cerebral artery

Cortical branches of posterior cerebral artery

Right vertebral artery

Basilar artery

Left vertebral artery

Posterior inferior cerebellar artery

1 Anterior cerebral artery distribution

Frontopolar artery

Middle cerebral artery
Anterior cerebral artery
Orbitofrontal artery
Internal carotid artery
Superior cerebellar artery
Anterior inferior cerebellar artery

2 Middle cerebral artery distribution

Fig. A-1-2.   Major cerebral arteries: distribution of blood supply.

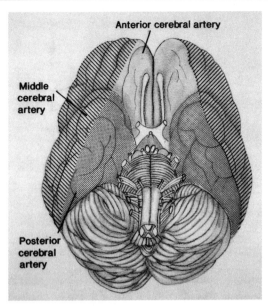

Fig. A-1-3. Major cerebral arteries: distribution of blood supply, view of base of the brain.

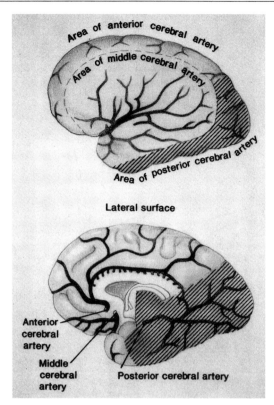

Lateral surface

Fig. A-1-4. Major cerebral arteries: distribution of blood supply, lateral views.

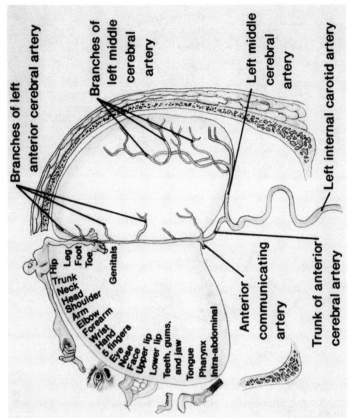

Fig. A-1-5. Anterior and middle cerebral artery distribution to sensory fibers.

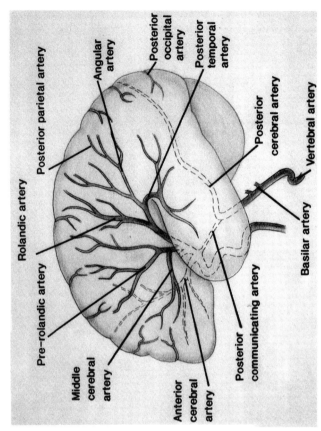

Fig. A-1-6.   Course and distribution of major supratentorial arteries, lateral view.

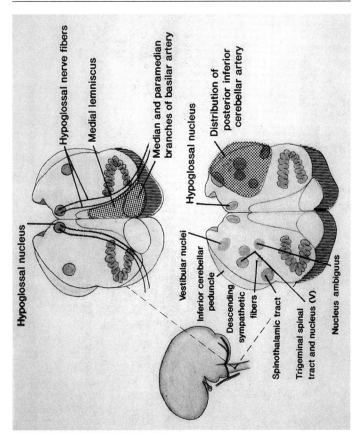

Fig. A-1-7.   Blood supply of medulla.

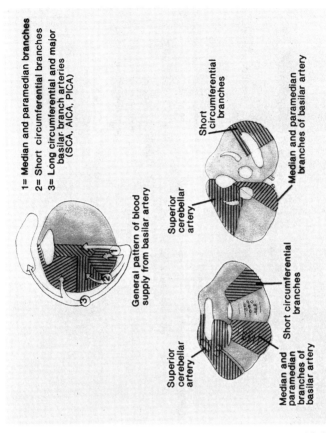

1= Median and paramedian branches
2= Short circumferential branches
3= Long circumferential and major basilar branch arteries (SCA, AICA, PICA)

General pattern of blood supply from basilar artery

Superior cerebellar artery

Median and paramedian branches of basilar artery

Short circumferential branches

Superior cerebellar artery

Short circumferential branches

Median and paramedian branches of basilar artery

Fig. A-1-8. Blood supply of pons and midbrain. AICA = anterior inferior cerebellar artery; PICA = posterior inferior cerebellar artery; SCA = superior cerebellar artery.

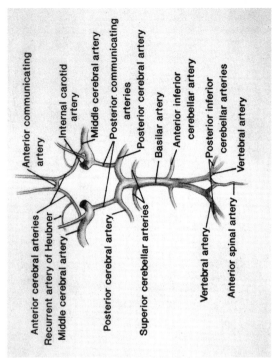

Fig. A-1-9. Circle of Willis.

Anterior communicating artery

Internal carotid artery

Middle cerebral artery

Posterior communicating arteries

Posterior cerebral artery

Basilar artery

Anterior inferior cerebellar artery

Posterior inferior cerebellar arteries

Vertebral artery

Anterior cerebral arteries

Recurrent artery of Heubner

Middle cerebral artery

Posterior cerebral artery

Superior cerebellar arteries

Vertebral artery

Anterior spinal artery

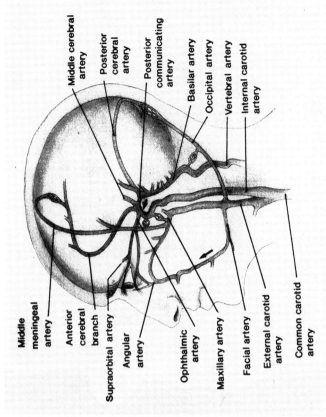

Fig. A-1-10. Collateral supply for intracranial circulation.

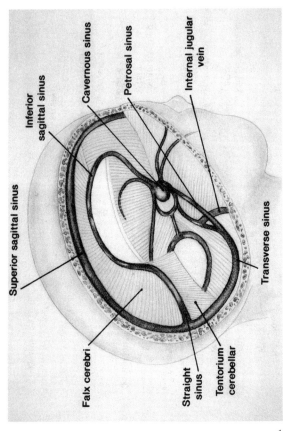

Fig. A-1-11.   Venous drainage system.
A. Dura mater and major venous sinuses.
B. Major venous sinuses and deep venous drainage.

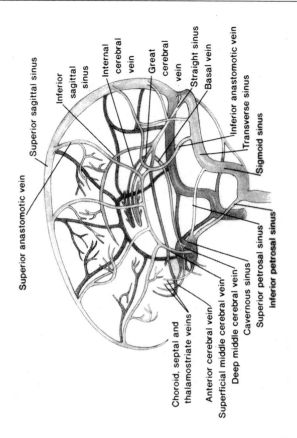

B

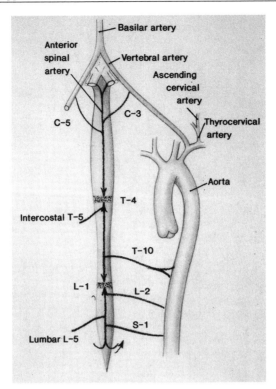

Fig. A-1-12.   Vascular supply to spinal cord.

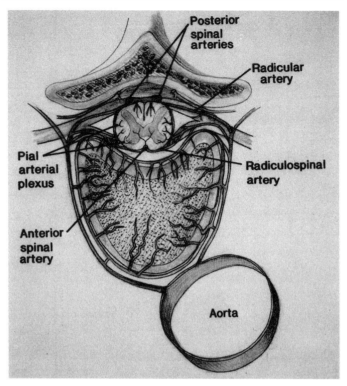

Fig. A-1-13. Vascular supply to spinal cord, axial view.

A-2.   Central nervous system ischemic vascular syndromes

Vessel	Major structure(s) supplied	Major clinical findings (syndromes)
Brachiocephalic trunk	Right side of head, arm	Lower blood pressure in ipsilateral arm, other findings as for ICA syndrome
Common carotid artery	Each side of head	Findings as for ICA syndrome; poorly conducted heart sound along ICA, absence of superficial temporal artery pulse
Internal carotid artery	All structures of frontal, parietal, and temporal lobes, medial surfaces of the two hemispheres	Contralateral hemiparesis, hemianesthesia, hemianopia, aphasia; global aphasia (DH) or denial or hemineglect (NDH)
Ophthalmic artery	Orbit, forehead, dura of anterior fossa	Ipsilateral monocular blindness or amaurosis fugax
Anterior choroidal artery	Optic tract, cerebellum peduncle, two-thirds of posterior limb of internal capsule, optic radiation	Findings as for middle cerebral artery syndrome (below), but language spared, pure motor or sensory stroke, ataxic hemiparesis, various intellectual deficits
Anterior cerebral artery	Medial aspects of cerebrum, superior border of frontal and parietal lobes	Weakness, clumsiness, and sensory loss affecting mainly distal contralateral leg
Small branches	Rostrum of corpus callosum, septum pellucidum, and lamina terminalis	Tactile anomia or ideomotor apraxia of limbs
Huebner's artery	Anterior limb of internal capsule, anterior portion of putamen, globus pallidum	Contralateral weakness of arm and face with or without rigidity or dystonia
Cortical branches	Major portion of mesial aspects of hemisphere, para-central lobule	Contralateral weakness and sensory loss in leg; if bilateral, behavior disturbances
Middle cerebral artery	Most of lateral surface of each hemisphere and deep structures of frontal and parietal lobes	Hemiplegia (face, arm, leg equally affected), hemi-anesthesia, hemianopia, aphasia (DH), hemineglect or dressing apraxia (NDH)
Upper division	Internal capsule (superior portion of anterior-posterior limb), corona radiata, external capsule, putamen, caudate nuclei (body)	Hemiplegia (face/arm more affected than leg), hemi-anesthesia or hemianopia, Broca's aphasia (DH) or spatial disorientation (NDH)

Lower division	Lateral surface of cerebral hemisphere at insula of lateral sulcus	Hemianopia or pure Wernicke's aphasia (DH) or other intellectual deficits (NDH)
Penetrating	Anterior limb of internal capsule, basal ganglia	Pure contralateral hemiplegia or hemiparesis
Cortical branches	Temporal, parietal, or frontal opercular surface of hemisphere	Monoparesis, discriminative and proprioceptive sensory loss, quadrantanopia, Broca's aphasia or Gerstmann's syndrome (DH), other intellectual deficits (NDH)
Vertebral artery	Midbrain, pons, medulla, and cerebellum	Various combinations of signs: ataxia, diplopia, vertigo, bulbar syndrome, facial weakness
Posterior-inferior cerebellar artery	Lateral medulla, cerebellum (posterior-inferior aspect), cranial nerves V, IX, X, vestibular nuclei, solitary nucleus/tract	Wallenberg's syndrome (alternating hemianesthesia, pharyngeal and laryngeal paralysis, dysphagia, hoarseness, decreased gag reflex, gait and ipsilateral limb ataxia), or Dejerine's syndrome
Anterior spinal artery	Caudal medulla (paramedian area), cranial nerve VII, solitary nucleus and tract, spinal cord (dorsolateral quadrants)	Radicular pain, loss of pain or temperature sensation, spastic weakness in legs with (cervical level) or without (below cervical level) focal atrophy and weakness of arms
Posterior spinal artery	Spinal cord (dorsal funiculus), dorsal gray horns	Loss of deep tendon reflexes and joint position sense, asterognosis at level involved
Basilar artery	Pons, midbrain, cerebellum, occipital lobe, part of temporal lobe	Diplopia, coma, bilateral motor and sensory signs, cerebellar and cranial nerve signs
Short paramedian arteries	Medial basal pons (pontine nuclei, corticospinal fibers, medial lemniscus)	Paraparesis, quadriparesis, dysarthria, dysphagia, tongue hemiparesis and atrophy, gaze paralysis, cranial nerve VI palsy, contralateral hemiparesis; Millard-Gubler-Foville, Raymond-Cestan, Marie-Foix syndromes
Internal auditory artery	Auditory and facial cranial nerves	Vertigo, nausea, vomiting, nystagmus
Anterior-inferior cerebellar artery	Lateral aspect of pons and anterior-inferior cerebellum	Ipsilateral facial paralysis, taste loss on half of tongue, deafness or tinnitus, limb ataxia, contralateral sensory loss over body

A-2. *(Continued)*

Vessel	Major structure(s) supplied	Major clinical findings (syndromes)
Superior cerebellar artery	Lateral midbrain, superior surface of cerebellum	Ipsilateral cranial nerve VI and VII palsy, gait and limb ataxia, cerebellar signs, contralateral hemiparesis
Posterior cerebral artery	Entire occipital lobe, inferior and medial portion of temporal lobe	Hemianopia, quadrantanopia (macular vision spared), Gerstmann's syndrome, or cortical blindness
Small perforating arteries	Midbrain, posterior thalamus	Midbrain (Weber's, Benedict's) or thalamic (Dejerine-Roussy) syndromes
Cortical arteries	Occipital lobe (medial surface), uncus, fusiform, temporal lobe (gyrus), occipital pole	Hemianopia or quadrantanopia with sparing of macular vision, alexia or color anomia (DH), cerebral blindness (if bilateral lesions)
Pial spinal arteries	Nerve roots and spinal cord	Anterior or posterior spinal artery syndromes

DH = dominant hemisphere; ICA = internal carotid artery; NDH = nondominant hemisphere.

A-3.   Symptoms of unruptured intracranial aneurysms

Artery affected and most common location	Major structure(s) involved (compressed)	Clinical findings*
Internal carotid artery		
Infraclinoid-intracavernous part	Cranial nerves III, IV, VI and pituitary fossa	Ipsilateral total ophthalmoplegia with small, poorly reactive pupil often associated with cranial nerve IV, V, VI palsy, facial pain or paresthesias or partial sensory loss, hypopituitarism, pulsatile noise in head
Supraclinoid part	Cranial nerves II, III, optic chiasm	Visual field defects associated with ipsilateral cranial nerve II palsy, decreased visual acuity, scotoma, optic atrophy or blindness; partial ophthalmoplegia due to cranial nerve III palsy
Middle cranial fossa, near petrous apex	Trigeminal ganglion, cranial nerves IV, VI	Raeder's paratrigeminal syndrome (unilateral oculosympathetic paresis—miosis and ptosis—associated with ipsilateral head, facial, or retroorbital pain and cranial nerve IV and VI palsy)
Ophthalmic artery	Cranial nerve II, optic foramen, pituitary fossa	Ipsilateral painless loss of vision, optic nerve atrophy, x-ray enlargement of optic foramen, hypopituitarism
Anterior cerebral artery (at junction with anterior communicating artery)	Olfactory tract, optic chiasm, frontal lobes	Ipsilateral anosmia, bitemporal hemianopia (may begin with lower bitemporal quadrants); large aneurysm can produce intellectual deficits
Middle cerebral artery (at level of lateral fissure)	Lateral surface of cerebral hemisphere, surface between frontal and temporal lobes	Ipsilateral pain in or behind eye and in low temple associated with contralateral focal motor seizures, hemiparesis, dysphasia (dominant hemisphere involvement), homonymous hemianopia or upper quadrantanopia

A-3. *(Continued)*

Artery affected and most common location	Major structure(s) involved (compressed)	Clinical findings*
Posterior communicating artery (at junction with internal carotid artery)	Cranial nerves III, VI	Painful palsy of cranial nerve III (pain typically occurs above brow and radiates back to ear) with or without ipsilateral nerve VI palsy (cranial nerve III paresis usually incomplete)
Vertebral artery (on surface of medulla)	Cranial nerves IX, X, XI, XII	Ipsilateral Collet-Sicard, Villaret, Schmidt, Jackson, or Tapia syndromes and occasionally paralysis of cranial nerve VIII
Basilar artery (upper border of pons)	Cranial nerve V	Ipsilateral facial pain with or without tic douloureux
Anterior-inferior cerebellar artery	Cranial nerve VII and brain stem structures	Ipsilateral paralysis of all facial muscles, loss of taste, occasionally signs of hydrocephalus
Superior cerebellar artery (at vertebro-basilar junction)	Cranial nerve III and brain stem structures	Homolateral focal headache, occipital or posterior cervical location, associated with ipsilateral ptosis, divergent strabismus, horizontal-vertical diplopia, pupil dilatation, ataxia
Posterior cerebral artery (proximal portion)	Midbrain structures	Focal ipsilateral headache (occipital or posterior cervical region), pseudobulbar signs, decreased level of consciousness

*Often mimic intracranial tumor at same location with slowly progressive focal neurologic signs. Aneurysms causing symptoms other than rupture are generally 7 mm or more in size.

A-4. Differential signs indicating hemispheric localization of intellectual deficits

Nondominant hemisphere	Dominant hemisphere	Bilateral hemispheric lesions
Prosopagnosia: inability to visually recognize well-known individuals	**Wernicke's aphasia:** difficulty understanding sentences when meaning depends on syntax, poor comprehension of spoken and written word, but fluent speech with, sometimes, jargon and impaired repetition	**Impairment of analytic and remote memory**
Impairment of spatial orientation		**Pseudobulbar palsy:** dysarthria, dysphagia, grasp, palmomental, sucking, snout, or rooting reflexes, increased jaw jerk, emotional lability, bulbar muscles spared
Anosognosia: ignores opposite hemiparetic side; denies weakness	**Broca's aphasia** (motor speech apraxia): good comprehension of spoken and written word, but poor repetition, naming, and writing, nonfluent agrammatic speech	
Constructional apraxia: inability to copy geometric pattern	**Conduction aphasia:** conversation relatively preserved, but cannot repeat words or sentences properly and makes phonemic, semantic, or paraphasic errors	**Akinetic mutism:** absence of any attempt at oral communication
Dressing apraxia: striking difficulty in dressing	**Transcortical sensory aphasia:** repeats words or sentences well but unable to understand meaning of spoken or written words	**Palilalia:** repetition of last word or words of speech
Amusia: inability to identify auditory characteristics of music or identify songs by listening to them	**Transcortical motor aphasia:** nonfluent speech, preserved auditory comprehension, near normal ability to repeat phrases spoken by examiner	**Apraxia of gait:** loss of coordinated walking movements in absence of weakness, cerebellar disease, or sensory loss
Motor impersistence: inability to concentrate on a task, with consequent motor or verbal impersistence (e.g., on instruction, cannot hold breath or hold arm up for more than a few seconds)	**Global aphasia:** nonfluent, agrammatic speech, or mute, with impaired comprehension and repetition	**Paratonia** (gegenhalten): "plastic rigidity"—muscle tone increases in proportion to speed and strength of movement across a joint
	Finger agnosia: inability to identify specific fingers named by examiner	
Spatial acalculia: impairment of spatial organization of numbers—misalignment of digits, visual neglect (e.g., 124 as 24), digit inversion (e.g., 9 interpreted as 6), and reversal errors (e.g., 23 interpreted as 32)	**Color agnosia:** inability to name colors or point to a color named by examiner	**Pure anarthria or aphonia:** muteness with sparing of writing ability
	Acalculia: difficulty performing arithmetic calculations	
	Gerstmann's syndrome: agraphia, acalculia, right-left confusion, finger agnosia	
	Agraphia: inability to write properly	
	Echographia: compulsive copying of words and phrases	
Sensory aprosodia: poor perception of emotional overtones of spoken language	**Apraxia of speech:** automatic or reactive speech spoken without errors, volitional speech contains substitutions, repetitions, prolongations	

Glasgow Coma Scale

Test	Response	Score
Eye opening	Spontaneous	4
	Opens eyes to verbal stimulus	3
	Opens eyes to painful stimulus	2
	No response to any stimulus	1
Verbalization (verbal response)	Fully alert and oriented	5
	Confused	4
	Inappropriate	3
	Incomprehensible	2
	None	1
Motor response of nonparalyzed side	Normal (obedience to command)	6
	Localizes painful stimulus	5
	Withdrawal response to pain	4
	Flexion response to pain	3
	Extension response to pain	2
	None	1

Functional Status Scales (Stroke Severity Scales)

C-1. Barthel index*

Function	Score	Description	
Feeding	10	Independent, able to apply any necessary device, eats in reasonable time	
	5	Needs help (e.g., cutting)	_____
Wheelchair or bed transfers	15	Independent, including placing locks of wheelchair and lifting footrests	
	10	Minimal assistance or supervision	
	5	Able to sit but needs maximal assistance to transfer	_____
Personal toilet (grooming)	5	Washes face, combs hair, brushes teeth, shaves (manages plug if using electric razor)	_____
Toilet transfers	10	Independent with toilet or bedpan, handles clothes, wipes, flushes, or cleans pan	
	5	Needs help for balance, handling clothes or toilet paper	_____
Bathing self	5	Able to use bathtub or shower or take complete sponge bath without assistance	_____
Walking	15	Independent for 50 yd, may use assistive devices, except for rolling walker	
	10	Walks with help for 50 yd	
	5	Independent with wheelchair for 50 yd, only if unable to walk	_____
Stairs, ascending and descending	10	Independent, may use assistive devices	
	5	Needs help or supervision	_____
Dressing and undressing	10	Independent, ties shoes, fastens fasteners, applies braces	
	5	Needs help, but does at least half of task within reasonable time	_____
Bowel control	10	No accidents, able to care for collecting device if used	
	5	Occasional accidents or needs help with enema or suppository	_____
Bladder control	10	No accidents, able to care for collecting device if used	
	5	Occasional accidents or needs help with device	_____
		Total score	_____

*The Barthel scale scores 10 functions on a scale from fully dependent to independent. If performance of the patient is inferior to that described, the score is 0; full credit is not given for an activity if the patient needs minimal help or supervision. Adapted from Mahoney FI, Barthel DW: Functional evaluation: The Barthel index. Md State Med J 14:61–65, 1965.

DEFINITION AND DISCUSSION OF BARTHEL INDEX SCORING

Feeding

10   Independent. The patient can feed self a meal from a tray or table when someone puts food within reach. Patient must put on an assistive device (if needed), cut up food, use salt and pepper, spread butter, etc. Patient must accomplish this in a reasonable time.

5   Some help is necessary (e.g., cutting food), as listed above.

Moving from Wheelchair to Bed and Return

15   Independent in all phases of this activity. Patient can safely approach bed in wheelchair, lock brakes, lift footrests, move safely to bed, lie down, come to a sitting position on the side of the bed, change position of the wheelchair (if necessary to transfer back into it safely), and return to wheelchair.

10   Some minimal help is needed in some steps of this activity or patient needs to be reminded or supervised for safety of one or more parts of this activity.

5   Patient can come to sitting position without help of second person but needs to be lifted out of bed or needs a great deal of help to transfer.

Doing Personal Toilet

5   Patient can wash hands and face, comb hair, clean teeth, and shave. Patient may use any kind of razor but must put in blade or plug in razor without help and take razor from drawer or cabinet. Female patients must put on own makeup, if used, but need not braid or style hair.

Getting on and off Toilet

10   Patient is able to get on and off toilet, fasten and unfasten clothes, prevent soiling of clothes, and use toilet paper without help. Patient may use wall bar or other stable object for support if needed. If necessary to use bedpan instead of toilet, patient must be able to place bedpan on a chair, empty bedpan and clean it.

5   Patient needs help because of imbalance or needs help handling clothes or in using toilet paper.

Bathing Self

5   Patient may use bathtub or shower or take complete sponge bath. Patient must be able to do all steps involved in whichever method is used without another person present.

Walking on a Level Surface

15   Patient can walk at least 50 yd without help or supervision. Patient may wear braces or prostheses and use crutches, canes, or walkerette but not rolling walker. Patient must be able to lock and unlock braces if used, assume standing position and sit down, place necessary mechanical aids into position for use, and dispose of them when sitting. (Putting on and taking off braces is scored under "dressing.")

10   Patient needs help or supervision in any of the above but can walk at least 50 yd with little help.

Propelling a Wheelchair

5   Patient cannot ambulate but can propel a wheelchair independently. Patient must be able to go around corners, turn around, maneuver the chair to a table, bed, toilet, etc. Patient must be able to push a chair at least 50 yd. (Do not score this item if patient receives score for walking.)

Ascending and Descending Stairs

10   Patient is able to go up and down a flight of stairs safely without help or supervision. Patient may (and should) use handrails, canes, or crutches when needed. Patient must be able to carry canes or crutches to ascend or descend stairs.

5   Patient needs help with or supervision of any of above items.

Dressing and Undressing

10   Patient is able to put on, remove, and fasten all clothing and shoelaces (unless necessary to use adaptions). Activity includes putting on, removing, and fastening corset or braces when these are prescribed. Special clothing such as suspenders, loafer shoes, or dresses that open in front may be used when necessary.

5   Patient needs help in putting on, removing, or fastening any clothing. Patient must do at least half the work. Patient must accomplish this in a reasonable time. (Women need not be scored on use of brassiere or girdle unless these are prescribed garments.)

Continence of Bowels

10   Patient is able to control bowels and has no accidents. Patient can use suppository or take enema when necessary (as for patients with spinal cord injury who have had bowel training).

5   Patient needs help in using suppository or taking enema or has occasional accidents.

Controlling Bladder

10   Patient is able to control bladder day and night. Patients with spinal cord injury who wear external device and leg bag must put them on independently, clean and empty the bag, and stay dry day and night.

5   Patient has occasional accidents or cannot wait for bedpan or get to the toilet in time or needs help with external device.

A score of 0 is given in all of the above activities when the patient cannot meet the criteria as defined above.

C-2.   Stroke Scale of National Institutes of Health–National Institute of Neurological Disorders and Stroke (NIH–NINDS)*

1. Date performed: __ __ / __ __ / __ __
   _{month   day   year}

2. (a) Level of consciousness:	Alert	( )	0
	Drowsy	( )	1
	Stuporous	( )	2
	Coma	( )	3
(b) Level of consciousness questions:	Answers both correctly	( )	0
	Answers one correctly	( )	1
	Incorrect	( )	2
(c) Level of consciousness commands:	Obeys both correctly	( )	0
	Obeys one correctly	( )	1
	Incorrect	( )	2
3. Best gaze:	Normal	( )	0
	Partial gaze palsy	( )	1
	Forced deviation	( )	2
4. Best visual:	No visual loss	( )	0
	Partial hemianopia	( )	1
	Complete hemianopia	( )	2
	Bilateral hemianopia	( )	3
5. Facial palsy:	Normal	( )	0
	Minor	( )	1
	Partial	( )	2
	Complete	( )	3
6. Best motor arm right:	No drift	( )	0
	Drift	( )	1
	Cannot resist gravity	( )	2
	No effort against gravity	( )	3
	No movement	( )	4
7. Best motor arm left:	No drift	( )	0
	Drift	( )	1
	Cannot resist gravity	( )	2
	No effort against gravity	( )	3
	No movement	( )	4
8. Best motor leg right:	No drift	( )	0
	Drift	( )	1
	Cannot resist gravity	( )	2
	No effort against gravity	( )	3
	No movement	( )	4
9. Best motor leg left:	No drift	( )	0
	Drift	( )	1
	Cannot resist gravity	( )	2
	No effort against gravity	( )	3
	No movement	( )	4
10. Limb ataxia:	Absent	( )	0
	Present in either upper or lower	( )	1
	Present in both upper and lower	( )	2
11. Sensory:	Normal	( )	0
	Partial loss	( )	1
	Dense loss	( )	2
12. Neglect:	No neglect	( )	0
	Partial neglect	( )	1
	Complete neglect	( )	2
13. Dysarthria:	Normal articulation	( )	0
	Mild to moderate dysarthria	( )	1
	Near unintelligible or worse	( )	2
14. Best language:	No aphasia	( )	0
	Mild to moderate aphasia	( )	1
	Severe aphasia	( )	2
	Mute	( )	3

*A high score signifies a worse clinical state.

Modified from Goldstein LB, Bertels C, Davis JN: Interrater reliability of the NIH stroke scale. Arch Neurol 46:660–662, 1989.

NIH–NINDS STROKE GLOSSARY

Level of Consciousness

0   Fully alert, immediately responsive to verbal stimuli, able to co-operate completely

1   Drowsy, consciousness slightly impaired, arouses when stimulated verbally or after shaking, responds appropriately

2   Stuporous, aroused with difficulty (often painful stimuli must be applied), arousal usually incomplete, responds inadequately, reverts to original state when not stimulated

3   Comatose, unresponsive to all stimuli or responds with reflex motor or autonomic effects

Level of Consciousness Questions

0   Patient knows age and month (only initial answer graded)

1   Patient answers one question correctly

2   Patient unable to speak or understand or answers incorrectly to both questions

Level of Consciousness Commands

0   Patient grips hand and closes or opens eyes to command

1   Patient does one correctly

2   Patient does neither correctly

Best Gaze

0   Normal

1   Partial gaze palsy, gaze abnormal in one or both eyes, but forced deviation or total gaze paresis is not present

2   Forced deviation or total gaze paresis not overcome by oculocephalic maneuver

Best Visual

0   Normal

1   Partial hemianopia, clear field cut

2   Complete hemianopia

3   Bilateral hemianopia

Facial Palsy

0   Normal

1   Minor (asymmetry with smiling and spontaneous speech, good volitional movement)

2   Partial (definite weakness but some movement remains)

3   Complete (no movement of entire half of face)

Right and Left Motor Arm

Patient is examined with arms outstretched at 90 degrees (if sitting) or at 45 degrees (if supine). Request full effort for 10 sec. If patient's consciousness or comprehension is abnormal, cue patient by actively lifting arms into position while giving request for effort.

0   No drift (limb holds 90 degrees for full 10 sec)

1   Drift (limb holds 90 degrees but drifts before end of 10 sec)

2   Cannot resist gravity (limb cannot hold 90 degrees for full 10 sec, but some effort against gravity)

3   No effort against gravity (limb falls, no resistance against gravity)

4   No movement

Right and Left Motor Leg
While supine, patient is asked to maintain the leg at 30 degrees for 5 sec. If patient's consciousness or comprehension is abnormal, cue patient by actively lifting leg into position while giving request for effort.

0   No drift (leg holds 30 degrees for 5 sec)

1   Drift (leg falls to intermediate position by end of 5 sec)

2   Cannot resist gravity (leg falls to bed by 5 sec, but some effort against gravity)

3   No effort against gravity (leg falls to bed immediately, no resistance against gravity)

4   No movement

Limb Ataxia
Finger-nose-finger and heal-to-shin tests are performed. Ataxia is scored only if clearly out of proportion to weakness. (Limb ataxia not testable in hemiplegia.)

0   Absent

1   Present in upper or lower limb

2   Present in both limbs

Sensory
Test with pin if patient's consciousness or comprehension is abnormal; score sensation normal unless deficit clearly recognized (e.g., clear-cut grimace asymmetry); without asymmetry, only hemisensory losses are counted as abnormal.

0   Normal, no loss of sensation

1   Mild/moderate (pinprick less sharp or dull on the affected side, or a loss of superficial pain with pinprick but patient aware of being tested)

2   Severe/total (patient unaware of being touched)

Neglect
0   None

1   Visual, tactile, or auditory hemi-inattention

2   Profound hemi-inattention to more than one modality

Dysarthria
0   Normal speech

1   Mild to moderate (slurs some words, understands with difficulty)

2   Unintelligible slurred speech (in the absence of, or out of proportion to, any dysphasia)

Best Language

0   Normal, no aphasia

1   Mild to moderate aphasia (word finding errors, naming errors, paraphasias or impairment of communication by comprehension or expression disability)

2   Severe aphasia (fully developed Broca's or Wernicke's aphasia or variant)

3   Mute or global aphasia

C-3.   Rankin disability scores

Grade I	No significant disability; able to carry out all usual activities of daily living (without assistance). Note: this does not preclude the presence of weakness, sensory loss, language disturbance, etc., but implies that these are mild and do not or have not caused patient to limit activities (e.g., if employed before, is still employed at same job).
Grade II	Slight disability; unable to carry out some previous activities, but able to look after own affairs without much assistance (e.g., unable to return to previous job; unable to do some household chores, but able to get along without daily supervision or help).
Grade III	Moderate disability; requires some help but able to walk without assistance (e.g., needs daily supervision, needs assistance with small aspects of dressing or hygiene, unable to read or communicate clearly). Note: ankle-foot orthosis or cane does not imply needing assistance.
Grade IV	Moderately severe disability; unable to walk without assistance and unable to attend to own bodily needs without assistance (e.g., needs 24-hr supervision and moderate to maximal assistance on several activities of daily living but still able to do some activities by self or with minimal assistance).
Grade V	Severe disability; bedridden, incontinent, and requires constant nursing care and attention.

Modified from Rankin J: Cerebral vascular accidents in patients over the age of 60: II. Prognosis. *Scott Med J* 2:200–215, 1957.

C-4. Clinical grades of subarachnoid hemorrhage

Hunt and Hess scale

Grade	Criteria
I	Asymptomatic or minimal headache or stiff neck
II	Moderate to severe headache, stiff neck, no neurologic deficit other than cranial nerve palsy
III	Drowsiness, confusion, or mild focal signs
IV	Stupor, moderate to severe hemiparesis, possibly early decerebrate signs
V	Deep coma

World Federation of Neurological Surgeons (WFNS) scale

WFNS grade	GCS score	Motor deficit
I	15	Absent
II	13–14	Absent
III	13–14	Present
IV	7–12	Present or absent
V	3–6	Present or absent

GCS = Glasgow Coma Scale.
From Hunt WE, Hess RM: Surgical risk as related to time of intervention in the repair of intracranial aneurysms. J Neurosurg 28:14–19, 1968; and from Drake CG: Report of World Federation of Neurological Surgeons Committee on a universal subarachnoid hemorrhage grading scale (letter). J Neurosurg 68:985–986, 1988.

Neurology Intensive Care
Unit Evaluation Form

| Name: | **CRITICAL** | Today's weight _____ kg | | Physician _____ | Date / / |
| Patient number: | **CARE** **FLOW** **SHEET** | Previous day's weight _____ kg
Preoperative weight _____ kg
Height _____ cm
Previous day fluid balance _____ | Diet _____ | Diagnosis _____
Operation _____ | Postoperative day # _____
Hospital day # _____ |

Time	2400	0100	0200	·····→	2100	2200	2300

Temperature scale:
T 40.0 ___
e 39.5 ___
m 39.0 ___   B
p 38.5 ___   l
e 38.0 ___   o   200
r 37.5 ___   o   190
a 37.0 ___   d   180
t 36.5 ___   170
u 36.0 ___   P   160
r 35.5 ___   r   150
e 35.0 ___   e   140
              s   130
              s   120
              u   110
              r
              e

• Temp

• Systolic (arterial)
• Diatolic (arterial)

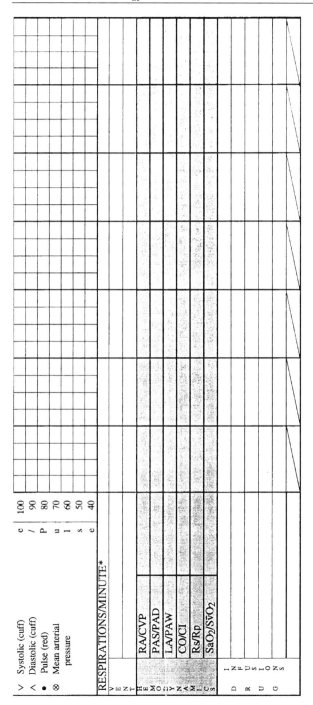

>	Systolic (cuff)
<	Diastolic (cuff)
●	Pulse (red)
⊗	Mean arterial pressure

P u l s e — 100 / 90 / 80 / 70 / 60 / 50 / 40

RESPIRATIONS/MINUTE*

VENT

HEMODYNAMICS
- RA/CVP
- PAS/PAD
- LA/PAW
- CO/CI
- Rs/Rp
- SaO$_2$/S$\bar{v}$O$_2$

INFUSIONS

DRUG

Oral or nasogastric

Subtotal

Blood

Subtotal

FLUID IN TOTAL

Urine

NG

Subtotal

FLUIDS IN

FLUIDS OUT

BLOOD

Subtotal							
FLUID OUT TOTAL							
FLUID BALANCE							
BLOOD BALANCE							
Electrocardiographic rhythm							
Pacer mode							
rate							
C Heart Sounds							
A Edema							
R Pulses (right/left)							
D							
I							
A Capillary Refill							
C Line Status							
S Color/Temperature							
K Incision							
I Dressing/Drainage							
N							

Time	2400	0100	0200	↑ ··········	2100	2200	2300
P Breath Sounds							
U Triflo/Voldyne							
L Chest physiotherapy							
M Cough							
O Suction/Secretions							
N Chest Tubes							
A							
R							
Y							
Level of consciousness							
Pupil Size R/L							
Pupil Reaction R/L							
N Finger Wiggle R/L							
E Gross Upper R/L							
U Toe Wiggle R/L							
R Gross Lower R/L							
O Dorsi Flexion R/L							
Plantar Flexion R/L							
Glasgow Coma Score							

		R/L										
	Extremity Sensation	R/L										
	Movement											
G	Bowel Sounds											
	Stool/Guaiac											
I	Nasogastrics: Color/pH											
R	Color/Character											
E	pH/Specific Gravity											
N	Keto/Diastick											
A												
L												
P	Activity/Turn											
E	Bath/Personal Care											
R	Siderails/Restraints											
S	Visits/MD Rounds											
O	TEDs/SCDs[†]											
N												
A												
L												

Tests/Labs								
O								
T								
H								
E								
R								
Level of Comfort								
Level of Sedation								

Nurse Initials/Signature

EQUIPMENT IN USE	COMMENTS
Specialty Bed	
Waffle Air Mattress	
Hypo/Hyperthermia Pad(s)	
Suction (type) Cont. x ____ Int. x ____	
Aqua K Pad	
Isolation Cart [ ] Initiated [ ] DC	
Pump (type) IMED x ____ PCA x ____	

TRAVENOL. x _____ KANGAROO x _____
Med Fusion x _____ AVI x _____
Other _____

STANDARDS

NEUROLOGICAL

EYES OPEN
4 = Spontaneous
3 = To Speech
2 = To Pain
1 = None

BEST VERBAL
5 = Oriented
4 = Confused
3 = Inapprop Speech
2 = Incompre Speech
1 = None

MOVEMENT
0 = Normal
-1 = Slightly Weak
-2 = Weak
-3 = Very Weak
-4 = No Movement

BEST MOTOR
6 = Obeys Command
5 = Localizes Pain
4 = Flexion Withdrawal
3 = Flexion Abnormal
2 = Extension to Pain
1 = None

PUPIL REACTION
0 = Normal
-2 = Sluggish
-4 = No Reaction

Pupil size scale:
pinpoint = .4
2 = -2
3 = 0
4 = 0
5 = 0
6 = 0
7 = +2
8 = +2
9 = +4

RESPONSE SCALE-LOC‡
1 = Alert
2 = Alert, confused
3 = Drowsy, responds to strong stim.
4 = Unconscious, localizes but does not ward off pain
5 = Unconscious, withdraws to pain
6 = Unconscious, abn. flexion/decorticate
7 = Unconscious, abn. extension/decerebrate
8 = Unconscious, flaccid

LEVEL OF COMFORT
0-10 Scale:
0 = No Pain
10 = Worst Pain

LEVEL OF SEDATION
0-5 Scale
1 = Wide Awake
2 = Drowsy
3 = Dozing Intermittently
4 = Mostly Sleeping
5 = Only Awakens When Aroused

SKIN TEMPERATURE
3 = Hot
2 = Normal
1 = Cool
0 = Cold

PERIPHERAL PULSES
4 = Normal
3 = Diminished
2 = Further Diminished
1 = Weak
0 = Absent
D = Doppler

SAFETY/SECURITY
2SR = 2 side rails up
4SR = 4 side rails up
WR = wrist restraints
AR = ankle restraints
JR = jacket restraints
C = call light

PERSONAL CARES
BB = Bed Bath
PB = Partial Bath
PC = Peri Care
SH = Shower
BC = Back Care
OC = Oral Care
T&R = Turn & Rub

COLOR
3 = Normal
2 = Cyanosis (Bluish)
1 = Rubor (Redness)
0 = Pallor

*RA/CVP, right atrium/central venous pressure; PAS/PAD, pulmonary artery peak systolic pressure/pulmonary artery end-diastolic pressure; LA/PAW, left atrium/pulmonary capillary wedge pressure; CO/CI, cardiac output/cardiac index; Rs/Rp, systemic vascular resistance/total pulmonary resistance; SaO_2/SvO_2, arterial oxygen saturation/venous oxygen saturation.
†SCDs, sequential compression devices.
‡Level of consciousness.

E

Neurologic Record Form

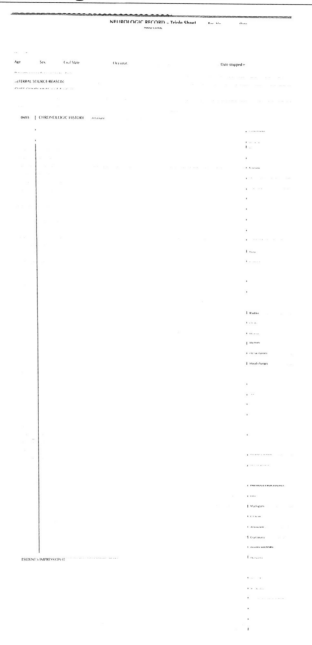

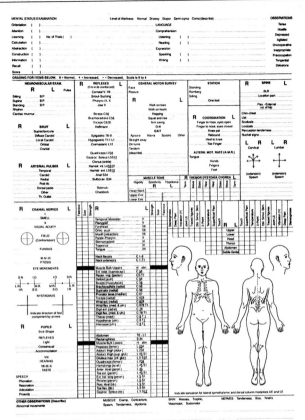

HANDWRITING (sample)

COMPREHENSIVE EXAMINATION REQUIRES COMPLETION OF ALL UNSHADED AREAS

NEUROLOGIC CONSULTATION

NEUROSURGICAL CONSULTATION

Lipid-Lowering Drugs: Indications (Effect on Lipids), Dosage, and Adverse Effects

Drug	Effect on lipids	Daily dosage (adults)	Adverse effects
Nicotinic acid (niacin)	Decrease LDL cholesterol and triglycerides and increase HDL cholesterol	Initial dosage 100 mg, 3 times/day increased by 100 mg, 3 times/day, each week until dosage of 1–2 g, 3 times/day is reached	Flushing (can be blocked by aspirin, 325 mg, before nicotinic acid), pruritus, GI distress, glucose intolerance, gout, rash, dizziness, liver dysfunction, atrial arrhythmias. *Monitoring:* hyperglycemia, hyperuricemia, and liver function abnormalities
Cholestyramine (Questran)	Decrease LDL cholesterol and maintain or increase triglycerides and increase HDL cholesterol	12–24 g	Constipation, bloating, nausea, diarrhea, gout, and binding of other drugs (other drugs should be administered 1 hr before or 4 hr after bile acid sequestrants)
Colestipol (Colestid)	Same as above	15–30 g	Same as above
Gemfibrozil (Lopid)	Decrease triglycerides and LDL cholesterol but increase HDL cholesterol	600–1200 mg	Myositis, possibly cholelithiasis or cholecystitis, GI distress
Lovastatin (Mevacor)	Decrease LDL cholesterol, maintain or decrease triglycerides, and maintain or increase HDL cholesterol	20–80 mg once daily in evening	Liver functional abnormalities, myositis
Pravastatin (Pravachol)	Same as above	10–20 mg once daily at bedtime	Contraindications: active liver disease or persistent elevations of liver function tests
Probucol (Lorelco)	Decrease LDL cholesterol, maintain triglycerides, and decrease HDL cholesterol	500–1000 mg	Diarrhea, prolonged QT interval, GI distress
Clofibrate (Atromid-S)	Decrease LDL cholesterol and triglycerides, maintain or increase HDL cholesterol	1–2 g	Cholelithiasis, myositis, possible increase in GI malignant lesions

F. *(Continued)*

Drug	Effect on lipids	Daily dosage (adults)	Adverse effects
Eicosapentaenoic acid (fish oils)	Increase, maintain, or decrease LDL cholesterol, decrease triglycerides, and maintain or increase HDL cholesterol	1–8 g	Weight gain, immune dysfunction

GI = gastrointestinal; LDL = low-density lipoprotein; HDL = high-density lipoprotein.

G

Commonly Prescribed Antihypertensive Drugs for Oral Use

Drug	Usual initial dose (mg/day)	Usual initial frequency (times/day)	Relative or absolute contraindications	Frequent or peculiar adverse reactions
β-Adrenergic blocker			Congestive heart failure, asthma, chronic bronchitis with bronchospasm, bradycardia/heart block, sick sinus syndrome, insulin-dependent diabetes mellitus, administration of MAO inhibitors, dyslipidemia (except labetalol, atenolol, metoprolol, acebutolol)	Bradycardia, atrioventricular block, reduced contractility, asthma, Raynaud's phenomenon, impotence in men, hypoglycemia, vivid dreams, and altered sleep patterns (propranolol, metoprolol, pindolol)
Atenolol	50	1		
Bisoprolol	5	1		
Nadolol	80	1		
Sotalol	80	2		
Acebutolol	400	2		
Alprenolol	200	2		
Metoprolol	100	2		
Propranolol	80	2–4*		
Timolol	10	2		
Pindolol	5	2		
Labetalol	100	2		
Oxprenolol	80	3		
α-Adrenergic blocker			None known	Dizziness, headache, drowsiness (rare)
Phenoxybenzamine	10	1–2		
Prazosin	1	2		
Ace inhibitor			Renal failure (reduction of dose required)	Hyperkalemia, leukopenia, pancytopenia, nephrotic syndrome, fever, rash, angioedema (rare)
Benazepril	10	1		
Captopril	12.5	2		
Enalapril	5	1		
Fosinopril	10	1		
Lisinopril	5	1		
Quinapril	5	1		
Ramipril	1.25	1		

G. *(Continued)*

Drug	Usual initial dose (mg/day)	Usual initial frequency (times/day)	Relative or absolute contraindications	Frequent or peculiar adverse reactions
Calcium antagonist				
Diltiazem	180	1	Acute myocardial infarction, atrial fibrillation/flutter, sick sinus syndrome, second- or third-degree atrioventricular block	Headache, flushing, dizziness, constipation, peripheral edema (rare)
Verapamil	80	3		
Amlodipine	2.5	1		
Felodipine	5	1		
Nifedipine (sustained release)	30	1		
Diuretic				
Hydrochlorothiazide	25	1–2	Diabetes mellitus, hyperuricemia, primary aldosteronism	Potassium depletion, hyperglycemia, hyperuricemia, hyperkalemia, diarrhea, gynecomastia, irregular menses, nausea, vomiting
Chlorthalidone	100	1	Renal failure	
Metolazone	0.5–1.0	1		
Spironolactone	25	2–4		
Amiloride	5	1		
Triamterene	50	1–2		
Furosemide	40	2–3		
Bumetanide	0.5	1		
Ethacrynic acid	50	1		

CA α^2-Agonist				
Clonidine	0.1	2	None known	Postural hypotension
Guanabenz	4	2	Pheochromocytoma, administration of MAO inhibitor	Postural hypotension, sedation, dry mouth, constipation
Methyldopa	250	2		
Guanfacine	1	1	None known	
PAA Antagonist				
Guanadrel	10	2	Pheochromocytoma, severe coronary artery disease, administration of MAO inhibitor, peptic ulcer, depression (reserpine, rauwolfia serpentina)	Postural hypotension, bradycardia, dry mouth, diarrhea, depression, nasal congestion
Guanethidine	10	1		
Rauwolfia serpentina	50	1		
Reserpine	0.05	1		
Direct Vasodilator				
Hydralazine	10	4	Lupus erythematosus, severe coronary artery disease	Headache, tachycardia, angina pectoris
Minoxidil	5	1		

ACE = angiotensin-converting enzyme; CA = centrally acting; MAO = monoamine oxidase; PAA = peripheral-acting adrenergic.
*Inderal LA, once daily.

Dosage, Routes, and Adverse Effects of and Precautions for Commonly Recommended Drugs for Treatment of Hypertensive Crisis and Malignant Hypertension*

Recommended drug	Dosage and method of administration	Onset	Duration	Adverse effects and precautions
Direct vasodilator				
Sodium nitroprusside	0.25–10 mg/kg as IV infusion; maximal dose for 10 min only	Instantaneous	2–3 min	Nausea, vomiting, muscle twitching; prolonged use may result in thiocyanate intoxication
Diazoxide	50–150 mg as IV bolus at 5–10 min intervals or 15–30 mg/min by IV infusion to maximum 600 mg	1–2 min	3–15 hr	Hypotension, tachycardia, aggravation of angina pectoris, nausea, vomiting, hyperglycemia with repeated injection; should be avoided in patients in whom aortic dissection is suspected (to prevent sodium retention, administer furosemide 20–80 mg, IV)
Hydralazine	10–30 mg/min as IV infusion	5–10 min	2–6 hr	Tachycardia, headache, vomiting, aggravation of angina pectoris; should be avoided in presence of myocardial ischemia or aortic dissection
	10–20 mg as IV bolus	10 min	2–6 hr	
	10–40 mg as IM agent	20–30 min	2–6 hr	
Nitroglycerin	5–100 mg/min as IV infusion	2–5 min	A few minutes	Headache, tachycardia, vomiting, flushing, methemoglobinemia; needs special delivery system because of drug binding to polyvinyl chloride
Enalaprilat	0.625–1.25 mg as IV infusion every 6 hr	50–60 min	6 hr	Renal failure in patients with bilateral renal artery stenosis, hypotension

377

H.   *(Continued)*

Recommended drug	Dosage and method of administration	Onset	Duration	Adverse effects and precautions
Direct vasodilator				
Minoxidil	5–20 mg PO 4 times/day	0.5–2 hr	2–4 hr	Tachycardia, aggravates angina, marked fluid retention
Adrenergic inhibitor				
Phentolamine	5–15 mg as IV bolus or 1 mg/min infusion	1–2 min	50–60 min	Tachycardia, orthostatic hypotension
Labetolol	10–80 mg as IV bolus every 10–20 min	5–10 min	2–6 hr	Bronchoconstriction, heart block, orthostatic hypotension
	2 mg/min as IV infusion 200–400 mg PO every 2–3 hr	0.5–2 hr	2–6 hr	
Prazosin	1–2 mg PO at 1 hr	0.25–1 hr	2–6 hr	Orthostatic hypotension
Ace inhibitor				
Captopril	25 mg PO, repeat at 35–45 min as required	15–30 min	2–6 hr	Hypotension, renal failure in bilateral renal artery stenosis
Calcium blocker				
Nifedipine	10–20 mg PO, repeat after 30 min as required (may be used sublingually)	15–30 min	2–6 hr	Rapid, uncontrolled hypotension may precipitate circulatory collapse in patients with aortic stenosis; headache

Ganglionic blocker

Trimethaphan camsylate	1–4 mg/min as IV infusion	1–5 min	5–10 min	Urinary retention, paresis of bowel and bladder, orthostatic hypotension, blurred vision, dry mouth

Sympatholytic agent

Clonidine	0.1–0.2 mg PO, at every hour as required to a total dose of 0.6 mg	0.5–1 hr	8–12 hr	Hypotension, drowsiness, dry mouth
Methyldopate	250–500 mg as IV infusion every 6 hr	0.5–1 hr	8–12 hr	Drowsiness

ACE = angiotensin-converting enzyme; IM = intramuscular; IV = intravenous; PO = oral.
*Administration of diuretics may be appropriate with any of these drugs.

A Stroke Risk Profile

I-1. Probability of stroke within 10 years for men aged 55–84 years and no previous stroke*

Risk factor	Points										
	0	1	2	3	4	5	6	7	8	9	10
Age (yr)	54–56	57–59	60–62	63–65	66–68	69–71	72–74	75–77	78–80	81–83	84–86
SBP (mm Hg)	95–105	106–116	117–126	127–137	138–148	149–159	160–170	171–181	182–191	192–202	203–213
Hyp Rx	No		Yes								
DM	No		Yes								
Cigs	No			Yes							
CVD	No			Yes							
AF	No				Yes						
LVH	No						Yes				

Points	10-yr probability (%)	Points	10-yr probability (%)	Points	10-yr probability (%)
1	2.6	11	11.2	21	41.7
2	3.0	12	12.9	22	46.6
3	3.5	13	14.8	23	51.8
4	4.0	14	17.0	24	57.3
5	4.7	15	19.5	25	62.8
6	5.4	16	22.4	26	68.4
7	6.3	17	25.5	27	73.8
8	7.3	18	29.0	28	79.0
9	8.4	19	32.9	29	83.7
10	9.7	20	37.1	30	87.9

AF = history of atrial fibrillation; Cigs = smokes cigarettes; CVD = history of cardiovascular disease (myocardial infarction, angina pectoris, coronary insufficiency, intermittent claudication, or congestive heart failure; DM = history of diabetes mellitus; Hyp Rx = under antihypertensive therapy; LVH = left ventricular hypertrophy on electrocardiogram; SBP = systolic blood pressure (mm Hg).

*Add points for risk factors listed (upper table), then add additional points for blood pressure level on antihypertensive therapy. Use lower table to obtain 10-year probability for stroke.

From Wolf PA, D'Agostino RB, Belanger AJ, Kannel WB: Probability of stroke: A risk profile. From the Framingham Study. Stroke 22:312–318, 1991.

I-2.   Probability of stroke within 10 years for women aged 55–84 years and no previous stroke*

Risk factor	Points										
	0	1	2	3	4	5	6	7	8	9	10
Age (yr)	54–56	57–59	60–62	63–65	66–68	69–71	72–74	75–77	78–80	81–83	84–86
SBP (mm Hg)	95–104	105–114	115–124	125–134	135–144	145–154	155–164	165–174	175–184	185–194	195–204
Hyp Rx	No (if yes, see below)										
DM	No			Yes							
Cigs	No			Yes							
CVD	No		Yes								
AF	No						Yes				
LVH	No				Yes						

If woman is currently under antihypertensive therapy, add points according to SBP:

Risk factor	Points										
	6	5	5	4	3	3	2	1	1	0	0
SBP (mm Hg)	95–104	105–114	115–124	125–134	135–144	145–154	155–164	165–174	175–184	185–194	195–204

I-2. *(Continued)*

Points	10-yr probability (%)	Points	10-yr probability (%)	Points	10-yr probability (%)
1	2.6	11	11.2	21	41.7
2	3.0	12	12.9	22	46.6
3	3.5	13	14.8	23	51.8
4	4.0	14	17.0	24	57.3
5	4.7	15	19.5	25	62.8
6	5.4	16	22.4	26	68.4
7	6.3	17	25.5	27	73.8
8	7.3	18	29.0	28	79.0
9	8.4	19	32.9	29	83.7
10	9.7	20	37.1	30	87.9

AF = history of atrial fibrillation; Cigs = smokes cigarettes; CVD = history of myocardial infarction, angina pectoris, coronary insufficiency, intermittent claudication, or congestive heart failure; DM = history of diabetes mellitus; Hyp Rx = under antihypertensive therapy; LVH = left ventricular hypertrophy on electrocardiogram; SBP = systolic blood pressure (mm Hg).

*Add points for risk factors listed (upper table), then add additional points for blood pressure level on antihypertensive therapy. Use lower table to obtain 10-year probability for stroke.

From Wolf PA, D'Agostino RB, Belanger AJ, Kannel WB: Probability of stroke: A risk profile. From the Framingham Study. Stroke 22:312–318, 1991.

Practice Guidelines for Management of Cerebrovascular Disease

J-1.   Guideline for initial evaluation by telephone of a patient with cerebrovascular disease

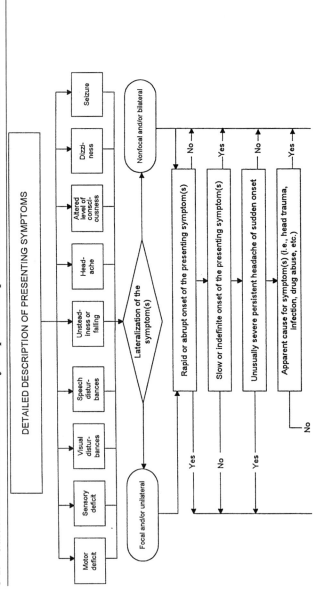

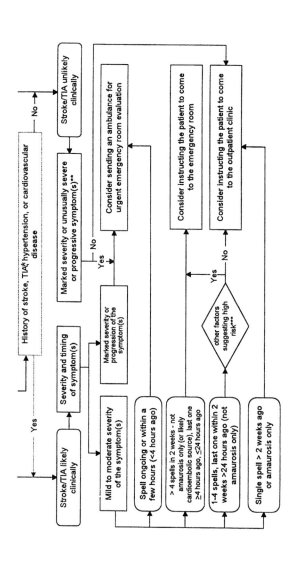

*TIA= transient ischemic attack.

**Including evidence of other serious medical disorders arising during the telephone interview.

***Probable cardioembolic source, or causative arterial stenosis.

J-2. Guideline for transient ischemic attack/reversible ischemic neurologic deficit/minor ischemic stroke

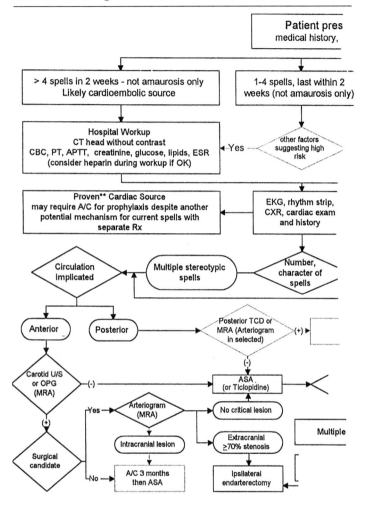

*TIA = transient ischemic attack; RIND = reversible ischemic neurologic deficit; MCI = minor cerebral infarction; ASA = acetylsalicylic acid (aspirin); EKG = electrocardiography; CT = computed tomography; TCD = transcranial Doppler ultrasonography; MRA = magnetic resonance angiography; OPG = ocular pneumoplethysmography; A/C = anticoagulation with warfarin; U/S = ultrasound; TEE = transesophageal echocardiography; CBC = complete blood count; ESR = erythrocyte sedimentation rate; PT = prothrombin time; APTT = activated partial thromboplastin time; Rx = therapy; CXR = chest x-ray; W/U = workup. Those actions and paths supported by reasonably good clinical or scientific evidence are indicated by

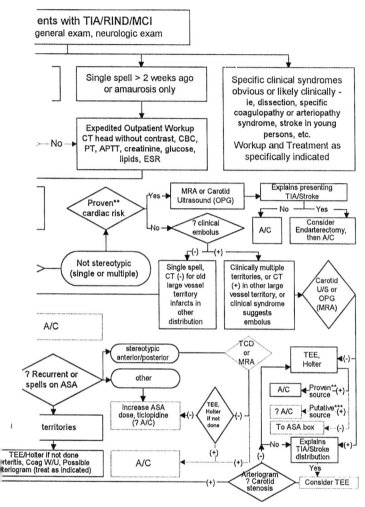

solid borders and lines; less rigorously supported data are denoted by hatched borders and lines.

**Proven cardiac risk factors for emboli include atrial fibrillation, mechanical valve, dilated cardiomyopathy, recent myocardial infarction, and intracardiac thrombus.

***Putative cardiac risk factors include sick sinus syndrome, patent foramen ovale, atherosclerotic debris in thoracic aorta, spontaneous echocardiographic contrast, myocardial infarction 2–6 months earlier, hypokinetic or akinetic left ventricular segment, and calcification of mitral annulus.

J-3. Guideline for major ischemic stroke

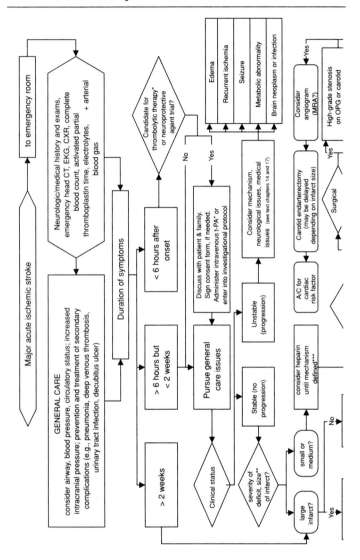

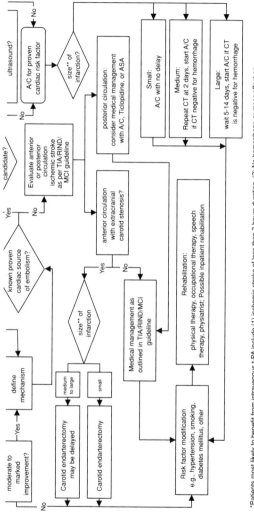

*Patients most likely to benefit from intravenous t-PA include (1) ischemic stroke of less than 3 hours duration, (2) No hemorrhage or mass effect on head CT, (3) absence of uncontrolled hypertension, (4) absence of rapidly improving deficit

**Infarct size categorization: small= subcortical only and less than 2 cm maximum diameter or less than one one-half lobe; medium=up to one lobe; large= larger than one lobe.

***Especially if (1) cardiac source of embolism is likely; (2) large vessel with near occlusion with stuttering onset; (3) progressing ischemic stroke; (4) hypercoagulable state responsive to heparin; (5) recurrent TIA or ischemic stroke before stroke event; (6) no hemorrhage on head CT scan.

C⁺= computed tomography; EKG= electrocardiography; CXR= chest x-ray; MRA= magnetic resonance angiography; A/C= anticoagulants; OPG= oculopneumoplethysmography; TIA= transient ischemic attack; RIND= reversible ischemic neurologic deficit; MCI= minor cerebral infarction; ASA= acetylsalicylic acid (aspirin).

J-4. Guideline for subarachnoid hemorrhage

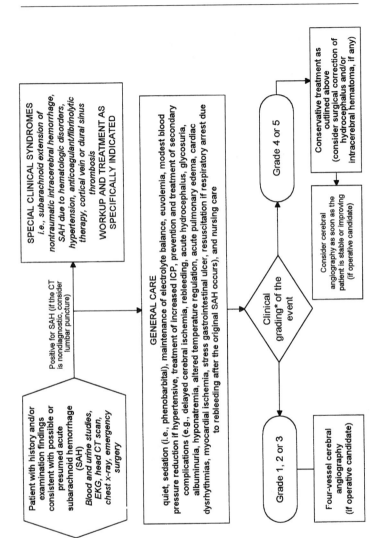

Patient with history and/or examination findings consistent with possible or presumed acute subarachnoid hemorrhage (SAH)
Blood and urine studies, EKG, head CT scan, chest x-ray, emergency surgery

Positive for SAH (if the CT is nondiagnostic, consider lumbar puncture)

SPECIAL CLINICAL SYNDROMES
i.e., subarachnoid extension of nontraumatic intracerebral hemorrhage, SAH due to hematologic disorders, hypertension, anticoagulant/fibrinolytic therapy, cortical vein or dural sinus thrombosis
WORKUP AND TREATMENT AS SPECIFICALLY INDICATED

GENERAL CARE
quiet, sedation (i.e., phenobarbital), maintenance of electrolyte balance, euvolemia, modest blood pressure reduction if hypertensive, treatment of increased ICP, prevention and treatment of secondary complications (e.g., delayed cerebral ischemia, rebleeding, acute hydrocephalus, glycosuria, albuminuria, hyponatremia, altered temperature regulation, acute pulmonary edema, cardiac dysrhythmias, myocardial ischemia, stress gastrointestinal ulcer, resuscitation if respiratory arrest occurs due to rebleeding after the original SAH occurs), and nursing care

Clinical grading* of the event

Grade 1, 2 or 3

Four-vessel cerebral angiography (if operative candidate)

Grade 4 or 5

Conservative treatment as outlined above (consider surgical correction of hydrocephalus and/or intracerebral hematoma, if any)

Consider cerebral angiography as soon as the patient is stable or improving (if operative candidate)

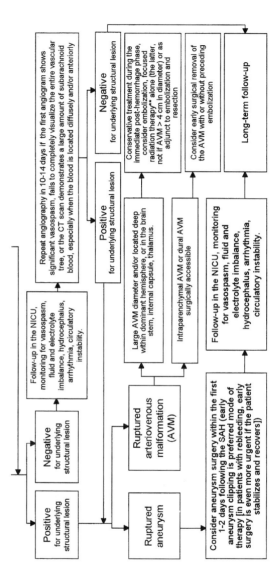

*Hunt and Hess clinical grades of SAH; TCD= transcranial Doppler ultrasonography; NICU= neurologic intensive care unit; EKG= electrocardiography; CT= computed tomography; ICP= intracranial pressure; AVM= arteriovenous malformation.

**Radiotherapy options for arteriovenous malformation treatment include gamma knife, linac, and proton beam.

J-5. Guideline for intracerebral/intraventricular hemorrhage

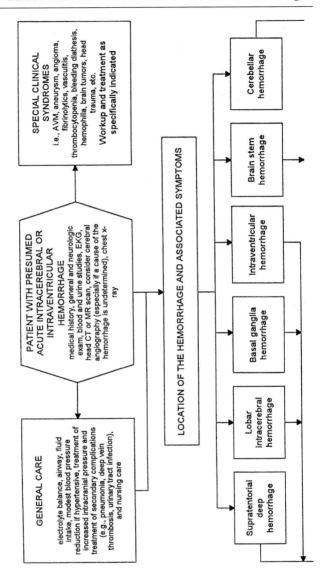

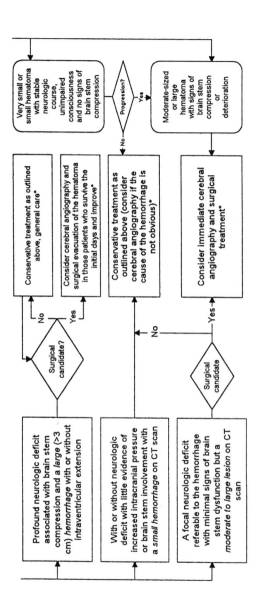

AVM= arteriovenous malformation; CT= computed tomography; MR= magnetic resonance; EKG= electrocardiography.
*Rehabilitation at a rehabilitation unit in the hospital, in the long-term facility, ambulatory, and/or at home; prevention of subsequent stroke (i.e., treatment of underlying disease, risk factor modification)

J-6. Guideline for asymptomatic carotid artery stenosis

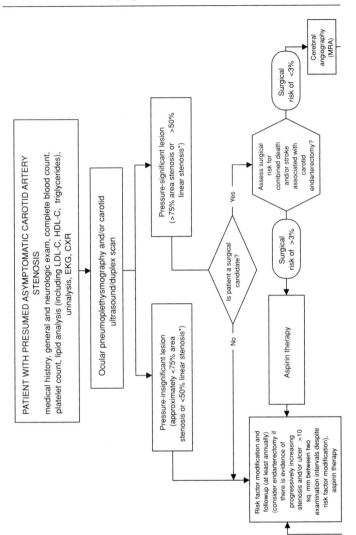

PATIENT WITH PRESUMED ASYMPTOMATIC CAROTID ARTERY STENOSIS
medical history, general and neurologic exam, complete blood count, platelet count, lipid analysis (including LDL-C, HDL-C, triglycerides), urinalysis, EKG, CXR

Ocular pneumoplethysmography and/or carotid ultrasound/duplex scan

Pressure-insignificant lesion (approximately <75% area stenosis or <50% linear stenosis*)

Pressure-significant lesion (>75% area stenosis or >50% linear stenosis*)

Is patient a surgical candidate?

Yes

No

Assess surgical risk for combined death and/or stroke associated with carotid endarterectomy?

Surgical risk of <3%

Surgical risk of >3%

Cerebral angiography (MRA)

Aspirin therapy

Risk factor modification and followup (at least annually) (consider endarterectomy if there is evidence of progressively increasing stenosis and/or ulcer >10 sq. mm between two examination intervals despite risk factor modification), aspirin therapy

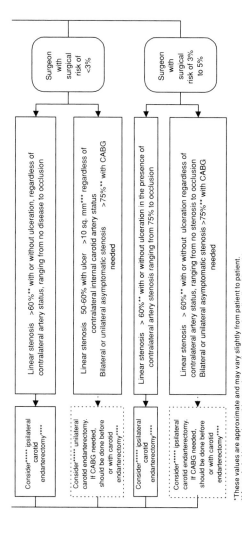

Surgeon with surgical risk of <3%

Surgeon with surgical risk of 3% to 5%

Linear stenosis >60%** with or without ulceration, regardless of contralateral artery status, ranging from no disease to occlusion

Linear stenosis 50-60% with ulcer >10 sq. mm*** regardless of contralateral internal carotid artery status
Bilateral or unilateral asymptomatic stenosis >75%** with CABG needed

Linear stenosis > 60%** with or without ulceration in the presence of contralateral artery stenosis ranging from 75% to occlusion

Linear stenosis > 60%** with or without ulceration regardless of contralateral artery status, ranging from no stenosis to occlusion
Bilateral or unilateral asymptomatic stenosis >75%** with CABG needed

Consider***** ipsilateral carotid endarterectomy****

Consider***** unilateral carotid endarterectomy. If CABG needed, should be done before or with carotid endarterectomy****

Consider***** ipsilateral carotid endarterectomy****

Consider***** ipsilateral carotid endarterectomy. If CABG needed, should be done before or with carotid endarterectomy****

*These values are approximate and may vary slightly from patient to patient.
**An occluded internal carotid artery is usually managed medically with aspirin.
***Ulcer size is defined by multiplying the length and width of the ulcer.
****Aspirin should be used before, during and after carotid endarterectomy, unless specifically contraindicated.
*****Available data suggest surgery is more beneficial in men than women. Other factors favoring surgery are absence of associated serious medical conditions, relatively local as opposed to diffuse atherosclerosis, and very high grade as opposed to high grade stenosis.
Actions and paths indicated by reasonably good clinical or scientific evidence are indicated by *solid borders and lines* less rigorously supported data are denoted by *dotted borders and lines.* Surgical risk is based on a combined estimate of the patient's general medical fitness to undergo surgery and the individual surgeon's risk of morbidity and mortality for patients with a specific surgical indication. ASA=acetylsalicylic acid (aspirin); LDL-C=low-density lipoprotein-cholesterol; HDL-C=high density lipoprotein-cholesterol; EKG=electrocardiography; CXR=chest x-ray; CABG=coronary artery bypass grafting.

K

Outline of Diets Low in Fat and Cholesterol and Table of Ideal Body Weight

K-1. Low-fat, low-cholesterol diet

Food	Anytime	Sometimes	Avoid
Fruits and vegetables	Any fresh, juiced, frozen, canned, or dried	Avocado, olives	Coconut; vegetables in cheese, cream, or butter; french-fried vegetables
Grains (breads, cereals, rice, pasta, and baked goods)	Bread, bagels, breadsticks, English muffins, pita bread, plain rolls, corn tortillas, hot and cold cereals, rice, bulgur, pasta, popcorn (plain or light microwave), pretzels, no-oil tortilla chips, fat-free and low-fat crackers and cookies	Biscuits, muffins (from mix), corn-bread, low-fat granola, pancakes, waffles, French toast, packaged rice mixes, popcorn (regular, microwave, or buttered), low-fat or reduced-fat snack foods	Doughnuts, croissants, sweet rolls, commercial muffins, granola, egg noodles, chow mein noodles, stuffing, regular chips, crackers, pies, cakes, cookies
Dairy products	Skim and 1%-fat milk, buttermilk, non-fat dry milk, fat-free yogurt and cheese, fat-free or low-fat cottage cheese	2%-fat milk, 4%-fat cottage cheese, reduced-fat and part-skim milk cheeses, low-fat yogurt, frozen yogurt, ice milk, sherbet	Whole milk, whole-milk yogurt and cheeses, ice cream (regular and gourmet)

K-1. *(Continued)*

Food	Anytime	Sometimes	Avoid
Meat, eggs, and meat substitutes	Any finfish or shellfish (except shrimp), water-packed tuna, surimi, poultry, ground turkey (without skin), USDA choice or select beef (round sirloin, tenderloin, flank, ground round), lamb (leg), pork (center-cut ham, loin chops, tenderloin), Canadian bacon, low-fat luncheon meats, dried beans and peas, lentils, egg substitutes, egg whites, tofu, tempeh, soy and textured protein meat substitutes, fat-free meat substitutes	Shrimp, oil-packed fish, fish sticks, poultry (with skin), ground beef (extra lean and lean), eggs (4/wk)	Fried fish or poultry, USDA prime beef, pork or lamb (rib, brisket, shoulder, porterhouse, T-bone), organ meats, regular ground beef, sausage, bacon, most regular luncheon meats, peanut butter, nuts
Fats	Polyunsaturated oils (corn, sunflower, soybean, sesame, cottonseed), monounsaturated oils (canola, olive, peanut), margarine, reduced-fat margarine, reduced-fat salad dressing, fat-free sour cream	Regular salad dressing, mayonnaise, reduced-fat sour cream, reduced-fat cream cheese, sour half-and-half	Coconut oil, palm and palm kernel oils, shortening, lard, butter, cream, half-and-half, sour cream, cream cheese, gravy, most nondairy creamers

From Medical Essay: Cholesterol. Mayo Clin Health Lett 11(6) (Suppl):1–8, 1993.

K-2.   Very low-fat, very low-cholesterol diet

Food	Anytime	Sometimes	Avoid
Fruits and vegetables	Any fresh, juiced, frozen, canned, or dried: apple, apricot, banana, blackberry, blueberry, cantaloupe, cherry, date, fig, grapefruit, grape, kiwi, nectarine, orange, peach, pear, pineapple, plum, prune, raisin, raspberry, strawberry, tangerine, watermelon Artichoke, bean (snap), beets, broccoli, brussels sprouts, cabbage, carrot, cauliflower, celery, corn, cucumber, eggplant, kale, lettuce, mushroom, onion, pea, pepper, potato (baked, mashed), spinach, squash, sweet potato (baked, mashed), tomato	Vegetables in fat-free cheese, cream sauce, or margarine	Avocado; olives; coconut; vegetables in cheese, cream sauce, or butter; fried vegetables
Grains (breads, cereals, rice, pasta, and baked goods)	Whole-grain breads and cereals (corn, oats, rye, wheat, barley, bulgur, millet, quinoa, buckwheat), bagels, English muffins, bread sticks, pita bread, plain roll, rice (brown, white, wild), macaroni and pasta, corn tortilla, popcorn (air-popped), pretzels, fat-free snack foods, fat-free crackers, fat-free cookies, fat-free muffins	Very low-fat snack foods	Doughnuts, croissants, sweet rolls, muffins, granola, egg noodles, chow mein noodles, stuffing, regular chips, snack foods, crackers, popcorn, cookies, cake, pies, reduced-fat or low-fat snack foods

K-2. *(Continued)*

Food	Anytime	Sometimes	Avoid
Dairy products and dairy product substitutes	Fat-free nondairy desserts	1 cup/day nonfat milk, nonfat yogurt, or nonfat dairy products (fat-free sour cream, cream cheese, fat-free cheese, fat-free cottage cheese)	Whole or 2%-fat milk, whole or reduced-fat yogurt and cheese, ice cream, cream, sour cream, cream cheese, cottage cheese
Meat, eggs, and meat substitutes	Beans (kidney, garbanzo, pinto, black, brown, white, great northern, mung, navy, red Mexican, lima), lentils, peas, (split, black-eyed), soybean products (tofu, tempeh, miso), Seitan (wheat gluten), egg whites, fat-free vegan burgers, fat-free veggie dogs	Textured vegetable protein, veggie burger, meatless breakfast strips, links, and patties, meatless hot dogs, meatless poultry and fish substitutes	All meats, poultry, fish, seafood, egg yolks, nuts, and seeds
Fats	Fat-free chocolate	Fat-free margarine, fat-free salad dressing, fat-free nondairy creamer, fat-free sour cream	All regular and reduced-fat oils, margarine, salad dressing, butter, lard, shortening, nondairy creamers, chocolate

K-3.   1983 Metropolitan Height and Weight Tables

Men[a]					Women[b]				
Height		Small frame	Medium frame	Large frame	Height		Small frame	Medium frame	Large frame
Ft	In.				Ft	In.			
5	2	128–134	131–141	138–150	4	10	102–111	109–121	118–131
5	3	130–136	133–143	140–153	4	11	103–113	111–123	120–134
5	4	132–138	135–145	142–156	5	0	104–115	113–126	122–137
5	5	134–140	137–148	144–160	5	1	106–118	115–129	125–140
5	6	136–142	139–151	146–164	5	2	108–121	118–132	128–143
5	7	138–145	142–154	149–168	5	3	111–124	121–135	131–147
5	8	140–148	145–157	152–172	5	4	114–127	124–138	134–151
5	9	142–151	148–160	155–176	5	5	117–130	127–141	137–155
5	10	144–154	151–163	158–180	5	6	120–133	130–144	140–159
5	11	146–157	154–166	161–184	5	7	123–136	133–147	143–163
6	0	149–160	157–170	164–188	5	8	126–139	136–150	146–167
6	1	152–164	160–174	168–192	5	9	129–142	139–153	149–170
6	2	155–168	164–178	172–197	5	10	132–145	142–156	152–173
6	3	158–172	167–182	176–202	5	11	135–148	145–159	155–176
6	4	162–176	171–187	181–207	6	0	138–151	148–162	158–179

[a]Weights at ages 25–59 years, based on lowest mortality. Weight in pounds, according to body frame (in indoor clothing weighing 5 lb, shoes with 1-in. heels).
[b]Weights at ages 25–59 years, based on lowest mortality. Weight in pounds, according to body frame (in indoor clothing weighing 3 lb, shoes with 1-in. heels).
From Metropolitan Life Foundation: Height and Weight, Table 1. Stat Bull Metrop Life Found 64:2–9, 1983.

Index